Atrial
Natriuretic
Peptides

Editors
Willis K. Samson, Ph.D.
Associate Professor
Department of Anatomy
University of Missouri
School of Medicine
Columbia, Missouri

Rémi Quirion, Ph.D.
Associate Professor and
Director of Research Laboratories
Department of Psychiatry
McGill University
Douglas Hospital Research Centre
Verdun, Québec, Canada

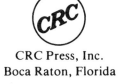

CRC Press, Inc.
Boca Raton, Florida

Library of Congress Cataloging-in-Publication Data

Atrial natriuretic peptides.

Includes bibliographies and index.
1. Atrial natriuretic peptides.   I. Samson, Willis
Kendrick, 1947-   . II. Quirion, Rémi, 1955-   .
[DNLM: 1. Natriuretic Peptides, Atrial.   QU 68 A882]
QP572.A86A88   1989   612'.1   89-486
ISBN 0-8493-6249-0

Direct all inquiries to CRC Press, Inc., 2000 Corporate Blvd., N.W., Boca Raton, Florida, 33431.

© 1990 by CRC Press, Inc.

International Standard Book Number 0-8493-6249-0

Library of Congress Card Number 89-486
Printed in the United States

PREFACE

The subject of a monograph such as this should be timely, somewhat controversial, of interest to a wide spectrum of basic and clinical scientists, and of sufficient potential therapeutic significance to merit the attention of primary care physicians as well. The atrial natriuretic peptides (ANPs) certainly fulfill all those criteria. Although their existence had been speculated upon for only a decade and indeed their structural identity has been known for just five years, in the short time since their identification a staggering literature has developed describing their physiologic and pharmacologic effects and a sizable volume of knowledge has been amassed on their presence and actions in human pathophysiology. Most satisfying to those of us who have been involved from the onset in the examination of the many sites of action and potential physiologic effects of ANP-like peptides is the continued interdisciplinary interest being expressed in these substances. Thus, while the molecular biologists continue to describe the control of ANP production and the post-translational processing which occurs prior to secretion, others interested in the sites and modes of secretion continue to expand our knowledge of the conditions under which the hormones are released and, in so doing, are providing interesting models for other hormonal systems. Studies on the mechanism of action of the peptides have had the unexpected reward of providing a tool for the understanding of second messenger systems in certain cell populations. At the same time the investigations into the physiology of ANP have recruited experts from many disciplines who have discovered common themes in the overall biologic effects of these hormones. As a result, an integrated physiology of the peptides has been revealed whereby central nervous system actions are coordinated with peripheral actions, and the interaction of ANP with other hormone systems involved in cardiovascular and renal control has become apparent. Investigators with a primarily clinical persuasion have been quick to focus not only on the potential for improvement of cardiac function that these peptides possess, but also have been able to relate many clinical findings to abnormal secretion of and/or response to endogenous ANP.

What we have attempted to do in this volume is to present, through the eyes of the scientists most intensely involved in the study of ANP, the breadth of knowledge that has accumulated and, via their willingness to speculate, the most promising avenues for future research on ANP. As with any monograph, not all of the many outstanding researchers in the field could be included and not all the diverse areas of study could be addressed. Additionally, in an attempt to avoid duplication of previous texts on the subject we decided to focus on more novel aspects of ANP physiology and have chosen not to review the earliest, most obvious observations.

Our goal was that this monograph would be an up-to-date review of the molecular biology, physiology, pharmacology, and pathology of the atrial natriuretic peptides. It has served also as a vehicle for many of us to speculate on the significance of our findings and the potential for these hormones. Hopefully, it will provide its readers with a sense of the excitement we have all felt in our attempts to dissect the integrative biological effects of a potent and novel hormonal system.

THE EDITORS

Willis Kendrick Samson, Ph.D., is an Associate Professor of Anatomy at the University of Missouri School of Medicine in Columbia, Missouri.

Dr. Samson received his B.A. degree in Chemistry from Duke University in 1968. After four years of service in the United States Army, he attended the California State University at Fresno, acquiring a second major in Biology. Dr. Samson then completed his dissertation studies and postdoctoral training as an N.I.H. fellow in the Neuroendocrine Group in Dallas, Texas. He accepted the position of Assistant Professor of Physiology at the University of Texas Health Sciences Center at Dallas in 1981.

Dr. Samson is a member of the American Physiological Society, the Endocrine Society, and the International Neuroendocrine Society and is a member of the editorial board of *Endocrinology*. He has been the recipient of grant awards from the National Institutes of Health, the American Heart Association, the American Cancer Society, the Olga Weed Cancer Fund, and private industry. He has presented numerous invited lectures at national and international conferences on his major research interests which include the central nervous system actions of atrial peptides, peptidergic control of prolactin secretion, and the development of cytotoxin methodologies for the creation of individual neuropeptide mutants. He is married to the former Suzanne Elizabeth Miller of St. Louis and they have twin sons Henry William and Charles Kendrick Samson.

Dr. Rémi Quirion, Ph.D., is Director of the Research Laboratories at the Douglas Hospital Research Centre and is Associate Professor in the Department of Psychiatry at McGill University, Montreal, Québec, Canada.

Dr. Quirion received his B.Sc. in Biology from the Université of Sherbrooke, Québec, in 1976, followed by M.Sc. and Ph.D. degrees in Pharmacology from the same University in 1977 and 1980, respectively. After completing his post-doctoral training from 1980 to 1983 at the NIMH in Bethesda, he joined the Douglas Hospital Research Centre and McGill University as an Assistant Professor in Psychiatry. He became an Associate Professor in 1989.

Dr. Quirion is a member of various scientific societies including the American Association for the Advancement of Sciences, the Society for Neuroscience, International Brain Research Organization (IBRO), and the International Society for Neurochemistry (ISN). He is also member of the Editorial Board of *Peptides, Synapse,* the *Canadian Journal of Physiology and Pharmacology* and the *Journal of Chemical Neuroanatomy*. He has received grants from various governmental agencies, lay organizations, and industries.

He has received various awards including pre- and post-doctoral fellowships from the Fonds de la Recherche en Santé du Québec (FRSQ) and the Medical Research Council of Canada (MRC). He is currently a "Chercheur-Boursier" of the FRSQ.

Dr. Quirion has presented multiple invited lectures at international meetings and universities. He has published more than 200 research papers in pharmacology, psychiatry, and the neurosciences. His current major research interests include neuropeptides and their receptors, aging and senile dementia, the modulation of brain cholinergic systems, and interactions between anxiolytics and antidepressants.

CONTRIBUTORS

John C. Burnett, M.D.
Department of Internal Medicine
Mayo Medical School
Rochester, Minnesota

Marc Cantin, M.D., Ph.D.
Director
Hypertension Group
Department of Pathobiology
Clinical Research Institute of Montreal
Montreal, Québec, Canada

Eero Castren, M.D.
Visiting Fellow
Laboratory of Clinical Science
National Institute of Mental Health
National Institutes of Health
Bethesda, Maryland

Jean-Guy Chabot, Ph.D.
Department of Psychiatry
Douglas Hospital Research Centre
Verdun, Québec, Canada

Jean R. Cusson, M.D., Ph.D.
Clinical Research Fellow
Laboratory of Clinical Pharmacology and
  Cardiovascular Physiology
Clinical Research Institute of Montreal
Montreal, Québec, Canada

Eric A. Espiner, M.D.
Professor
Department of Endocrinology
Princess Margaret Hospital
Christchurch, New Zealand

Jacques Genest, M.D.
Consultant
Clinical Research Institute of Montreal
Montreal, Québec, Canada

Christopher C. Glembotski, Ph.D.
Professor
Department of Biology
San Diego State University
San Diego, California

Kenneth L. Goetz, Ph.D.
Director of Research, and Head
Division of Experimental Medicine
St. Luke's Hospital
Kansas City, Missouri

Jorge Silvio Gutkind, Ph.D.
Visiting Fellow
National Institute of Dental Research
National Institutes of Health
Bethesda, Maryland

Pavel Hamet, M.D., Ph.D.
Director
Laboratory of Molecular Pathophysiology
Clinical Research Institute of Montreal
Montreal, Quebec, Canada

Bernd Hamprecht, Ph.D.
Professor
Institute of Physiological Chemistry
University of Tübingen
Tübingen, West Germany

Jing Ru Hu, Ph.D.
Department of Pharmacology
University of Heidelberg
Heidelberg, West Germany

Teruaki Imada, Ph.D.
Research Associate
Department of Biochemistry
Vanderbilt University
Nashville, Tennessee

Hiroo Imura
Professor
Department of Medicine
Kyoto University Faculty of Medicine
Kyoto, Japan

Tadashi Inagami, Ph.D.
Professor
Department of Biochemistry
Vanderbilt University
Nashville, Tennessee

Mitsuhiro Kawata, M.D.
Associate Professor
Department of Anatomy
Kyoto Prefectural University of Medicine
Kyoto, Japan

Masaki Kurihara, Ph.D.
Research Assistant
Department of Neurosurgery
Nagasaki Medical School
Nagasaki, Japan

Rudolph, E. Lang, M.D.
Professor
Department of Pharmacology
University of Heidelberg
Heidelberg, West Germany

Pierre LaRochelle, M.D., Ph.D.
Director
Laboratory of Clinical Pharmacology and
  Cardiovascular Physiology
Clinical Research Institute of Montreal
Montreal, Québec, Canada

Dale C. Leitman, Ph.D.
Department of Biological Chemistry
University of California, Davis
School of Medicine
Davis, California

John A. Lewicki, Ph.D.
Vice President and Director
Research Department
California Biotechnology Inc.
Mountain View, California

Ferid Murad, M.D.
Vice-President
Discovery
Abbott Laboratories
Abbott Park, Illinois

Kazuwa Nakao
Assistant Professor
Department of Medicine
Kyoto University Faculty of Medicine
Kyoto, Japan

Mitsuhide Naruse, M.D.
Assistant Professor
Department of Medicine
Tokyo Women's Medical College
Tokyo, Japan

Adil J. Nazarali, Ph.D.
Guest Researcher
Section on Pharmacology
National Institute of Mental Health
National Institutes of Health
Bethesda, Maryland

Jorge E. B. Pinto, Ph.D.
Associate Professor
Department of Physiology
University of Buenos Aires
Buenos Aires, Argentina

Rémi Quirion, Ph.D.
Director
Research Laboratories
Department of Psychiatry
Douglas Hospital Research Centre
Verdun, Québec, Canada

Georg Reiser, Ph.D.
Institute of Physiological Chemistry
University of Tübingen
Tübingen, West Germany

A. Mark Richards, M.D.
Physician
Department of Cardiology
Princess Margaret Hospital
Christchurch, New Zealand

Juan M. Saavedra, M.D.
Chief, Section on Pharmacology
Laboratory of Clinical Science
National Institute of Mental Health
National Institutes of Health
Bethesda, Maryland

Willis K. Samson, Ph.D.
Associate Professor
Department of Anatomy
University of Missouri School of Medicine
Columbia, Missouri

Yutaka Sano, M.D.
Professor
Department of Anatomy
Kyoto Prefectural University of Medicine
Kyoto, Japan

R. M. Scarborough, Ph.D.
Staff Scientist
California Biotechnology Inc.
Mountain View, California

Paul P. Shields, Ch.E.
Doctoral Candidate
Department of Biochemistry
University of Pennsylvania
Philadelphia, Pennsylvania

Kazuo Shizume, M.D.
Professor
Department of Medicine
Tokyo Women's Medical College
Tokyo, Japan

Gaétan Thibault, Ph.D.
Associate Director
Laboratory of Pathobiology of Hypertension
Clinical Research Institute of Montreal
Montreal, Québec, Canada

Johanne Tremblay, Ph.D.
Associate Director
Laboratory of Molecular Pathophysiology
Clinical Research Institute of Montreal
Montreal, Québec, Canada

Nick C. Trippodo, Ph.D.
Section Head
Department of Pharmacology
Squibb Institute for Medical Research
Princeton, New Jersey

Rudiger von Harsdorf, M.D.
Department of Pharmacology
University of Heidelberg
Heidelberg, West Germany

TABLE OF CONTENTS

Chapter 1

MOLECULAR BIOLOGY OF THE ATRIAL NATRIURETIC PEPTIDES

John A. Lewicki and Robert M. Scarborough

TABLE OF CONTENTS

I. INTRODUCTION

Atrial natriuretic peptide (ANP) is a peptide hormone synthesized in the cardiac atria of normal mammals that regulates blood pressure and extravascular fluid volume.[1-6] Since the initial discovery of ANP by deBold and the subsequent determination of its amino acid sequence, innumerable investigations have probed the role of this hormone in the maintenance of cardiovascular homeostasis. Studies that utilize modern techniques of molecular biology have been preeminent in these investigations. Molecular biological approaches have been used to define the basic structure of the gene that encodes ANP, to address fundamental matters pertaining to the biosynthesis and processing of ANP, to study the regulation of ANP gene expression in atrial and extra-atrial tissues, and, most recently, to study the structure of ANP receptors. Thus, studies of the ANP gene and the regulation of its expression have promoted our understanding of the contribution of this hormonal system to both normal physiological and pathophysiological regulatory states. It is the objective of this chapter to review the current status of investigations employing the disciplines of molecular biology to study the ANP hormonal system.

II. STRUCTURE OF THE ANP cDNA AND GENE

The amino acid sequence of the ANP prohormone (pre-proANP) from various species has been determined from nucleotide sequences of cloned cDNAs encoding pre-proANP. The first identification of DNA complements of pre-proANP mRNA followed the successful purification of multiple species of ANP from mammalian atria. A series of ANP forms ranging from 21 to 73 amino acids in length were purified from both rat and human atria.[6-10] Each of these peptides contained a common amino acid core sequence. This observation, along with findings that both high and low molecular weight forms of ANP can be extracted from atria, implied a precursor-product relationship.[7,10,11]

A common strategy undertaken to clone the ANP precursor utilized oligonucleotide probes based on the amino acid sequence of ANP to screen cDNA libraries complementary to atrial mRNA. Using this approach, cDNAs which encode rat, human, dog, and rabbit pre-proANP have been cloned.[12-19] Full-length cDNAs of about 850 base pairs in length contain 5' and 3' untranslated regions and a region of about 456 base pairs which encodes a pre-prohormone (pre-proANP) of 152 amino acids (151 in human) (see Figure 1). The sequence of the first 24 amino acids of pre-proANP resembles that commonly found in eukaryotic signal peptides. The signal peptide is removed from pre-proANP as the polypeptide is transported across the endoplasmic reticulum. This results in the generation of proANP. ProANP is 126 to 128 amino acids in length, depending upon the species.[18] The sequence of the circulating form of bioactive ANP comprises the carboxyl terminal 28 amino acids of proANP.[19-24] ProANP is cleaved naturally to yield the bioactive 28-amino-acid ANP molecule and a single 98-amino-acid amino terminal fragment that also circulates (Figure 1). Thus, it is likely that the heterogeneity in length of the ANPs isolated originally from atria resulted from artifactual proteolytic processing during isolation.

As shown in Figure 2, the deduced amino acid sequences of pre-proANP cDNAs of various species reveal that this prohormone is highly conserved.[25] The amino acid sequence homology among the proANP molecules from various species is about 75%. The sequence of the mature 28-amino-acid ANP is invariant, except for an isoleucine at residue 12 of the rat, rabbit, and mouse ANPs which is replaced by a methionine residue in the human, bovine, and dog forms of ANP. Various regions of the prohormone domain, excluding the ANP region, are also highly conserved (see Figure 2). The conservation of amino acid sequence in this ''desANP'' prohormone region raises the possbility that the polypeptide might have another important biological function.[26] A genetic construct encoding this 98-amino-acid

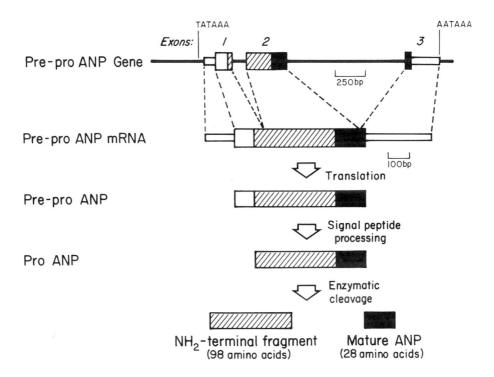

FIGURE 1. A schematic representation of the human pre-proANP gene and corresponding mRNA, as revealed by cDNA sequences. The steps involved in translation and subsequent protein processing are outlined.

NH$_2$-terminal fragment of proANP has been expressed in the bacterium, *Eschericia coli*.[27] The "desANP" prohormone was purified and infused into Sprague-Dawley rates at concentrations up to 10 μg/kg/min. No detectable hemodynamic, endocrine, or renal effects were elicited by the molecule. Thus, the function and role of the proANP amino terminal fragment remains obscure at present.

Genomic clones containing DNA encoding pre-proANP have been isolated and sequenced from human,[28-30] rat,[31] mouse,[30] and bovine[25] genomic libraries. It has been determined that the pre-proANP gene is present once per haploid genome in each species. The pre-proANP gene, which is similar structurally between species, is comprised of three exons and two intervening sequences (Figure 1). Each gene contains a TATAAAA sequence approximately 30 bases upstream of the major transcription start site. This TATA-box homolog dictates the position of transcriptional initiation. Appropriate splice signals (GT-AT) are apparent at intron-exon junctions. The first exon of the gene encodes the 5′ untranslated region, the signal peptide, and the first 16 amino acids of mature proANP. The bulk of the coding region is contained within the second exon. An intervening sequence of 1093 base pairs in the human gene and 527 base pairs in the mouse gene separates the penultimate arginine residue of mature ANP from the carboxyl terminal tyrosine residue, which is encoded by the third exon along with the 3′ untranslated region. Although this tyrosine residue is followed by codons for arginine-arginine-stop (CGAAGATAA) in the rodent genes, it is followed by codons for stop-arginine-stop (TGAAGATAA) in the human gene, the result of a single base change within this codon.[30] The arginine-arginine dipeptide at the carboxyl terminus of the rodent proANP sequence is removed during processing as it has not been observed in any ANP form isolated to date. Several natural allelic variations within the human pre-proANP gene have been identified using restriction fragment-length polymorphism analysis.[32-34] It is not known whether these polymorphisms are linked to a disease state and their significance is currently unknown.

```
                                        10
HUMAN   Met Ser Ser Phe Ser Thr Thr Thr Val Ser Phe Leu Leu Leu Leu Ala Phe Gln Leu
BOVINE      Gly         Ser Ala --- Ile                 Phe
MOUSE       Gly                 --- Ile     Leu Gly         Phe     Val         Trp
RAT         Gly                 --- Ile     Lys Gly     Phe         Phe         Trp

        20                              30
HUMAN   Leu Gly Gln Thr Arg Ala|Asn Pro Met Tyr Asn Ala Val Ser Asn Ala Asp Leu Met
BOVINE  Pro         Gly             Val     Gly Ser
MOUSE   Pro     His Ile Gly         Val     Ser             Thr
RAT     Pro     His Ile Gly         Val     Ser             Thr

            40                              50
HUMAN   Asp Phe Lys Asn Leu Leu Asp His Leu Glu Glu Lys Met Pro Leu Glu Asp Glu Val
BOVINE                          Arg         Asp                                 Ala
MOUSE                                           Val
RAT                                             Val

            60                              70
HUMAN   Val Pro Pro Gln Val Leu Ser Asp Pro Asn Glu Glu Ala Gly Ala Ala Leu Ser Pro
BOVINE          Ser             Glu Gln                             Pro
MOUSE   Met             Ala     Glu Gln Thr                                     Ser
RAT     Met             Ala     Glu Gln Thr Asp                                 Ser

                80                              90
HUMAN   Leu Pro Glu Val Pro Pro Trp Thr Gly Glu Val Ser Pro Ala Gln Arg Asp Gly Gly
BOVINE      Ser     Met             Met         Asn                 Glu
MOUSE                               Ser         Pro Leu                 Ser
RAT                                 Ser         Pro                     Ser

                100                             110
HUMAN   Ala Leu Gly Arg Gly Pro Trp Asp Ser Ser Asp Arg Ser Ala Leu Leu Lys Ser Lys
BOVINE  Val                         Glu
MOUSE       Ser Arg     Ser             Pro
RAT                                     Pro

                    120                             130
HUMAN   Leu Arg Ala Leu Leu Thr Ala Pro Arg Ser Leu Arg Arg Ser Ser Cys Phe Gly Gly
BOVINE                                      _____
MOUSE                       Ala Gly
RAT                         Ala Gly

                    140                             150
HUMAN   Arg Met Asp Arg Ile Gly Ala Gln Ser Gly Leu Gly Cys Asn Ser Phe Arg Tyr  -
BOVINE  _____ Arg
MOUSE       Ile
RAT         Ile

HUMAN    -
BOVINE  Arg
MOUSE
RAT
```

FIGURE 2.   Comparison of the pre-proANP amino acid sequence derived from the human gene with the bovine, rat, and mouse sequences. The bovine, rat, and mouse sequences are shown only where they differ from the human sequence. The signal peptidase cleavage site (|) and biologically active ANP region (——) are indicated.

Several additional features of the pre-proANP gene have been identified which may affect the expression of the gene. For instance, the second intron of the human pre-proANP gene contains nucleotide sequences homologous to putative glucocorticoid regulatory elements (GRE) of the mouse mammary tumor virus and human metallothionein II genes,[35] consistent with observations that the gene is regulated by glucocorticoid hormones[36] (see below). In addition, the human and mouse genes contain nucleotides in the 5′ flanking region, approximately 250 base pairs upstream of the transcriptional start site, which are homologous to the SV40 enhancer sequences.

A comparison of the rat pre-proANP gene sequence with that of the human pre-proANP gene reveals a higher degree of homology in the 5′ flanking sequences than in the introns or 3′ flanking regions. This may reflect a conservation of important regulatory sequences. Several studies have been undertaken recently to characterize the 5′ regulatory sequences of the pre-proANP gene which control high-level tissue-specific expression. The studies have utilized chimeric genes in which the 5′ regulatory regions of the pre-proANP gene have been fused to a foreign gene such as chloramphenicol acetyltransferase (CAT). It has been observed that a contiguous stretch of 3500 nucleotides, all immediately upstream of the transcriptional start site of the rat pre-proANP gene, can direct the specific expression of the foreign CAT gene in cultured atrial cardiocytes derived from adult rats and in cultured atrial and ventricular cardiocytes from fetal rats.[37] The same fusion gene has been introduced into the mouse gene line and the transgene is expressed dominantly in the atria, although low-level expression is observed in the ventricle and brain of these animals.[37] This pattern of tissue-specific expression of CAT mirrors the expression of the ANP gene in normal animals. It is not known whether this DNA sequence controls the regulated expression of the gene in response to hormones, neurotransmitters, or physical factors. In a study of comparable design, Field has recently reported that a 500-base-pair fragment derived from the 5′ flanking region of the human pre-proANP gene directs the tissue-specific expression of large T-antigen in the atria of transgenic mice.[38] Expression of large T-antigen was not observed in any other tissue. The expression of large T-antigen leads to hyperplasia in the right atria of the transgenic mice. The significance of this effect remains to be elucidated. Nevertheless, the studies imply that *cis*-acting DNA sequences in close proximity to the transcriptional start site of the pre-proANP gene direct the tissue-specific expression of this gene. Similar approaches of fusing both control and mutant regulatory regions of the ANP gene to reporter genes and assessing expression of these genes in various cells and tissues will enhance our ultimate understanding of the regulation of pre-proANP gene expression.

III. BIOSYNTHESIS AND PROCESSING OF ANP

ANP has been localized to secretory granules of the adult atria.[39] These secretory granules were first identified several decades ago.[40] It has been proposed that the peptide hormone is stored in these granules, transported to the cell membrane, and released into the extracellular milieu in response to appropriate stimuli. Numerous groups have pursued an understanding of the complete biosynthetic cascade and this topic is reviewed in detail in this chapter. The successful cloning of pre-proANP cDNAs and genes has provided a foundation for sophisticated studies of ANP biosynthesis and processing of the proANP precursor into the predominant bioactive ANP forms.

The pre-proANP mRNA species is the most abundant mRNA species in the mammalian atria. It comprises approximately 0.5 to 2% of the total atrial mRNA pool. The steady-state level of an mRNA species is a function of both biosynthesis and degradation rates. Atrial pre-proANP mRNA is abundant because its gene is transcribed actively in this tissue and the pre-proANP mRNA is relatively stable ($t^1/_2$ = 18 h).[41]

Following translation of the pre-proANP mRNA and cleavage of the signal peptide by signal peptidase, the resulting product is the 126-amino-acid ANP prohormone (proANP). ProANP represents greater than 95%, if not all, of the ANP found in atrial granules.[18,42] Despite the fact that proANP is the major atrial storage form of the hormone, proANP cannot be detected reproducibly in plasma.[42] Rather, as noted above, the principal circulating peptides are the products of proANP processing, namely, the mature 28-amino-acid ANP and the 98-amino-acid des-ANP amino terminal fragment.

The above findings have prompted speculation as to the sites and mechanisms of proANP conversion to ANP. Primary cultures of neonatal rat cardiocytes release predominantly proANP into the culture medium.[43] This is true for both atrial cardiocytes, which store the proANP in granules and secrete the peptide through a regulated pathway, and ventricular cardiocytes, which release newly synthesized proANP through a constitutive pathway.[44] These data suggest the possibility that a rapid conversion of proANP to ANP might occur following the release of proANP into the circulation. Consistent with this possibility is the observation that proANP can be converted to mature ANP by serum or "thrombin-like" proteases.[45-47] A serum enzyme which specifically converts proANP to ANP has been purified.[48] However, the physiological relevance of this enzyme has been disputed. Several groups have demonstrated that neither plasma nor whole blood is capable of processing the precursor molecule.[27,45,46] Furthermore, we have determined that recombinant proANP is not converted to the 28-amino-acid mature ANP form upon infusion of this molecule into anesthetized

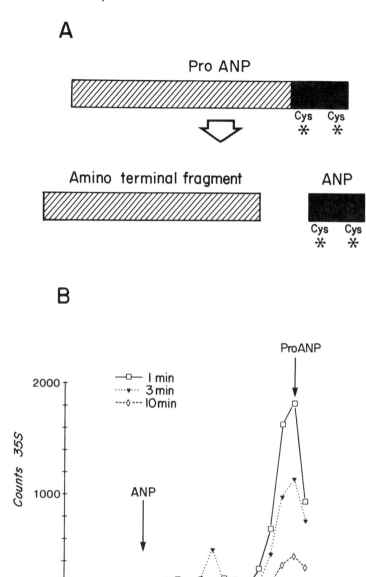

FIGURE 3.   (A) A schematic representation of the proANF molecule and the products of proANP processing. The positions of ^{35}S-cysteine (*) residues are shown. (B) The distribution of ^{35}S-cysteine-labeled protein fragments after injection of pure [^{35}S]-cysteine-labeled proANP into anesthetized rabbits. Pure human recombinant ^{35}S-proANP was injected into rabbits via the femoral vein. Blood was removed at indicated times from the femoral artery and was fractionated into plasma. Plasma samples were chromatographed on high-pressure liquid chromatography and fractions were monitored for ^{35}S. The migratory positions of ANP and proANP are shown.

rabbits.[45] In these studies, outlined in Figure 3, recombinant ANP was radiolabeled biosynthetically with ^{35}S-cysteine. Since the only cysteines of proANP are in the mature ANP domain, this intervention places the radiolabel in this region of the molecule (Panel A). Pure ^{35}S-proANP was infused into the femoral vein of anesthetized rabbits and arterial samples were removed over time and analyzed by high-pressure liquid chromatography for the distribution of ^{35}S-labeled products. As shown in Figure 3B, although proANP was degraded with a half-life of about 5 min, specific conversion of this protein to mature ANP was not detected. These data suggest that conversion of proANP to mature ANP takes place prior to entering the circulation, either within the secretory granule as it is targeted for secretion or in the extracellular milieu immediately upon release. Imada and co-workers[49] have recently isolated an enzyme from atrial tissue which appears to be capable of correctly processing the proANP molecule to ANP. This "atriopeptidase" has been partially purified and its enzymatic properties are currently being studied. If this enzyme plays a physiological role in converting proANP to ANP, then assignment of this enzyme activity to specific cells or subcellular fractions should help to define the mechanisms involved in the generation of the mature ANP peptide.

IV. REGULATION OF ANP GENE EXPRESSION IN ATRIAL AND EXTRA-ATRIAL TISSUES

As denoted by its name, ANP was identified initially in cardiac atria. Early attempts to detect this peptide by bioassay in cardiac ventricles failed and it was presumed that expression of the pre-proANP gene was limited to atrial tissue.[1-6] Following the generation of antibodies directed to ANP, specific radioimmunoassay and immunocytochemical analysis led to the detection of ANP-like immunoreactivity in extra-atrial tissues, including the hypothalamus of the brain,[50-52] pituitary,[52] kidney,[52,53] and adrenal.[52] These studies did not discriminate between ANP-like immunoreactivity which resulted from contamination or uptake from blood and ANP-like material that was synthesized locally. Furthermore, since ANP-like immunoreactive material is present in quite small amounts in these tissues, the precise identity of this material could not be established. In an attempt to achieve clarification of these issues, we embarked on a series of collaborative studies with Dr. David Gardner which demonstrated that the pre-proANP gene is transcribed in a number of extra-atrial tissues.[54] These data provided the requisite evidence that ANP can be biosynthesized locally in tissues other than the atrium.

Using specific DNA probes, pre-proANP mRNA can be detected in the cardiac ventricle, lung, pituitary, aortic arch, and hypothalamus of the brain. The abundance of pre-proANP mRNA in these extra-atrial tissues is reduced substantially relative to the atria; the atrium contains about 100 times more pre-proANP mRNA than the ventricle or lung and only trace amounts of pre-proANP mRNA can be detected in the hypothalamus. However, it has been demonstrated recently by Bloch and co-workers that fetal rat ventricle contains about as much pre-proANP mRNA as the atrium.[44] Thus, the ANP gene appears to be actively transcribed in both the atria and ventricles of the fetus. Ventricular pre-proANP mRNA levels are increased dramatically following experimentally induced ventricular hypertrophy and in patients exhibiting moderate to severe congestive heart failure.[55,56] Thus, the pre-proANP gene is a member of an emerging family of genes that are expressed quite actively in the fetal ventricle and in the adult ventricle following cardiac stress and/or hypertrophy. Ventricular ANP is not packaged in secretory-like granules; rather, it appears to be secreted constitutively.[44] It is likely that ANP from the ventricle may contribute significantly to the elevated circulatory pool of ANP during hypertrophy and heart failure.

The pre-proANP transcripts in extra-atrial tissues are identical to the atrial gene transcripts in overall size and have similar 5′ and 3′ termini. The techniques of primer extension analysis and S$_1$ nuclease mapping were used to establish the similarity of the pre-proANP mRNA in the atria, ventricle, lung, and hypothalamus.[54,57] While the major atrial storage form of the peptide is proANP, shorter peptide fragments, proANP(102—126) and proANP(103—126) are stored in the central nervous system.[58] To eliminate the possibility that these different peptides arise from distinct mRNA species, we cloned a hypothalamic pre-proANP cDNA.[57]

The partial-length hypothalamic cDNA is identical to the atrial pre-proANP cDNA at each of its 612 bases. This result supports the hypothesis that, following transcription and RNA processing, an identical pre-proANP mRNA species exists in all tissues which express the gene. Differences in the peptide structure and routes of secretion result from tissue-specific variations in the processing of the proANP molecule.

The role of ANP in extra-atrial tissues is unknown at present. Within the brain, ANP has been localized to neurons of the anterolateral border of the third ventricle (A3V3) and to the hypothalamus, two regions involved in the regulation of the cardiovascular system.[50,51] In the aortic arch, the distribution of ANP mirrors that of aortic baroreceptors, suggesting a role for the peptide in modulation of these receptors.[59] Finally, it is plausible to speculate that ANP may serve as an autocrine factor with a local regulatory role in tissues such as the lung.[54] Further investigations will test these possibilities.

Since ANP is a member of an intricate network of factors which affect cardiovascular homeostasis, it is anticipated that the expression of the pre-proANP gene is regulated in a complex manner. To date, investigations of the regulation of the pre-proANP gene have not been extensive. However, it is already clear that the gene is affected by divergent factors, including hormones, neurotransmitters, and physical factors such as atrial stretch and changes in intravascular volume.

Several groups have documented that pre-proANP gene expression is increased by glucocorticoid hormones.[36,55] *In vivo* administration of dexamethasone to rats results in a two- to fivefold increase in pre-proANP mRNA; this effect is most pronounced following adrenalectomy, which removes the influence of endogenous steroid hormones on this gene. The effect of dexamethasone appears to involve a direct influence on the transcription of the pre-proANP gene. In addition, the dexamethasone-induced increase in pre-proANP mRNA can be reproduced in primary cultures of neonatal rate cardiocytes. These data indicate that the pre-proANP gene is regulated directly by glucocorticoids in the rat and imply that glucocorticoid-responsive regulatory elements identified previously in the human pre-proANP gene are also present in the rat gene.

Mineralocorticoid hormones also appear to affect pre-proANP gene expression. The continuous administration of exogenous mineralocorticoids results in transient renal sodium retention, followed by a return to normal sodium balance within a few days. Increased expression of ANP has been implicated in this "escape" from mineralocorticoid-induced sodium retention.[60] Administration of pharmacological doses of the mineralocorticoid, desoxycorticosterone acetate (DOCA), to the rat results in a 2.5-fold increase in circulating immunoreactive ANP levels 12 to 24 h after administration. Concomitant with the elevation of plasma ANP, pre-proANP mRNA levels in atria are increased 12 h after DOCA administration and remain elevated for at least 72 h in the rat.[60] Similarly, in the conscious dog, atrial pre-proANP mRNA is increased five- to sevenfold following 10 d of administration of DOCA.[61] These data support a role for ANP as a contributing factor to the escape phenomena.

Finally, it has been demonstrated that pre-proANP gene expression is also increased by thyroid hormone.[62] The thyroid hormone agonist, thyroxine, increases the levels of pre-proANP mRNA both in primary cultures of neonatal cardiocytes and intact rats. The effect of thyroxine is contingent upon the volume status of the animals. While thyroxine has no effect on pre-proANP mRNA levels in hydrated rats, a threefold increase in pre-proANP mRNA is observed in dehydrated animals. Baseline levels of pre-proANP mRNA are reduced in the dehydrated controls when compared to euvolemic animals: thus, the effect of thyroxine was to restore mRNA levels to control volumes. The reported alteration of pre-proANP mRNA during dehydration, salt loading, and volume expansion,[17] taken together with the effects of hormones like glucocorticoids, mineralocorticoids, and thyroid hormones, provides initial insights into the complex regulation of the gene. The data support a broad role for ANP in the maintenance of fluid and electrolyte balance and as a mediator of various stimuli.

V. PURIFICATION, CLONING, AND EXPRESSION OF ANP RECEPTORS

The diverse biological actions of ANP result from the high-affinity binding of the peptide to specific membrane-associated receptors of target organs. Specific ANP receptors have been identified in numerous tissues, including endothelial and smooth muscle cells of the vasculature, epithelial and mesangial cells of the renal glomerulus, renal papilla, lung, adrenal, pituitary, and various regions of the brain.[63] A widespread role for the peptide in regulating cardiovascular homeostasis is implied by this broad distribution of receptors.

As with most other hormones and neurotransmitters, it is now apparent that the ANP receptor population is heterogenous.[64-67] Pharmacological studies have revealed the existence of at least two different ANP receptor subpopulations. One receptor is tightly coupled to the stimulation of particulate guanylate cyclase, leading to increases in intracellular cyclic GMP accumulation. This receptor probably mediates many of the biological effects of ANP.[68] Structure-activity studies have revealed that, in general, minor modifications of the ANP molecule lead to markedly diminished potency for stimulating cyclic GMP.[64] These results demonstrate that ANP receptors are coupled to the stimulation of cyclic GMP accumulation and are quite sensitive to changes in the amino acid sequence of ANP. These receptors have been termed B-ANP receptors to denote their implicit role in transducing the biological effects of ANP.[69]

In contrast to this finding, a second ANP receptor pool is remarkably tolerant to changes in the ANP amino acid sequence.[70,71] ANP analogs, truncated at the carboxyl and/or amino termini, or containing deletions of amino acids from within the 17-membered disulfide-bridged core of ANP, bind to this site with high affinity, but are unable to increase cyclic GMP accumulation or to antagonize the ability of full-length ANP to increase intracellular cyclic GMP.[70,71] Thus, these analogs are selective for receptors which are not coupled to cyclic GMP metabolism. Receptor-selective analogs have been used as probes to discern the function of the cyclic GMP uncoupled receptor pool.[69] Based on results of *in vitro* and *in vivo* studies, our group has obtained substantial evidence that these receptors function in the metabolic clearance of circulating ANP. A classical "ANP-like" pharmacological effect cannot be ascribed to this receptor. These receptors have been termed C-ANP receptors to denote their role as clearance receptors.[69] Similar "Class II" clearance receptors have been described for other polypeptides.

Delineation of the physiological and molecular relationship between B-ANP receptors, coupled to the stimulation of particulate guanylate cyclase and C-ANP receptors involved in the metabolic clearance of the hormone, requires purification, cloning, and functional expression of the gene(s) encoding the receptors. A structural correlate to the two populations of ANP receptors defined by binding studies was obtained by cross-linking radio-iodinated ANP to tissue and cell preparations. These studies demonstrated specific ANP binding to two membrane-associated proteins of about 60,000 and 130,000 Da, respectively.[72-75] Kuno and co-workers reported recently that ANP binding and particulate guanylate cyclase activity copurify from lung and that both activities reside in a single polypeptide chain of 130,000 Da.[76] These data imply that the 130,000-Da ANP binding protein is the receptor which is coupled to the stimulation of particulate guanylate cyclase (B-ANP receptor). Additional support for this hypothesis has been reported recently by Takayanagi et al.[77] These investigators have purified two distinct ANP receptor proteins from adrenal tissues. The larger receptor form, comprised of a single subunit of about 130,000 Da, contains constitutive guanylate cyclase activity. Furthermore, only native ANP sequences, which stimulate cyclic GMP accumulation, bind to this 130,000-Da receptor species.[77]

At the present time, several groups have purified an ANP receptor with a subunit molecular mass of 60,000 Da.[77-79] The identification of this receptor as the C-ANP receptor

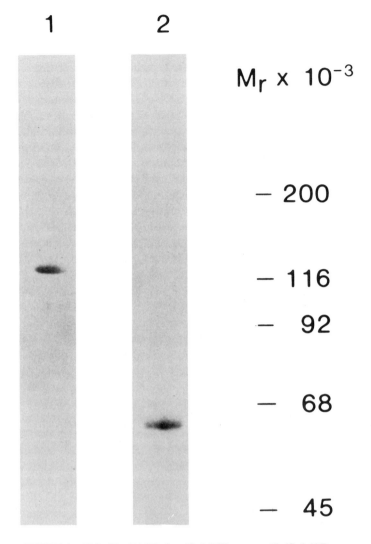

FIGURE 4. NaDodSo$_4$/PAGE of purified ANP receptor. Purified ANP receptor (1 μg) was suspended in 30 μg of buffer containing either no dithiothreitol (lane 1) or 10 mM dithiothreitol (lane 2). Proteins were visualized by silver staining. The migration positions of standard proteins are shown at the right.

was established by examining the binding and functional activities of a series of ANP analogs selective for this protein. To achieve purification of this receptor, cultured bovine aortic smooth muscle (BASM) cells were used by our group as a source of starting material.[78] These cells contain an abundant population of the C-ANP receptor.[79] Solubilization of the receptor protein from cellular membranes, followed by affinity chromatography on ANP-Sepharose, led to a preparation of C-ANP receptor greater than 90% pure, as judged by SDS-polyacrylamide electrophoresis. As shown in Figure 4, the purified receptor migrates as a single band of 60,000 Da, upon SDS-PAGE electrophoresis in the presence of reducing agent, and migrates at 120,000 Da following electrophoresis in the absence of reducing agent. Based on these data, it has been concluded that the C-ANP holoreceptor is a 120,000-Da homodimer.[78,80]

Recently, a cDNA encoding the C-ANP receptor has been cloned and expressed in our laboratories.[81,82] Amino-terminal sequence analysis of the purified C-ANP receptor defined

A

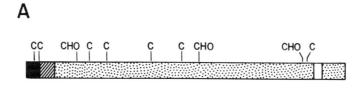

B

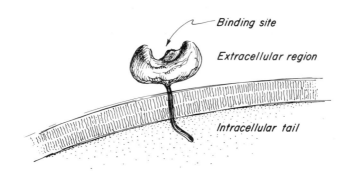

Binding site

Extracellular region

Intracellular tail

FIGURE 5. (A) A schematic representation of the C-ANP receptor based upon
the nucleotide sequence of a cloned cDNA. The signal peptide (■), proreceptor
(▨), extracellular (▦), transmembrane (□) and cytoplasmic (▦) domains are
outlined. C implies the location of cysteine residues and CHO represents putative
glycosylation sites. (B) A pictorial representation of the C-ANP receptor inserted
into a cellular membrane.

a 32-amino-acid segment which was used for the design of oligonucleotide probes. The
oligonucleotide probes were used to screen a cDNA library complementary to BASM-derived
mRNA. Positive clones were sequenced and determined to encode the C-ANP receptor. A
total cDNA of about 3500 base pairs contains a 5′ untranslated region of 465 base pairs,
an open reading frame of 1614 base pairs, and a long 3′ untranslated stretch. The C-ANP
receptor cDNA thus encodes a protein of 537 amino acids. Based on the deduced amino
acid sequence of the protein, several prominent structural features are apparent. These are
depicted in Figure 5A. The first 21 amino acids of the protein are highly hydrophobic and
characteristic of an eukaryotic signal peptide. This region is followed by a stretch of 20
amino acids which appear to represent a proreceptor domain that is removed during intracellular processing of the protein. The mature c-ANP receptor isolated from BASM cells
begins at amino acid residue 42 and is 496 amino acids in length. The mature receptor can
be subdivided into an extracellular domain (437 amino acids), a hydrophobic transmembrane-
spanning region (20 amino acids), and a short cytoplasmic tail (39 amino acids). The predicted
molecular mass of 55,701 Da agrees well with the subunit molecular mass of 60,000 Da
for the purified receptor, particularly since the cDNA predicts three putative glycosylation
sites in the mature receptor sequence.

Examination of the amino acid sequence suggests little sequence homology between this
receptor and other classes of hormone receptors. Nevertheless, the structural arrangement
of this protein, which includes a short, COOH-terminally oriented cytoplasmic domain and
a single transmembrane-spanning region, is similar to the growth-factor receptor family[83,84]
and other receptors involved in ligand transport, such as the LDL,[85] transferrin,[86] asialo-

glycoprotein,[87] and the recently cloned IGF-II/mannose 6-phosphate receptor.[88-90] (Figure 5B).

The five cysteines predicted for this receptor all occur in the extracellular domain and illustrate a major difference from the growth-factor receptors, which are quite rich in cysteine.[83,84] The low abundance of cysteine residues in this receptor is similar to the IL-2 and transferrin receptors.[86,91,92] Interestingly, the transferrin receptor is also a disulfide-linked homodimer.

Several lines of evidence confirm that the cloned cDNA encodes the C-ANP receptor. First, *in vitro* translation of mRNA prepared from the cDNA leads to the biosynthesis of a 58,000-Da protein which reacts specifically with anti-C-ANP receptor antisera.[93] Injection of the mRNA into *Xenopus* oocytes elicits specific, saturable binding of ^{125}I-ANP to membranes prepared from these oocytes. No binding is observed in mock injected oocytes. A series of ANP analogs, specific for C-ANP receptors, also bind with high affinity to the receptor expressed in *Xenopus* oocytes. Finally, vaccinia virus constructs containing engineered DNA sequences encoding the C-ANP receptor have been used to direct expression of the C-ANP receptors in a variety of host mammalian cell lines.[93] Once again, specific, saturable, high-affinity binding of C-ANP receptor-specific ligands to membrane-associated receptors is observed in cells infected only with the viral vector containing DNA sequences that encode the complete receptor. Using this same approach, the extracellular domain of the C-ANP receptor has also been expressed without its membrane anchor. The mutant receptor protein is secreted outside of the cell into the extracellular media. This secreted receptor also binds C-ANP receptor-selective ligands in a specific and saturable manner. The affinity of C-ANP ligands for the secreted receptor is identical to the membrane-associated receptor.[93] In summary, these data demonstrate that expression of the cloned DNA sequence encoding the C-ANP receptor imparts a specific ligand-binding function that appears identical to the native receptor *in situ*. These approaches, when combined with successful cloning and expression of the Mr = 130,000 guanylate cyclase-coupled receptor (B-ANP receptor), should afford a detailed understanding of the structural and biological relationship of these two, and perhaps additional, ANP receptors.

VI. SUMMARY

In the 7 years since the initial discovery of ANP, progress toward a detailed understanding of the physiological, biochemical, and clinical relevance of this hormone has been enormous. Achievements during this period include, but are not limited to, (1) isolation and sequence determination of ANP and proANP, (2) cloning of the gene that encodes this polypeptide, (3) identification of fundamental mechanisms regulating ANP biosynthesis, processing, and release, (4) investigation into the physiological and pharmacological properties of the hormone in both experimental animals and in man, and (5) identification of ANP receptors and relevant second messenger systems. Numerous advances, which include the application of modern techniques of molecular biology, have been fundamental to these discoveries.

In the upcoming months and years, we can anticipate that many additional investigators will apply the methods of modern molecular biology to the study of the ANP hormonal system. This approach, when combined with other scientific achievements, will add to our preexisting base of understanding of ANP and will open new avenues for further exploration. We should anticipate continuing rapid scientific progress in this exciting research field.

REFERENCES

1. **deBold, A. J.**, Atrial natriuretic factor: a hormone produced by the heart, *Science*, 230, 767, 1985.
2. **Ballerman, B. J. and Brenner, B. M.**, Biologically active atrial peptides, *J. Clin. Invest.*, 76, 2041, 1985.
3. **Lang, R. E., Tholken, H., Ganten, D., Luft, F. C., Ruskoaho, H., and Unger, T.**, Atrial natriuretic factor — a circulating hormone stimulated by volume loading, *Nature (London)*, 314, 264, 1985.
4. **Maack, T., Camargo, M. J. F., Kleinert, H. D., Laragh, J. H., and Atlas, S. A.**, Atrial natriuretic factor: structure and functional properties, *Kidney Int.*, 27, 607, 1985.
5. **Cantin, M. and Genest, J.**, The heart and the atrial natriuretic factor, *Endocrine Rev.*, 6, 107, 1985.
6. **Currie, M. G., Geller, D. M., Cole, B. R., Siegel, N. R., Fok, K. F., Adams, S. P., Eubanks, S. R., Galluppi, G. R., and Needleman, P.**, Purification and sequence analysis of bioactive atrial peptides (atriopeptins), *Science*, 221, 67, 1983.
7. **Seidah, N. G., Lazure, C., Chretien, M., Thibault, G., Garcia, R., Cantin, M., Genest, J., Nutt, R. F., Brady, S. F., Lyle, T. A., Paleveda, W. S., Colton, C. D., Ciccarone, T. M., and Veber, D. F.**, Amino acid sequence of homologous rat atrial peptides: natriuretic activity of native and synthetic forms, *Proc. Natl. Acad. Sci. U.S.A.*, 81, 2640, 1984.
8. **Atlas, S. A., Kleinert, H. D., Camargo, M. J. F., Januszewicz, A., Sealey, J. E., Laragh, J. H., Schilling, J. W., Lewicki, J. A., Johnson, L. K., and Maack, T.**, Purification, sequencing and synthesis of natriuretic and vasoactive rat atrial peptide, *Nature (London)*, 309, 717, 1984.
9. **Flynn, T. G., deBold, M. L., and deBold, A. J.**, The amino acid sequence of an atrial peptide with potent diuretic and natriuretic properties, *Biochem. Biophys. Res. Commun.*, 117, 859, 1983.
10. **Kangawa, K. and Matsuo, H.**, Purification and complete amino acid sequence of α-human atrial natriuretic polypeptide (α-hANP), *Biochem. Biophys. Res. Commun.*, 118, 131, 1984.
11. **Kangawa, K., Fukuda, A., Kubota, I., Hayashi, Y., and Matsuo, H.**, Identification in rat atrial tissue of multiple forms of natriuretic polypeptides of about 3,000 daltons, *Biochem. Biophys. Res. Commun.*, 121, 585, 1984.
12. **Yamanaka, M., Greenberg, B., Johnson, L., Seilhamer, J., Brewer, M., Friedemann, T., Miller, J., Atlas, S., Laragh, J., Lewicki, J., and Fiddes, J.**, Cloning and sequence analysis of the cDNA for the rat ANF precursor, *Nature (London)*, 309, 719, 1984.
13. **Maki, M., Takayanagi, R., Misono, K. S., Pandey, K. M., Tibbetts, C., and Inagami, T.**, Structure of rat ANF precursor deduced from cDNA sequence, *Nature (London)*, 309, 722, 1984.
14. **Seidman, C., Duby, A., Choi, E., Graham, R., Haber, E., Homcy, C., Smith, J., and Seidman, J.**, Structure of rat pre-proatrial natriuretic factor as defined by a complementary DNA clone, *Science*, 225, 324, 1984.
15. **Zivin, R., Condra, J., Dixon, R., Seidah, M., Chretien, M., Nemer, M., Chamberland, M., and Drouin, J.**, Molecular cloning and characterization of DNA sequences encoding rat and human ANF, *Proc. Natl. Acad. Sci. U.S.A.*, 81, 6325, 1984.
16. **Oikawa, S., Imai, M., Ueno, A., Tanaka, S., Noguchi, T., Nakazato, H., Nangawa, K., Fukuda, A., and Matsuo, H.**, Cloning and sequence analysis of cDNA encoding a precursor for human ANP, *Nature (London)*, 309, 724, 1984.
17. **Nakayama, K., Ohkubo, H., Hirose, T., Inayama, S., and Nakanishi, S.**, mRNA sequence for human cardiodilatin-atrial natriuretic factor precursor and regulation of precursor mRNA in rat atria, *Nature (London)*, 310, 699, 1984.
18. **Kangawa, K., Tawaragi, Y., Oikawa, S., Mizuno, A., Sakuragawa, Y., Nakazato, H., Fukuda, A., Minamino, N., and Matsuo, H.**, Identification of rat gamma-atrial natriuretic polypeptide and characterization of the c-DNA encoding its precursor, *Nature (London)*, 312, 152, 1984.
19. **Oikawa, S., Imai, M., Inuzuka, C., Tawaragi, Y., Nakazato, H., and Matsuo, H.**, Structure of dog and rabbit precursors of atrial natriuretic polypeptides deduced from nucleotide sequence of cloned cDNA, *Biochem. Biophys. Res. Commun.*, 132, 892, 1985.
20. **Schwartz, D., Geller, D. M., Manning, P. T., Siegel, N. R., Fok, F., Smith, C. E., and Needleman, P.**, Ser-Leu-Arg-Arg-Atriopeptin III: the major circulating form of atrial peptide, *Science*, 229, 397, 1985.
21. **Vuolteenaho, O., Arjamaa, O., and Ling, N.**, Atrial natriuretic polypeptides (ANP): rat atria store high molecular weight precursor but secrete processed peptides of 25-35 amino acids, *Biochem. Biophys. Res. Commun.*, 129, 82, 1985.
22. **Theiss, G., John, A., Morich, F., Neuser, D., Schroder, W., Stasch, J.-P., and Wohlfeil, S.**, α-hANP is the only form of circulating ANP in humans, *FEBS Lett.*, 218, 159, 1987.
23. **Thibault, G., Lazure, C., Schiffrin, E. L., Gutkowska, J., Chartier, L., Garcia, R., Seidah, N. G., Chretien, M., Genest, J., and Cantin, M.**, Identification of a biologically active circulating form of rat atrial natriuretic factor, *Biochem. Biophys. Res. Commun.*, 130, 981, 1985.

24. **Yandle, T., Crozier, I., Nicholls, G., Espiner, E., Carne, A., and Brennan, S.,** Amino acid sequence of atrial natriuretic peptides in human coronary sinus plasma, *Biochem. Biophys. Res. Commun.*, 146, 832, 1987.

25. **Vlasuk, G., Miller, J., Bencen, G., and Lewicki, J.,** Structure and analysis of the bovine atrial natriuretic peptide precursor gene, *Biochem. Biophys. Res. Commun.*, 136, 396, 1986.

26. **Winters, C. J., Sallman, A. L., Meadows, J., Rico, D. M., Vesely, D. L.,** Two new hormones: prohormone atrial natriuretic peptides 1-30 and 31-67 circulate in man, *Biochem. Biophys. Res. Commun.*, 150, 231, 1988.

27. **Vlasuk, G., Scarborough, R. M., and Lewicki, J. A.,** unpublished observation, 1985.

28. **Greenberg, B., Bencen, G., Seilhamer, J., Lewicki, J., and Fiddes, J.,** Nucleotide sequence of the gene encoding human ANF precursor, *Nature (London)*, 312, 656, 1984.

29. **Maki, M., Parmentier, M., and Inagami, T.,** Cloning of the genomic DNA for human ANF, *Biochem. Biophys. Res. Commun.*, 125, 797, 1984.

30. **Seidman, C., Bloch, K., Klein, K., Smith, J., and Seidman, J.,** Nucleotide sequences of the human and mouse atrial natriuretic factor genes, *Science*, 226, 1206, 1984.

31. **Argentin, S., Nemer, M., Drouin, J., Scott, G., Kennedy, B., and Davies, P.,** The gene for rat atrial natriuretic factor, *J. Biol. Chem.*, 260, 4568, 1985.

32. **Frossard, P. M., Gonzalez, P. A., Greenberg, B., Fiddes, J. C., and Atlas, S. A.,** *Bgl*II dimorphism at the human atrial natriuretic peptide (ANP) gene locus, *Nucleic Acids Res.*, 14, 5121, 1986.

33. **Frossard, P. M. and Coleman, R. T.,** Human atrial natriuretic peptides (ANP) gene locus, *Bgl*I RFLP, *Nucleic Acids Res.*, 14, 9223, 1986.

34. **Frossard, P. M., Coleman, R. T., and Morrison, N. A.,** Human natriuretic peptides (ANP) gene locus: *Bsm*I RFLP, *Nucleic Acids Res.*, 15, 7656, 1987.

35. **Karin, M., Haslinger, A., Holtgreve, H., Richards, R. I., Krautre, P., Westphal, W. M., and Beato, M.,** Characterization of DNA sequences through which cadmium and glucocorticoid hormones induce human metallothionein II gene, *Nature (London)*, 308, 513, 1984.

36. **Gardner, D. G., Hane, S., Trachewsky, D., Schenk, D. B., and Baxter, J. D.,** Atrial natriuretic peptide mRNA regulated by glucocorticoids *in vivo*, *Biochem. Biophys. Res. Commun.*, 139, 1047, 1986.

37. **Seidman, C. E., Fenton, R., Zeller, R., Bloch, K. D., Lee, R. T., Wong, D. W., and Seidman, J. G.,** The molecular basis for atrial natriuretic factor gene expression, *J. Cell. Biochem. Suppl.*, 12A, 3, 1988.

38. **Field, L. J.,** Atrial natriuretic factor — SV40 T antigen transgenes produce tumors and cardiac arrhythmias in mice, *Science*, 239, 1029, 1988.

39. **Cantin, M., Gutkowska, J., Thibault, G., Milne, R. W., Ledoux St. Min Li, S., Chapeau, C., Garcia, R., and Genest, J.,** Immunocytochemical localization of atrial natriuretic factor in the heart and salivary glands, *Histochemistry*, 87, 113, 1984.

40. **Jamieson, J. D. and Palade, G. E.,** Specific granules in atrial muscle, *J. Cell. Biol.*, 23, 151, 1964.

41. **Gardner, D., DeSchepper, C., Gertz, B., and Kim, D.,** The gene for rat ANP is regulated by glucocorticids *in vitro*, *J. Clin. Invest.*, 82, 1275, 1989.

42. **Miyata, A., Kangawa, K., Toshimori, T., Hatoh, T., and Matsuo, H.,** Molecular forms of atrial natriuretic polypeptides in mammalian tissues and plasma, *Biochem. Biophys. Res. Commun.*, 129, 248, 1985.

43. **Bloch, K. D., Scott, J. A., Zisfein, J. B., Fallon, J. T., Margolis, M. N., Seidman, C. E., Matsueda, G. R., Homcy, C. J., Graham, R. M., and Seidman, J. G.,** Biosynthesis and secretion of proatrial natriuretic factor by cultured rat cardiocytes, *Science*, 230, 1168, 1985.

44. **Bloch, K. D., Seidman, J. G., Naftilan, J. D., Fallon, J. T., and Seidman, C. E.,** Neonatal atria and ventricles secrete atrial natriuretic factor via tissue-specific secretory pathways, *Cell*, 47, 695, 1986.

45. **Hilliker, S., Vlasuk, G., Borden, L., Hancock, N., Scarborough, R., Schwartz, K., and Lewicki, J.,** Fate of the atrial natriuretic peptide precursor in the circulation, in Program 1st World Conf. Biologically Active Peptides, Abstr. 90A, New York, May 31 to June 1, 1986.

46. **Michener, M. L., Gierse, J. K., Seetharam, R., Fok, K. F., Olins, P. O., Mai, M. S., and Needleman, P.,** Proteolytic processing of atriopeptin prohormone, *Mol. Pharmacol.*, 30, 552, 1986.

47. **Gibson, T. R., Shields, P. P., and Glembotski, C. C.,** The conversion of atrial natriuretic peptide ANP-(1-126) to ANP-(99-126) by rat serum: contribution to ANP cleavage in isolated perfused rat hearts, *Endocrinology*, 120, 764, 1987.

48. **Zisfein, J. B., Graham, R. M., Dreskin, S. V., Wildey, G. M., Fischman, A. J., and Homcy, C. J.,** Characterization and purification of a protease in serum that cleaves proatrial natriuretic factor (ProANP) to its circulating forms, *Biochemistry*, 26, 8690, 1987.

49. **Imada, T., Takayanagi, R., and Inagami, T.,** Identification of a peptidase which processes atrial natriuretic factor precursor to tis active form with 28 amino acid residues in particulate fractions of rat atrial homogenate, *Biochem. Biophys. Res. Commun.*, 143, 587, 1987.

50. **Jacobowitz, D. M., Skofitsch, G., Keiser, H. R., Eskay, R. L., and Zamir, N.**, Evidence for the existence of atrial natriuretic factor-containing neurons in the rat brain, *Neuroendocrinology*, 40, 92, 1985.

51. **Saper, C. B., Standaert, D. G., Currie, M. G., Schwartz, D., Geller, D. M., and Needleman, P.**, Atriopeptin-immunoreactive neurons in the brain: presence in cardiovascular regulatory areas, *Science*, 227, 1047, 1985.

52. **McKenzie, J. C., Tanaka, I., Misono, K. S., and Inagami, T.**, Immunocytochemical localization of atrial natriuretic factor in the kidney, adrenal medulla, pituitary and atrium of the rat, *J. Histochem. Cytochem.*, 33, 828, 1985.

53. **Sakamoto, M., Nakao, K., Kihara, M., Morii, N., Sugawara, A., Suda, M., Shimokura, M., Kiso, Y., Yamori, Y., and Imura, H.**, Existence of atrial natriuretic polypeptide in kidney, *Biochem. Biophys. Res. Commun.*, 128, 1281, 1985.

54. **Gardner, D. G., Deschepper, C. F., Ganong, W. F., Hane, S., Fiddes, J., Baxter, J. D., and Lewicki, J.**, Extra-atrial expression of the gene for atrial natriuretic factor, *Proc. Natl. Acad. Sci. U.S.A.*, 83, 6698, 1986.

55. **Day, M. L., Schwartz, D., Wiegand, R. C., Stockman, P. T., Brunnert, S. R., Tolunay, H. E., Currie, M. G., Standaert, D. G., and Needleman, P.**, Ventricular atriopeptin: unmasking of mRNA and peptide synthesis by hypertrophy or dexamethasone, *Hypertension*, 9, 485, 1987.

56. **Lattion. A.-L., Michel, J.-B., Arnauld, E., Corvol, P., and Sombrier, F.**, Myocardial recruitment during ANF mRNA increase with volume overload in the rat, *Am. J. Physiol.*, 251, H890, 1986.

57. **Gardner, D. G., Vlasuk, G. P., Baxter, J. D., Fiddes, J. C., and Lewicki, J. A.**, Identification of atrial natriuretic factor gene transcripts in the central nervous system of the rat, *Proc. Natl. Acad. Sci. U.S.A.*, 84, 2175, 1987.

58. **Shiono, S., Nakao, K., Morii, N., Yamada, T., Itoh, H., Sakamoto, M., Sugawara, A., Saito, Y., Katsuura, G., and Imura, H.**, Nature of atrial natriuretic polypeptide in rat brain, *Biochem. Biophys. Res. Commun.*, 135, 728, 1986.

59. **Gardner, D. G., Deschepper, C. F., and Baxter, J. D.**, The gene for the atrial natriuretic factor is expressed in the aortic arch, *Hypertension*, 9, 103, 1987.

60. **Ballerman, B. J., Bloch, K. D., Seidman, J. G., and Brenner, B. M.**, Atrial natriuretic peptide transcription, secretion and glomerular receptor activity during mineralocorticoid escape in the rat, *J. Clin. Invest.*, 78, 840, 1986.

61. **Metzler, C. H., Gardner, D. G., Keil, L. C., Baxter, J. D., and Ramsay, D. J.**, Increased synthesis and release of atrial peptide during mineralocorticoid escape in conscious dogs, *Am. J. Physiol.*, 252, R188, 1987.

62. **Gardner, D. G., Gertz, B. J., and Hane, S.**, Thyroid hormone increases ANP mRNA accumulation *in vivo* and *in vitro*, *Mol. Endocrinol.*, 1, 260, 1987.

63. **Jacobs, J. W., Vlasuk, G. P., and Rosenblatt, M.**, Atrial natriuretic factor receptors, in *Endocrinology and Metabolism Cinics of North America*, Vol. 16 (No. 1), Rosenblatt, M. and Jacobs, J. W., Eds., W.B. Saunders, Philadelphia, 1987.

64. **Scarborough, R. M., Schenk, D. B., McEnroe, G. A., Arfsten, A., Kang, L.-L., Schwartz, K., and Lewicki, J. A.**, Truncated atrial natriuretic peptide (ANP) analogs: comparison between receptor binding affinity and cyclic GMP stimulation in cultured aortic smooth muscle cells, *J. Biol. Chem.*, 261, 12960, 1986.

65. **Leitman, D. C. and Murad, F.**, Comparison of binding and cyclic GMP accumulation by atrial natriuretic peptides in endothelial cells, *Biochim. Biophys. Acta*, 885, 74, 1986.

66. **Takayanagi, R., Snajdar, R. M., Imada, T., Tamura, M., Pandey, K. N., Misono, D. S., and Inagami, T.**, Purification and characterization of two types of atrial natriuretic factor receptors from bovine adrenal cortex: guanylate cyclase-linked and cylase-free receptors, *Biochem. Biophys. Res. Commun.*, 144, 244, 1987.

67. **Leitman, D. C. and Murad, F.**, Atrial natriuretic factor receptor heterogeneity and stimulation of particulate guanylate cyclase and cyclic GMP accumulation, in *Endocrinology and Metabolism Clinics of North America: Atrial Natriuretic Factor*, Vol. 16, Rosenblatt, M. and Jacobs, J. W., Eds., W.B. Saunders, Philadelphia, 1987, 79.

68. **Murad, F.**, Cyclic guanosine monophosphate as a mediator of vasodilation, *J. Clin. Invest.*, 78, 1, 1986.

69. **Maack, T., Suzuki, M., Almeida, F. A., Nussenzveig, D., Scarborough, R. M., McEnroe, G. A., and Lewicki, J. A.**, Physiological role of silent receptors of atrial natriuretic factor, *Science*, 238, 675, 1987.

70. **Scarborough, R. M., McEnroe, G., Kang, L.-L., Arfsten, A., Schwartz, K., Almeida, F., Maack, T., and Lewicki, J.**, Receptor interactions of atrial natriuretic peptide ring deletion analogs, in Program 2nd World Congr. Biologically Active Atrial Peptides, Abstr. b173, New York, May 20 to 21, 1987.

71. **McEnroe, G., Scarborough, R., Schwartz, K., Arfsten, A., Kang, L., Lappe, R., Silver, P., Wendt, R., and Lewicki, J.,** Unique requirements for interaction of ANP analogs with guanylate cyclase-coupled and uncoupled ANP binding components, in 2nd World Congr. Biologically Active Atrial Peptides, Abstr. b171 New York, May 20 to 21, 1987.

72. **Schenk, D. B., Phelps, M., Porter, J. G., Scarborough, R. M., McEnroe, G. A., and Lewicki, J.,** Identification of the receptor for atrial natriuretic factor in cultured vascular cells, *J. Biol. Chem.,* 260, 14887, 1985.

73. **Vandlen, R. L., Arcuri, K. E., and Napier, M. A.,** Identification of a receptor for atrial natriuretic factor in rabbit aorta membranes by affinity cross-linking, *J. Biol. Chem.,* 260, 14887, 1985.

74. **Hirose, S., Akiyama, F., Shinjo, M., Ohno, H., and Murakami, K.,** Solubilization and molecular weight estimation of atrial natriuretic factor receptor from bovine adrenal cortex, *Biochem. Biophys. Res. Commun.,* 130, 574, 1985.

75. **Leitman, D. C., Andresen, J. W., Kuno, T., Kamisaki, Y., Chang, J.-K., and Murad, F.,** Identification of multiple binding sites for atrial natriuretic factor by affinity crosslinking in cultured endothelial cells, *J. Biol. Chem.,* 261, 11650, 1986.

76. **Kuno, T., Andersen, J. W., Kamisaki, Y., Waldman, S. A., Chang, L. Y., Saheki, S., Leitman, D. C., Nakane, M., and Murad, F.,** Co-purification of an atrial natriuretic factor receptor and particulate guanylate cyclase from rat lung, *J. Biol. Chem.,* 261, 5817, 1986.

77. **Takayanagi, R., Inagami, T., Snajdar, R. M., Imada, T., Tamura, M., and Misono, K. S.,** Two distinctive forms of receptors for atrial natriuretic factors in bovine adrenocortical cells, *J. Biol. Chem.,* 262, 12104, 1987.

78. **Schenk, D. B., Phelps, M. N., Porter, J. G., Fuller, F., Cordell, B., and Lewicki, J. A.,** Atrial natriuretic peptide receptor: purification and elucidation of its structural subunit composition, *Proc. Natl. Acad. Sci. U.S.A.,* 84, 1521, 1987.

79. **Schenk, D. B., Johnson, L. K., Schwartz, K., Sista, H., Scarborough, R. M., and Lewicki, J. A.,** Distinct atrial natriuretic factor receptor sites on cultured bovine aortic smooth muscle and endothelial cells, *Biochem. Biophys. Res. Commun.,* 127, 433, 1985.

80. **Shimonaka, M., Saheki, T., Hagiwara, H., Ishido, M., Hogi, T. F., Wakita, K., Inada, Y., Kondo, J., and Hirose, S.,** Purification of atrial natriuretic peptide receptor from bovine lung, *J. Biol. Chem.,* 262, 5510, 1987.

81. **Schenk, D., Porter, G., Fuller, F., Arfsten, A., and Lewicki, J.,** Cloning and expression of the receptor for atrial natriuretic factor, in *Program 2nd World Congr. Biologically Active Atrial Peptides,* New York, May 20 to 21, 1987, 190.

82. **Fuller, F., Porter, J. G., Arfsten, A., Miller, J., Schilling, J., Scarborough, R. M., Lewicki, J., and Schenk, D. B.,** Atrial natriuretic peptide C-receptor: complete sequence and functional expression of cDNA clones, *J. Biol. Chem.,* 263, 9395, 1988.

83. **Ullrich, A., Coussens, L., Hayflick, J. S., Dull, T. S., Gray, H., Tam, A. W., Lee, J., Yarden, Y., Libermann, T. A., Schlessinger, J., Downwand, J., Mayes, E. L. U., Whittle, N., Waterfield, M. D., and Seeburg, P. H.,** Human epidermal growth factor receptor cDNA sequence and aberrant expression of the amplified gene in A431 epidermoid carcinoma cells, *Nature (London),* 309, 418, 1984.

84. **Yarden, Y., Escobedo, J. A., Kuang, W.-J., Yang-Feng, T. L., Daniel, T. O., Tremble, P. M., Chen, E. Y., Ando, M. E., Harkins, R. N., Franke, Y., Fried, V. A., Ullrich, A., and Williams, L. T.,** Structure of the receptor for platelet-derived growth factor helps define a family of closely related growth factor receptors, *Nature (London),* 323, 226, 1986.

85. **Yamamoto, T., Davis, C. G., Brown, M. S., Schneider, W. J., Casey, M. L., Goldstein, J. L., and Russell, D. W.,** The human LDL receptor: a cysteine-rich protein with multiple alu sequences in its mRNA, *Cell,* 39, 27, 1984.

86. **McClelland, A., Kuhn, L. C., and Ruddle, F. H.,** The human transferrin receptor gene: genomic organization, and the complete primary strucutre of the receptor deduced from a cDNA sequence, *Cell,* 39, 267, 1984.

87. **Ashwell, G. and Harford, J.,** Carbohydrate-specific receptors of the liver, *Annu. Rev. Biochem.,* 51, 531, 1982.

88. **Morgan, D. O., Edman, J. C., Standring, D. N., Fried, V. A., Smith, M. C., Roth, R. A., and Rutter, W. J.,** Insulin-like growth factor II receptor as a multifactorial binding protein, *Nature (London),* 329, 301, 1987.

89. **Roth, R. A.,** Structure of the receptor for insulin-like growth factor II: the puzzle amplified, *Science,* 239, 1269, 1988.

90. **Macdonald, R. G., Pfeffer, S. R., Coussens, L., Tepper, M. A., Brocklebank, C. M., Mole, J. E., Anderson, J. K., Chen, E., Czech, M. P., and Ullrich, A.,** A single receptor binds both insulin-like growth factor II and mammose-6-phosphate, *Science,* 239, 1134, 1988.

91. Leonard, W. J., Depper, J. M., Crabtree, G. R., Rudikoff, S., Pumphrey, J., Robb, R. J., Kronke, M., Suetlik, P. B., Peffer, N., Waldmann, J. A., and Greene, W. C., Molecular cloning and expression of cDNAs for the human interleukin-2 receptor, *Nature (London)*, 311, 626, 1984.

92. Nikaido, T., Shimizu, A., Ishida, N., Sabe, H., Teshigawa, K., Maeda, M., Uchiyama, T., Yodoi, H., and Hongo, T., Molecular cloning of cDNA encoding human interleukin-2 receptor, *Nature (London)*, 311, 631, 1984.

93. Porter, J. G., Wang, Y., Schwartz, K., Arfsten, A., Spratt, K., Dale, B., Schenk, D., Fuller, F., Scarborough, R. M., and Lewicki, J. A., C-ANP receptor structure and expression, *Am. J. Hypertens*, 1(No. 3, Part 2), 123A, 1988.

Chapter 2

THE WHOLE HEART IS AN ENDOCRINE GLAND

M. Cantin and J. Genest

TABLE OF CONTENTS

I. INTRODUCTION

The atria in mammals are an endocrine gland,[1-4] secreting, in the rat, atrial natriuretic factor (ANF), a 28-amino-acid peptide (Ser_{99}-Tyr_{126})[5] which is diuretic, natriuretic, vasodilatory, and inhibitory of aldosterone, cortisol, arginine vasopressin, and renin release. In the rat, the N-terminal moiety (Asn_1-Arg_{98}) of the propeptide (Asn_1-Tyr_{126}) is also present in the circulation.[6] The presence of ANF mRNA[7] and of immunoreactive IR-ANF in ventricular cardiocytes[8,9] and the secretion of IR-ANF by cultured rat ventricular cardiocytes[10] indicate that, in mammals, these cells, like their counterparts in nonmammalian vertebrates,[11] contain and release ANF. Previous studies have demonstrated that the plasma levels of IR-ANF are markedly increased in an experimental model of congestive heart failure, the cardiomyopathic hamster.[8,9] In these animals, the ratio of IR-ANF between atria and ventricles, which is 132:1 in control animals, becomes 4:1 in animals with severe heart failure because of a decrease in atrial levels and a concomitant increase in ventricular levels.[8] The aim of the present study was threefold: (1) to assess whether the levels of cardiac ANF mRNA and of IR-ANF in Brattleboro rats are different from those of control Long-Evans rats and to correlate the changes observed at the electron microscopic level in atrial and ventricular cardiocytes of these animals, (2) to assess whether IR-ANF levels in atria and ventricles of cardiomyopathic hamsters reflect changes in gene expression, as well as in secretory activity, by measuring ANF mRNA and by evaluating the respective contribution of atria and ventricles to plasma IR-ANF levels by measuring ANF release in the Langendorff preparation, and (3) to assess the presence of ANF in the entire conduction system of the rat heart and in the false tendons (chordae tendinae spuriae, CTS) of the rabbit.[12]

A. ANF IN THE HEART OF BRATTLEBORO RATS

The plasma levels of IR-ANF were not significantly different in Brattleboro rats (33.6 ± 4.1 pg/ml) than in their Long-Evans controls (29.4 ± 4.6 pg/ml).[13] ANF mRNA levels[13] were significantly higher in the left, but not in the right, atrium of Brattleboro rats, as compared to their Long-Evans controls. Both right and left atrial IR-ANF concentrations were significantly higher in Brattleboro than in Long-Evans rats. In the ventricles, ANF mRNA and IR-ANF concentrations were about twofold higher in Brattleboro than in Long-Evans rats. The number of secretory granules was increased in the Brattleboro rat right atrium, as compared to their Long-Evans controls, but not significantly so. Typical secretory granules, as revealed by immunocytochemistry using the immunogold technique, were present in ~10% of the ventricular cardiocytes dispersed throughout the thickness of the ventricular wall. Such secretory granules were not seen in Long-Evans rats.

B. VENTRICLES ARE A MAJOR SITE OF ANF SYNTHESIS AND RELEASE IN CONGESTIVE HEART FAILURE

As already demonstrated,[8] the plasma levels of the C-terminal moiety of ANF were higher in hamsters with moderate heart failure (114.8 ± 2.3 fmol/ml) than in controls (8.9 ± 0.7 fmol/ml). In severe heart failure, the levels were lower (71.4 ± 16.1 fmol/ml) than in moderate heart failure, but higher than in controls. The levels of the N-terminal moiety of ANF[6] were higher in moderate heart failure (1309.3 ± 208.1 fmol/ml) than in controls (151.8 ± 9.5) and still higher (1907.0 ± 70.2 fmol/ml) in severe heart failure.

In rats with the Langendorff preparation, the levels of IR-ANF expressed per milliliter of effluent for the first 10-min period following equilibration was in the nanogram range in the case of the whole heart (490.0 ± 83 fmol/ml), which is 50 times higher than the levels found in the coronary effluent of isolated ventricles (9.8 ± 2.9 fmol/ml). These values, in each case, tended to decrease with time (120 min), but not in a significant manner. The ratio of the total amount secreted within 2 h by whole heart and isolated ventricles, respectively, is thus 28:1, which corresponds to a participation of 3.4% by the ventricles.

In control hamsters, the level of IR-ANF released by the whole heart during the first 10 min of the perfusion period following equilibration was significantly smaller (26.2 ± 2.5 fmol/ml) than that released by the rat heart. The amount released in the same conditions by the isolated ventricles of control animals was 7.1 ± 0.4 fmol/ml, which is significantly less than for the whole heart, but about equal to the amount released by the control rat isolated ventricles. The amount released by the whole hearts of cardiomyopathic hamsters in moderate heart failure during the first 10 min of perfusion (134.0 ± 9.2 fmol/min) is significantly higher than the amount found in the effluent of control hamsters for the same period while, here again, the amount released by the isolated ventricles reveals, as compared to the whole heart, a significant drop (16.6 ± 4.0 fmol/min), which is, nevertheless, significantly higher than that originating from control rat and hamster ventricles. Here again, the levels of IR-ANF released by whole heart or by isolated ventricles tended to decrease with time, but not to a significant degree. In severe heart failure, the amount released by the whole heart (40.4 ± 7.1 fmol/min) during the same time period was significantly less than in moderate heart failure, but the isolated ventricles of the former animals released significantly more (41.2 ± 5.1 fmol/ml) than did those of the latter. All these values tended to decrease with perfusion time, particularly those of the ventricular effluent of hamsters with severe heart failure, but not in a significant manner. The ratio of the total amount of IR-ANF released by the whole heart as compared to ventricles, which is 3:1 in control hamsters, became 6:1 in moderate heart failure and 1.3:1 in severe heart failure. Thus, while the ventricles contributed 35.8% of the total amount of released IR-ANF in control hamsters, the amount released by the ventricles in moderate heart failure decreased to 17.5% and reached 73.9% in severe heart failure.

The HPLC pattern of rat plasma IR-ANF revealed two main peaks of immunoreactivity corresponding to the C- and N-terminal moieties. In addition, a small peak corresponding to the whole propeptide, as visualized by the IRMA (immunoradiometric assay)[14] technique utilizing a double antibody technique to detect the whole ANF propeptide, was also recognized by the C- and N-terminal antibodies. The HPLC pattern of the Langendorff effluent from the whole heart was almost identical to that of plasma, while that of the ventricular effluent was very different: the greater part of the released form was the propeptide, with smaller peaks of the C- and N-terminal peptides.

The HPLC pattern of IR-ANF in control hamster plasma was slightly different from that of the rat. Most of the plasma peptides eluted as the N terminal, with a smaller peak of C-terminal ANF. No high Mr form corresponding to the propeptide was found in plasma. In the Langendorff effluent of the whole heart, both C- and N-terminal forms were found again with a predominance of the N terminal and a very small peak of the propeptide. In the effluent from ventricles, the amount of the propeptide was slightly higher than that of the C terminal, with a predominance again of the N terminal.

The HPLC pattern of plasma IR-ANF from animals in moderate heart failure was essentially similar to that of control animals, except for the presence of a small peak of the propeptide recognized by the IRMA technique and by the two antibodies. This small peak was also present in the effluent of the whole heart, as in control animals, and increased markedly in the ventricular effluent.

In severe heart failure, plasma contained a small amount of the propeptide. The amount of the propeptide was markedly increased in the effluent from the whole heart and particularly from ventricles.

C. ANF IN THE CONDUCTION SYSTEM

As determined by RIA, the amount of C-terminal ANF (Ser_{99}-Tyr_{126}) present in the superior vena cava was 148 times (per mg protein) lower than in the atria, while it was only 22 times less in the supradiaphragmatic portion of the vena cava. The amount of ANF present in the subdiaphragmatic vena cava was found to be negligible. The CTS were enriched 10 times in IR-ANF, as compared to the ventricular septum. HPLC showed that most IR-ANF in the superior vena cava, supradiaphragmatic vena cava, and CTS was of the high Mr form (Asn_1-Tyr_{126}), as in the atria[15] and ventricles.[9] The amount of ANF mRNA present in CTS was commensurate with ANF levels. Using β/γ nonmuscle actin mRNA as an internal standard, the amount of ANF mRNA in CTS was found to be ~10 times higher than in the interventricular septum.

D. IMMUNOHISTOCHEMISTRY

1. Superior Vena Cava

The whole wall of the superior vena cava is made up of cells having the same dimensions, general morphology, and immunohistochemical reactivity as transitional cells of the atrio-ventricular node (*vide infra*). These cells have a weak or absent immunoreactivity. A few of the cells, dispersed in the wall of the vein, have a much higher immunoreactivity. The lumen of the vena cava is lined with endothelial cells which either abut directly on transitional or atrial-like cells or are in contact with rare smooth muscle cells. Arterioles and venules are found in the wall of the "vein".

2. Supradiaphragmatic Vena Cava

The superior half of this portion of the vena cava is made up of cells having an immunoreactivity as intense as in the atria. A valve (Eustachian valve), also made up of intensely reactive cells covered with endothelium, separates the lumen of the vena cava from the lumen of the right atrium. The inferior portion of the vein contains very few typical atrial cardiocytes admixed with fibroblasts, collagen, and smooth muscle cells.

3. Sino-Atrial Node

The sino-atrial node is a horseshoe-shaped structure with the convex, middle portion facing the heart. The nodal cells and the transitional cells which surround them on all sides show a variable immunoreactivity: while some are not reactive at all, some are lightly reactive and some show a moderate immunoreactivity. A nodal artery with arteriolar branches surrounded by nodal cells courses through the entire node.

4. Atrio-Ventricular Node

The most posterior portion of the node is almost completely located in the lower portion of the atrial septum. It then slides down on the right side of the interventricular septum before passing on the right side of the central fibrous body to form the His bundle and then the right and left branches. The node and the His bundle are also surrounded on all sides by layers of transitional cells which, for the most part, have a weak immunoreactivity. The nodal cells themselves are as reactive as ventricular cardiocytes. The "true" atrial cells of the interatrial septum are as reactive as those of the right and left atrium. The cells of the central portion of the His bundle are as reactive as ventricular cardiocytes, while the cells of the right and left branches are almost as intensely reactive as atrial cardiocytes.

5. Intraventricular Conduction System

Two types of cells constitute the rat CTS: the majority (~70%) (Purkinje type I cells) are intensely immunoreactive, while the remainder (Purkinje type II cells) show a finely granular reactivity. The subendocardial Purkinje network is also made up of these two cell types. In these locations, Purkinje type I cells form cable-like structures, while Purkinje type II cells are either located beneath the former or abut directly on the endocardium. The latter are not separated from working ventricular cardiocytes by connective tissue septa. Coronary arteries and arterioles are surrounded by a cushion of Purkinje type II cells which blend with the surrounding myocardium.

E. ULTRASTRUCTURE

1. Superior Vena Cava

The entire wall of the superior vena cava is made up of cells having all the ultrastructural characteristics of atrial cardiocytes, but most do not contain secretory-like granules and can thus be categorized as "transitional" cells. Most of these cells contain a relatively large Golgi complex and their peri Golgi cytoplasm contain vacuoles, suggesting, as does their low immunoreactivity, that, like ventricular cardiocytes, they secrete ANF by the constitutive pathway. Some of these cardiocytes contain typical secretory-like granules identical to those of atrial cardiocytes and, in fact, cannot be distinguished from atrial cardiocytes by any criteria. Many of these cells contain two types of mitochondria: large ones similar in structure to those of atrial cardiocytes and slender ones made up of a single crista with a doughnut shape. No granule could be seen within their pale matrix. They occur either singly or in groups of 5 to 20, often located in the paranuclear Golgi area. The subendothelial area contains collagen bundles and rare smooth muscle cells.

2. Supradiaphragmatic Inferior Vena Cava

The superior portion of the vein wall is made up almost entirely of cells identical to atrial cardiocytes. They contain numerous secretory-like granules and have a large Golgi complex in a paranuclear position. Smaller Golgi complexes surrounded by a few secretory-like granules are often found close to the sarcolemma. In the inferior portion of the vein, atrial-like cells make up about half the cell population of the vein wall, which also contains fibroblasts, collagen, and smooth muscle cells.

3. Subdiaphragmatic Vena Cava

Atrial-like cardiocytes are practically never seen. The vein wall is made up of irregularly arrayed smooth muscle cells.

4. Sino-Atrial Node

The node is made up of small cells containing a disorganized contractile apparatus. A relatively large Golgi complex is often present close to the nucleus. Secretory-like granules are present in several of these cells. The nodal cells are located close to the sinus artery or off one of its branches and are surrounded on all sides by larger cells (transitional) which make up the whole wall of the superior vena cava and extend between the node and the wall of the right atrium, as well as externally on the lateral side of the vena cava.

5. Atrio-Ventricular Node

The node is made up of very numerous small nodal cells which possess many of the morphological characteristics of the nodal cells in the sino-atrial node. Several of these cells contain secretory-like granules, but the granulated cells are not as numerous as in the sino-atrial node itself. Transitional cells surround the nodal cells on all sides and at some point make up practically the whole inferior portion of the interatrial septum.

6. His Bundle

Most of the cells of the central portion of the His bundle are similar to nodal cells and, like these cells, also contain secretory-like granules. The superior portion is in contact with numerous nerve bundles.

Right and left branches of the His bundle — These cells are the longest and largest of the whole conduction system in the rat. They are almost identical to atrial cardiocytes and practically all of them contain numerous secretory-like granules not only in the paranuclear Golgi region, but also throughout their cytoplasm. The Golgi complex is long, occupies a paranuclear position, and resembles its atrial counterpart.

F. INTRAVENTRICULAR CONDUCTION SYSTEM
1. CTS

Two populations of cells were found in CTS. In both cases, the cells were surrounded by connective tissue sheaths covered by endothelium. Fibroblasts, nerve terminals, Schwann cells, and a few mast cells were present in the matrix of collagen and elastic fibers. The majority of CTS were made up of cells resembling atrial cardiocytes (Purkinje type I cells). They had a large Golgi complex comprised of saccules and vesicles, often containing protogranules occupying the central paranuclear zone and numerous secretory-like granules. The secretory-like granules were of two types: either small (79 nm) and dense or large (180 nm) and pale. The myofilaments generally occupied the peripheral part of the cells. They often lacked the typical parallel arrangement of their atrial and ventricular counterparts and were characterized by abnormalities in Z-band organization and localization. Complexes of thick and thin filaments in close apposition to polyribosomes were often found in the peripheral regions of the cells. No T-system was detected.

Another population of CTS was made up of cells identical to working ventricular cardiocytes, except for their smaller size (7.0 vs 10 μm in transverse diameter for working ventricular cardiocytes), absence of a T-system, and the presence of a very extensive paranuclear Golgi complex comprised of small vesicles that often contained protogranules. The secretory-like granules were smaller (75 nm), of the dense type, few in number, and almost always located in the immediate Golgi periphery. Bundles of intermediate filaments and myofilament-polyribosome complexes were not seen and the Z-bands were smaller than, but otherwise similar in morphology and localization to, those of working ventricular cardiocytes. Here again, no T-system was found. In both types of Purkinje cells, two kinds of mitochondria were noted: large ones similar to those of working ventricular cardiocytes and slender ones made up of a single crista with a doughnut shape.

G. SUBENDOCARDIAL CELLS

Cells with almost the same ultrastructural features as those found in the false tendons were present throughout the subendocardial myocardium. Purkinje type I cells formed cable-like structures immediately beneath the endocardium. These cell bundles were surrounded by thick layers of collagen and elastic fibers. Cells resembling Purkinje type II cells were present in the subendocardium beneath the Purkinje type I cells. These cells were not embedded in connective tissue and were of the same size and ultrastructure as working ventricular cardiocytes, except for a large paranuclear Golgi complex made up of numerous saccules and a few protogranules. Sparse, small (80 nm), and dense secretory-like granules were present around the Golgi area. The same type of cells were also present immediately beneath the endocardium in several areas devoid of Purkinje type I cells. They had the same ultrastructure.

H. PERIVASCULAR AREAS

Purkinje type II cells formed a cushion around coronary arteries and arterioles. Here again, they were identical to working ventricular cardiocytes, except for a large paranuclear Golgi complex containing a few small (78.1 nm), dense, secretory-like granules.

I. IMMUNOCYTOCHEMISTRY
1. Vena Cava

Superior vena cava — Numerous cells in the superior vena cava contained secretory granules which were covered with gold particles after exposure to one of the three affinity-purified antibodies (C- and N-terminal polyclonal and C-terminal monoclonal)[16] and the immunogold technique.

Supradiaphragmatic vena cava — Practically all the cells in the upper and lower portion of the supradiaphragmatic vena cava were typical atrial-like cardiocytes which contained numerous secretory granules decorated with gold particles after exposure to one of the three antibodies.

Sino-atrial node — Several nodal and transitional cells were found to contain secretory-like granules which were decorated with gold particles in the same conditions as above.

Atrio-ventricular node — Several of the nodal cells and many of the transitional cells contained secretory-like granules which were decorated with gold particles after exposure to one of the three antibodies.

2. CTS

The secretory granules of Purkinje type I and II cells from the CTS were decorated with gold particles after exposure to one of the three antibodies.

3. Subendocardial Cells

Here again, Purkinje type I and II cells contained secretory granules which were immunostained with the three antibodies.

4. Perivascular Cells

Secretory granules of periarterial and periarteriolar cells were also decorated with gold particles with the three antibodies.

J. ANF IN RABBIT CTS
1. Biochemistry

As determined by RIA, the amount of IR-ANF (C terminal) present in rabbit CTS (from both ventricles) was ~39 times lower (per milligram protein) than in the atria. HPLC analysis revealed that almost equal parts of the eluted peptides correspond to the C- and N-terminal portion of the molecule and to the propeptide of ANF.

2. Immunohistochemistry

All CTS conduction cells reacted more strongly than ventricular cardiocytes with the three antibodies.

3. Ultrastructure

The CTS of rabbits, as already described,[17] contain Purkinje cells embedded in connective tissue and surrounded by endothelium. The Purkinje cells contain a central nucleus, with a relatively large Golgi complex often seen at both poles. Small Golgi vesicles, a few lysosome-like structures, and a few secretory-like granules are present. The complexity of the peripheral contractile apparatus of these cells has been described.[17]

4. Immunocytochemistry

IR-ANF could not be detected in the immunostained fine sections embedded in Lowicryl K$_4$M. In fine frozen sections (immunocryo-ultramicrotomy),[18] however, Golgi saccules and the few secretory granules present in these cells were decorated with gold particles after exposure of the sections to antibodies, indicating that these structures contain IR-ANF.

II. DISCUSSION

A number of conditions are now known to produce an elevation of both IR-ANF and ANF mRNA in atria and ventricles.[8,9,19-21] Glucocorticoid-stimulated IR-ANF synthesis is accompanied by an increase in ANF mRNA in the rat atria.[22] In primary cultures of rat atria, dexamethasone, testosterone, and triiodothyronine markedly stimulate both the synthesis and secretion of IR-ANF.[23] Dexamethasone has also been shown to increase both

ANF and ANF mRNA in rat ventricles *in vivo*[19] and the same finding has been reported in primary cultures of rat ventricular cardiocytes.[24] Testosterone and triiodothyronine have comparable effects on both IR-ANF levels and secretion in cultures of rat ventricular cardiocytes.[24] Sodium administration can also enhance atrial ANF release and atrial ANF content,[25] particularly when it is associated with an increase in plasma volume.[26] An elevation of ventricular ANF mRNA and IR-ANF has also been associated with hypertrophy in either cardiomyopathic hamsters,[8,9] volume-overloaded rats,[20] or ventricular hypertrophy in humans.

In both cardiomyopathic hamsters and humans, the increase in gene expression is accompanied by the presence of an enlarged Golgi complex and typical secretory granules containing IR-ANF in ~20% of cardiocytes.[8,9] While the stimulation to these changes in the ventricular cardiocytes during hypertrophy may be tentatively attributed to heightened telediastolic pressure and wall stretch,[8,9] such a situation does not occur in Brattleboro rats which are euvolemic.[27,28] Likewise, although Brattleboro rats have a 5% elevation in plasma osmolality and sodium content,[29] this is unlikely to lead to the observed increase in IR-ANF and ANF mRNA in the atria since their excessive drinking behavior normalizes their plasma volume.[28,29] Furthermore, one would expect such increases to elevate plasma ANF levels and to decrease atrial ANF concentrations.[25,26] Brattleboro rats are not known to exhibit increased secretion of glucocorticoids,[30] sex steroids,[31] or thyroid hormone.[32] These results thus raise the possibility that the increased synthesis and storage of ANF in both atria and ventricles of Brattleboro rats are related to a decrease in the response of the heart to hemodynamic changes in the absence of vasopressin, which would act as a modulatory or conditioning factor for release. Such a hypothesis has already been suggested since, in conscious rats, the effect of AVP on the release of ANF at near-plasma physiological levels depends on the blood volume.[33] Thus, AVP may be necessary for the atrial secretory response to occur following atrial stretch. Since ventricular cardiocytes release ANF in culture[10] and in the Langendorff preparation, even at times when they do not harbor secretory granules, their constitutive pathway of secretion may also be conditioned by AVP.

In control hamsters, the ratio of atrial to ventricular IR-ANF (132:1)[8,9] is analogous to the ANF mRNA ratio (100:1). In cardiomyopathic hamsters with severe congestive heart failure, atrial IR-ANF levels are decreased by 50%,[8,9] while ANF mRNA is decreased by 40%. At the ultrastructural level, the atrial cardiocytes of these animals show a pattern of intense secretory activity.[9] These findings are compatible with the hypothesis of maximally stimulated cells where gene expression is not increased to a level commensurate with demand and suggest that gene expression is uncoupled from secretory activity. Whether the decrease in gene expression is due to a negative feedback effect of increased plasma ANF levels remains to be determined. In severe heart failure, IR-ANF levels in ventricles are increased 32-fold,[9] while ANF mRNA is increased 100-fold. These results tend to indicate that ventricular cardiocytes in severe heart failure are maximally stimulated and that the discrepancy between the 32-fold increase in IR-ANF and the 100-fold increase in ANF mRNA may be due to lower hormone accumulation in ventricular cardiocytes related to the overall constitutive nature of ANF secretion in these cells.

The amount of C-terminal IR-ANF released by the whole heart of hamsters in moderate and severe congestive heart failure is in agreement with the plasma levels of IR-ANF observed in these animals: in both cases, they are higher in moderate than in severe congestive heart failure.[8,9] This suggests that the results of perfusion in the Langendorff preparation may serve as a useful estimate of the *in vivo* situation. The relative proportion of C-terminal IR-ANF released by the isolated ventricles vs. the whole heart is very small (3.5%) in the rat heart and is much higher (35.8%) in the control hamster. In moderate heart failure, the amount released by the ventricles is relatively smaller (17.5%), whereas it reaches 73.9% in severe congestive heart failure. Thus, the contribution of atria vs. ventricles to plasma

ANF may be more important in moderate heart failure than in control hamsters and the reverse may be true in the severe stage of the disease.

HPLC analysis revealed that a small amount of the propeptide is found in rat plasma and in the effluent from the whole heart. The cleavage of ANF by the isolated rat ventricles is different since the major portion is recognized as the propeptide by the IRMA technique and by both C- and N-terminal antibodies. Almost identical patterns emerge from the analysis of control and cardiomyopathic hamster hearts, thus indicating that the relative absence of maturation of the propeptide by ventricular cardiocytes is not markedly increased in heart failure. It is thus likely that the small amount of the propeptide in plasma originates from the ventricles. The absence of the propeptide in control hamster plasma may be due to cleavage in the circulation, as is possibly the case for the small fragments surrounding the C- and N-terminal peaks. In control rat plasma, for instance, ~10% of ANF is in the form of Ser_{103}-Tyr_{126}.[34] In rat plasma, analysis by HPLC at different time intervals after prohormone injection revealed nonspecific hydrolysis of the pro-ANF molecule.[6] Analysis of cardiomyopathic hamster plasma by a different HPLC method has also shown the presence of a small amount of high Mr ANF.[9] These results indicate that ventricular cardiocytes from both control and cardiomyopathic animals cleave only a variable portion of the secretory product. This is at variance with other cell types where constitutively secreted proteins like albumin from hepatocytes[35,36] or α-mating factor from yeast[37] are properly cleaved. These observations raise the possibility that the ANF released by atrial cardiocytes in culture, which is predominantly in the propeptide form,[38,39] is constitutively secreted.[40]

These results suggest that in experimental congestive heart failure, secretion from atrial and ventricular cardiocytes is maximally stimulated. This is accompanied by decreased gene expression in atrial cardiocytes and markedly increased gene expression in ventricular cardiocytes. Thus, in atrial cardiocytes, gene expression and secretory activity are apparently uncoupled, while they proceed conjointly in ventricular cardiocytes. The increase in plasma ANF observed in moderate congestive heart failure is mainly due to atrial hypersecretion, whereas ventricular secretion is much more important in severe heart failure. While the propeptide is properly cleaved by atria, a relatively large portion of pro-ANF is released as such by the ventricles, whether from control or cardiomyopathic animals. This leads to the presence of a small quantity of the propeptide in the circulation, while the remainder is nonspecifically hydrolyzed.

The present results also indicate that the whole intrathoracic portion of the superior vena cava is mostly made up of transitional cells and atrial-like cardiocytes. The level of IR-ANF present in the tissue is much higher than in cardiac ventricular tissue and HPLC analysis indicates that most of the ANF, as in the atria[15] and ventricles,[9] corresponds to pro-ANF (Asn_1-Tyr_{126}). These results are confirmed by immunohisto- and cytochemistry. In the supradiaphragmatic portion of the vena cava, the amount of IR-ANF is the most important found to date outside of the atria. Here again, the HPLC pattern is that of the propeptide of ANF and this is confirmed by immunocytochemistry. This correlates well with the intense immunoreactivity of these cells and the presence of numerous secretory granules harboring ANF in the atrial-like cells which make up the wall of the vein. Even the valve at the junction of the supradiaphragmatic vena cava and right atrium is made up of the same type of atrial-like granulated cells. The presence of ''cardiac muscle'' in the vena cava has already been described in several mammalian species,[41-44] including man.[44] The same type of cell has also been described in the pulmonary veins[45-47] and the presence of ''nodal'' cells has been described in their walls.[48]

The present results also indicate that the whole impulse-conduction system of the rat, from the sino-atrial node to the last intraventricular cells, contains a number of features encountered in peptide-secreting endocrine cells. The localization of the sino-atrial node has already been established in the rat[46-52] and its ultrastructural features have also been described.[50,51,53] We have now established that many nodal cells and transitional cells of the sino-atrial node harbor ANF-containing secretory granules. The whole intrathoracic portion of the superior vena cava can be considered as part of the sino-atrial node since the transitional cells immediately surrounding the node are identical to those forming the whole vein wall and are in anatomical continuity with them.

The localization and histological organization of the atrio-ventricular node in the rat[54-57] is similar to those described in other mammalian species.[58] Here again, several nodal cells, as well as transitional cells, contain typical secretory granules harboring IR-ANF. The cells of the His bundle in the rat are tightly packed and arranged in longitudinal arrays. This organization is different from the one which has been described in other species.[59,60] The left and right His bundles show as intense an immunoreactivity as the atrial cardiocytes and ultrastructurally are giant atrial cells, many times longer and larger than their atrial counterpart, but with a similar ultrastructure. Again, these cells have a large Golgi complex and numerous secretory granules harboring IR-ANF.

A complex network of ANF-producing cells corresponding to Purkinje cells is also present within the ventricular myocardium of the rat. These cells have ultrastructural similarities with either atrial[61] (Purkinje type I) or ventricular (Purkinje type II) working cardiocytes. All these cells possess the morphological characteristics of endocrine cells and the IR-ANF contained in their secretory granules is recognized by antibodies against the C-terminal (Ser_{99}-Tyr_{126}) and the N-terminal (Asn_1-Arg_{98}) moieties of the molecule. It is thus evident that, as confirmed by HPLC analysis, the secretory granules of all these cell types, as in atrial cardiocytes, contain the whole ANF propeptide.

In Purkinje type I cells, the secretory granule population, as in atrial cardiocytes, is heterogenous, while it is made up of a single granule type in Purkinje type II cells. The presence of Purkinje type II cells in the CTS of other species, as far as we are aware, has not been described. From their localization and their junction with subendocardial cells of the same type, it may be deduced that they are involved in the regulation of ventricular contraction. The presence of nodal cells in close proximity to CTS Purkinje type II cells strengthens this possibility. The small doughnut-shaped mitochondria in these two cell types, as in all other cell types of the rat conduction system and in the vena cava, as in the Purkinje cells of several animal species,[62-64] are also an indication of their belonging to the same general type of structure.

The presence of Purkinje type II cells around the coronary vasculature is not surprising. Although not previously described in mammals, perivascular Purkinje cells are well-defined features of the avian conduction system.[65,66] Since ANF has been shown to possess either a vasodilatory effect on human coronary arteries[67] or a vasoconstrictive effect on guinea pig coronaries,[68] the presence of ANF-containing cells in close proximity suggests a paracrine role for these cells in the control of coronary artery tone.

The cells of the vena cava and of the entire conduction system which harbor ANF-containing secretory granules are regulated, their secretion is by definition secretagogue-dependent,[39] and the effects possibly autocrine. This situation may be analogous to that occurring in the central nervous system, where ANF-containing neurons[69,70] and ANF-binding sites[71] are present and where the inhibitory effects of the peptide on their firing rate have been described.[72]

Although ANF is present in granule form in several nodal and transitional cells of the conduction system, many of these cells do not possess such a feature. Most of them, however, exhibit a low immunoreactivity and practically all possess a relatively well-developed Golgi complex, numerous small vesicles and saccules of rough endoplasmic reticulum, and numerous small secretory-like vesicles which may form the ultrastructural basis of ANF secretion by the constitutive pathway.[36] Since ANF is produced by ventricular working cardiocytes, even in the presence of a rudimentary secretory apparatus, it may as well be the case for the cells of the conduction system.

Although well-defined ANF-containing secretory granules have now been described in porcine[73] and rat Purkinje cells, they do not seem to be a feature of the Purkinje cells of several other mammalian species.[64] The large paranuclear space of the Purkinje cells in all these species and the presence of a well-defined Golgi complex and numerous peripheral small vesicles may indicate that ANF again is present and that secretion is constitutive. In the rabbit Purkinje cells, as revealed by HPLC, RIA, and immunohistochemistry, ANF is present and a few typical secretory granules containing IR-ANF are revealed by immuno-cryoultramicrotomy.

Since ANF is known to inhibit adenylate cyclase and decrease cAMP[74] and to stimulate particulate guanylate cyclase and increase intracellular cGMP levels,[75] it may have similar effects in Purkinje fibers. In these cells, cAMP is able to produce a positive inotropic effect and to induce arrythmia,[76-78] while cGMP depresses the slow response action potential and prevents isoproterenol-induced arrythmia.[79] Analogous effects of cAMP and cGMP have also been observed in sinus node cells.[80-82] The presence of ANF throughout the conduction system and its possible effects on second messengers may, at least partially, explain the episodes of bradycardia and even sinus arrest which have been described in man infused with relatively large amounts of ANF.[83,84]

REFERENCES

1. **Cantin, M. and Genest, J.,** The heart and the atrial natriuretic factor, *Endocrine Rev.,* 6, 641, 1985.
2. **De Bold, A. J.,** Atrial natriuretic factor: a hormone produced by the heart, *Science,* 230, 767, 1985.
3. **Genest, J. and Cantin, M.,** *Reviews of Physiology, Biochemistry and Pharmacology,* Vol. 110, Springer-Verlag, Berlin, 1988, 1.
4. **Needleman, P. and Greenwald, J. E.,** Atriopeptin: a cardiac hormone intimately involved in fluid, electrolyte and blood pressure homeostasis, *N. Engl. J. Med.,* 314, 828, 1986.
5. **Thibault, G., Lazure, C., Schiffrin, E. L., Gutkowska, J., Chartier, L., Garcia, R., Seidah, N. G., Chrétien, M., Genest, J., and Cantin, M.,** Identification of a biologically active circulating form of rat atrial natriuretic factor, *Biochem. Biophys. Res. Commun.,* 130, 981, 1985.
6. **Thibault, G., Murthy, K. K., Gutkowska, J., Seidah, N. G., Lazure, C., Chrétien, M., and Cantin, M.,** NH_2-terminal fragment of rat pro-atrial natriuretic factor in the circulation: identification, radioimmunoassay and half-life, *Peptides,* 9, 47, 1988.
7. **Nemer, M., Lavigne, J. P., Drouin, J., Thibault, G., Gannong, G., and Antakly, T.,** Expression of atrial natriuretic factor gene in heart ventricular tissue, *Peptides,* 7, 1147, 1986.
8. **Cantin, M., Thibault, G., Ding, J., Jasmin, G., Hamet, P., and Genest, J.,** ANF in experimental congestive heart failure, *Am. J. Pathol.,* 130, 552, 1988.
9. **Ding, J., Thibault, G., Gutkowska, J., Garcia, R., Karabatsos, T., Jasmin, G., Genest, J., and Cantin, M.,** Cardiac and plasma atrial natriuretic factor (ANF) in experimental congestive heart failure, *Endocrinology,* 121, 248, 1987.
10. **Cantin, M., Ding, J., Thibault, G., Gutkowska, J., Salmi, L., Garcia, R., and Genest, J.,** Immunoreactive atrial natriuretic factor is present in both atria and ventricles, *Mol. Cell. Endocrinol.,* 52, 105, 1987.
11. **Chapeau, C., Gutkowska, J., Schiller, P. W., Milne, R. W., Thibault, G., Garcia, R., Genest, J., and Cantin, M.,** Localization of immunoreactive atrial natriuretic factor (ANF) in the heart of various animal species, *J. Histochem. Cytochem.,* 33, 541, 1985.
12. **Kjorell, V., Thornell, L. E., Lehto, V. P., Virtanen, I., and Whalen, R. G.,** A comparative analysis of intermediate filament proteins in bovine heart Purkinje fibers, *Eur. J. Cell. Biol.,* 44, 68, 1987.
13. **Lavigne, J. P., Drouin, J., Ding, J., Thibault, G., Nemer, M., and Cantin, M.,** Atrial natriuretic factor (ANF) gene expression in the Brattleboro rat, *Peptides,* in press.
14. **Thibault, G., Milne, R. W., and Cantin, M.,** A two-site immunoradiometric assay for proatrial natriuretic factor. Application to tissue extracts, *Peptides,* in press.
15. **Thibault, G., Garcia, R., Gutkowska, J., Bilodeau, J., Lazure, C., Seidah, N. G., Chrétien, M., Genest, J., and Cantin, M.,** The propeptide (Asn 1-Tyr 126) is the storage form of rat atrial natriuretic factor, *Biochem. J.,* 241, 265, 1987.

16. **Milne, R. W., Gutkowska, J., Thibault, G., Schiller, P., Charbonneau, C., Genest, J., and Cantin, M.,** A murine monoclonal antibody against rat atrial natriuretic factor (ANF) which cross-reacts with mouse ANF, *Mol. Immunol.,* 24, 147, 1987.

17. **Thornell, L. E.,** Myofilament-polyribosome complexes in the conduction system of hearts from cow, rabbit and cat, *J. Ultrastruct. Res.,* 41, 579, 1972.

18. **Griffith, G., Simons, K., Warren, G., and Tokuyasu, K. T.,** Immunoelectron microscopy using thin, frozen sections: application to studies of the intracellular transport of Semliki forest virus spike glycoproteins, *Methods Enzymol.,* 96, 466, 1983.

19. **Day, M. L., Schwartz, D., Wiegand, R. C., Stockman, P. T., Brunnert, S. R., Tolunay, H. E., Currie, M. G., Standaert, D. G., and Needleman, P.,** Ventricular atriopeptin. Unmasking of messenger RNA and peptide synthesis by hypertrophy or dexamethasone, *Hypertension,* 9, 485, 1987.

20. **Lattion, A. L., Michel, J. B., Arnauld, E., Corvol, P., and Soubrier, F.,** Myocardial recruitment during ANF mRNA increase with volume overload in the rat, *Am. J. Physiol.,* 251, H890, 1986.

21. **Takayanagi, R. T., Imada, T., and Inagami, T.,** Synthesis and presence of atrial natriuretic factor in rat ventricles, *Biochem. Biophys. Res. Commun.,* 142, 483, 1987.

22. **Gardner, D. G., Hane, S., Trachewsky, D., Shenk, S., and Baxter, J. D.,** Atrial natriuretic peptide mRNA is regulated by glucocorticoids *in vivo, Biochem. Biophys. Res. Commun.,* 139, 1047, 1986.

23. **Matsubara, H., Hirata, Y., Yoshimi, H., Takata, S., Takagi, Y., Iida, T., Yamane, Y., Umeda, Y., Nishikawa, M., and Inada, M.,** Effects of steroid and thyroid hormones on synthesis of atrial natriuretic peptide by cultured atrial myocytes of rat, *Biochem. Biophys. Res. Commun.,* 145, 336, 1987.

24. **Matsubara, H., Hirata, Y., Yoshimi, H., Takata, S., Takagi, Y., Yamane, Y., Umeda, Y., Nishikawa, M., and Inada, M.,** Ventricular myocytes from neonatal rats are more responsive to dexamethasone than atrial myocytes in synthesis of atrial natriuretic peptide, *Biochem. Biophys. Res. Commun.,* 148, 1030, 1987.

25. **Takayanagi, R., Tanaka, I., Maki, M., and Inagami, T.,** Effects of changes in water-sodium balance on levels of atrial natriuretic factor messenger RNA and peptide in rats, *Life Sci.,* 36, 1843, 1985.

26. **Schwartz, D., Katsube, M. C., and Needleman, P.,** Atriopeptin release in conditions of altered salt and water balance in the rat, *Biochem. Biophys. Res. Commun.,* 137, 922, 1986.

27. **Conrad, K. P., Gellei, M., North, W. G., and Valtin, H.,** Influence of oxytocin on renal hemodynamics and electrolyte and water excretion, *Am. J. Physiol.,* 251, F290, 1986.

28. **Kinter, L. B.,** Water balance in the Brattleboro rat: considerations for hormone replacement therapy, *Ann. N.Y. Acad. Sci.,* 394, 448, 1982.

29. **Dlouha, A., Krecek, J., and Zicha, J.,** Postnatal development and diabetes insipidus in Brattleboro rat, *Ann. N.Y. Acad. Sci.,* 394, 10, 1982.

30. **Milne, O. C., Baiment, M. R. I., Henderson, I. W., Mosley, W., and Jones, I. C.,** Adrenocortical function in the Brattleboro rat, *Ann. N.Y. Acad. Sci.,* 394, 230, 1982.

31. **Sokol, H. W. and Zimmerman, E. A.,** The hormonal status of the Brattleboro rat, *Ann. N.Y. Acad. Sci.,* 394, 535, 1982.

32. **Galton, V. A., Valtin, H., and Johnson, D. G.,** Thyroid function in the absence of vasopressin, *Endocrinology,* 78, 1224, 1966.

33. **Itoh, H., Nakao, K., Yamada, T., Morii, N., Shiono, S., Sugawara, A., Sato, Y., Mukoyama, M., Arai, H., Katsuura, G., Eigyo, M., Matsushita, M., and Imura, H.,** Modulatory role of vasopressin in secretion of atrial natriuretic polypeptide in conscious rats, *Endocrinology,* 120, 2186, 1987.

34. **Schwartz, D., Geller, D. M., Manning, P. T., Siegel, N. R., Fok, K. F., Smith, C. E., and Needleman, P.,** Ser-Leu-Arg-Arg-atriopeptin III: the major circulating form of atrial peptide, *Science,* 229, 397, 1985.

35. **Edwards, K., Fleischer, B., Dryburg, H., Fleischer, S., and Schreider, G.,** The distribution of albumin precursor protein and albumin in the liver, *Biochem. Biophys. Res. Commun.,* 72, 310, 1976.

36. **Ikehara, Y., Oda, K., and Kato, K.,** Conversion of proalbumin into serum albumin within secretory vesicles of rat liver, *Biochem. Biophys. Res. Commun.,* 72, 319, 1976.

37. **Julius, D., Schekman, R., and Thornor, R.,** Glycosylation and processing of preproalpha-factor through the yeast secretory pathway, *Cell,* 36, 309, 1984.

38. **Bloch, K. D., Scott, J. A., Zisfein, J. B., Fallon, J. T., Margolies, N. M., Seidman, C. E., Matsueda, G. R., Homcy, C. J., Graham, R. M., and Seidman, J. G.,** Biosynthesis and secretion of proatrial natriuretic factor by cultured rat cardiocytes, *Science,* 230, 1168, 1985.

39. **Glembotski, C. C. and Gibson, T. R.,** Molecular forms of immunoreactive atrial natriuretic peptide released from cultured rat atrial myocytes, *Biochem. Biophys. Res. Commun.,* 132, 1008, 1985.

40. **Burgess, T. L. and Kelly, R. B.,** Constitutive and regulated secretion of proteins, *Annu. Rev. Cell. Biol.,* 3, 243, 1987.

41. **Asai, J., Nakazato, M., Toshimori, H., Matsukura, S., Kangawa, K., and Matsuo, M.,** Presence of atrial natriuretic polypeptide in the pulmonary vein and vena cava, *Biochem. Biophys. Res. Commun.,* 146, 1465, 1987.

42. **Carrow, R. and Calhoun, M. L.,** The extent of cardiac muscle in the great vein of the dog, *Anat. Rec.,* 150, 249, 1964.

43. **Karrer, H. E.,** The striated musculature of blood vessels. I. General cell morphology, *J. Biophys. Biochem. Cytol.,* 6, 383, 1959.

44. **Spach, M. S., Barr, R. C., and Jewett, P. H.,** Spread of excitation from the atrium into thoracic veins in human beings and dogs, *Am. J. Cardiol.,* 30, 844, 1972.

45. **Ludatscher, R. M.,** Fine structure of the muscular wall of rat pulmonary veins, *J. Anat.,* 103, 345, 1968.

46. **Springall, D. R., Bhatnagha, M., Wharton, J., Hamid, Q., Gulbenkian, S., Hedges, M., Meleagros, L., Bloom, S. R., and Polak, J. M.,** Expression of the atrial natriuretic peptide gene in the cardiac muscle of rat extra-pulmonary and intrapulmonary veins, *Thorax,* 43, 44, 1988.

47. **Stieda, L.,** Ueber Quergestre ifte muskelfasern in der wand der lungevenen, *Arch. Mikrosk. Anat.,* 14, 243, 1877.

48. **Masani, F.,** Node-like cells in the myocardial layer of the pulmonary veins of the rat: an ultrastructural study, *J. Anat.,* 145, 133, 1986.

49. **Halpern, M. H.,** The sino-atrial node of the rat heart, *Anat. Rec.,* 123, 425, 1955.

50. **Melax, H. and Leeson, T. S.,** Fine structure of the impulse-conducting system in rat heart, *Can. J. Zool.,* 48, 837, 1970.

51. **Merrillees, N. C. A.,** The fine structure of the sinus node in the rat, *Adv. Cardiol.,* 12, 34, 1974.

52. **Muir, A. R.,** The sino-atrial node of the rat heart, *Q. J. Exp. Physiol.,* 40, 378, 1955.

53. **Taylor, I. M.,** Observation on the sinoatrial nodal artery of the rat, *J. Anat.,* 130, 821, 1980.

54. **Bompiani, C. D., Rouiller, Ch., and Hatt, P. Y.,** Le tissu de conduction du coeur chez le rat. Etude au microscope électronique, *Arch. Mal. Coeur Vaiss.,* 52, 1257, 1959.

55. **Moravec, J. and Moravec, M.,** Intrinsic nerve plexus of mammalian heart: morphological basis of cardiac rhythmical activity, *Int. Rev. Cytol.,* 106, 89, 148, 1987.

56. **Moravec, M. and Moravec, J.,** Some morphological aspects of the atrioventricular junction in the rat heart, *Pathol. Biol.,* 29, 266, 1981.

57. **Viragh, S. Z. and Porte, A.,** Structure fine du tissu vecteur dans le coeur du rat, *Z. Zellforsch. Mikrosk.,* 55, 263, 1961.

58. **Anderson, R. H., Becker, A. E., Brechenmacher, C., Davis, M. J., and Rossi, L.,** The human atrioventricular junctional area: a morphological study of the A-V node and bundle, *Eur. J. Cardiol.,* 3/1, 11, 1975.

59. **James, T. N. and Sherf, L.,** Fine structure of the His bundle, *Circulation,* 44, 9, 1971.

60. **James, T. N., Sherf, L., and Urthaler, F.,** Fine structure of the bundle branches, *Br. Heart J.,* 36, 1, 1974.

61. **Cantin, M., Benchimol, S., Castonguay, Y., Berlinguet, J. C., and Huet, C.,** Ultrastructural cyto-chemistry of atrial muscle cells. Characterization of the specific granules in the human left atrium, *J. Ultrastruct. Res.,* 52, 179, 1975.

62. **Bencosme, S. A., Trillot, A., Alanis, J., and Benitez, P.,** Correlative ultrastructural and electrophysiologic study of the Purkinje system of the heart, *J. Electrocardiol.,* 2, 27, 1969.

63. **Martinez-Palomo, A., Alanis, J., and Benitez, P.,** Transitional cardiac cells of the conductive system of the dog heart. Distinguishing morphological and electrophysiological features, *J. Cell. Biol.,* 47, 1, 1970.

64. **Sommer, J. R. and Jennings, R. B.,** Ultrastructure of cardiac muscle, in *The Heart and Cardiovascular System,* Fozzard, H. A., Jennings, R. B., Haber, E., Katz, A. M., and Morgan, H. E., Eds., Raven Press, New York, 1986, 61.

65. **Hirakow, R.,** Fine structure of Purkinje fibers in the chick heart, *Arch. Histol. Jap.,* 27, 485, 1966.

66. **Mizuhira, V., Hirukow, R., and Uzawa, H.,** Fine structure of Purkinje fibers in the avian heart, in *Electrophysiology and Ultrastructure of the Heart,* Sano, T., Mizuhira, V., and Matsuda, K., Eds., Grune and Stratton, New York, 1967, 15.

67. **Wangler, R. D., Breuhans, B. A., Otero, H. O., Hastings, D. H., Holzman, M. D., Saneii, H. H., Sparks, D. V., and Chimoskey, J. F.,** Coronary vasoconstrictor effect of atriopeptin II, *Science,* 230, 558, 1985.

68. **Rapoport, R. M., Ginsberg, R., Waldman, S. A., and Murad, F.,** Effect of atriopeptin on relaxation and cyclic cGMP levels in human coronary artery in vitro, *Eur. J. Pharmacol.,* 124, 193, 1986.

69. **Jacobowitz, D. M., Skofitsch, G., Keiser, H. R., Eskay, R. L., and Zamir, N.,** Evidence for the existence of atrial natriuretic factor containing neurons in the rat brain, *Neuroendocrinology,* 40, 92, 1985.

70. **Kawata, M., Nakao, K., Morii, N., Kiso, Y., Yamashita, H., Imura, H., and Sano, Y.,** Atrial natriuretic polypeptide: topographical distribution in the rat brain by radioimmunoassay and immunohistochemistry, *Neuroscience,* 16, 521, 1985.

71. **Bianchi, C., Gutkowska, J., Ballak, M., Thibault, G., Garcia, R., Genest, J., and Cantin, M.,** Radioautographic localization of ^{125}I-atrial natriuretic factor binding sites in the brain, *Neuroendocrinology,* 4, 365, 1986.

72. **Okuya, S. and Yamashita, Y.,** Effect of atrial natriuretic polypeptide in rat hypothalamic neurons in vitro, *J. Physiol.,* 389, 717, 1987.

73. **Toshimori, H., Toshimori, K., Oura, C., and Matsuo, H.,** Immunohistochemistry and immunocyto-chemistry of atrial natriuretic polypeptide in porcine heart, *Histochemistry,* 86, 595, 1982.

74. **Anand-Srivastava, M. B. and Cantin, M.,** Atrial natriuretic factor receptors are negatively coupled to adenylate cyclase in cultured atrial and ventricular cardiocytes, *Biochem. Biophys. Res. Commun.,* 138, 427, 1986.

75. **Hamet, P., Tremblay, J., Pang, S. C., Skuherska, R., Schiffrin, E. L., Garcia, R., Cantin, M., Genest, J., Palmour, R., Ervin, F. R., Martin, S., and Goldwater, R.,** Cyclic GMP as mediator and biological marker of atrial natriuretic factor, *J. Hypertens.,* 4, S49, 1986.

76. **Pecker, M. S., Wook-Bin, I. M., Sonn, J. K., and Lee, C. O.,** Effect of norepinephrine and cyclic AMP in intracellular sodium ion activity and contractile force in canine cardiac Purkinje fibers, *Circ. Res.,* 59, 390, 1986.

77. **Podzuweit, T.,** Catecholamine-cyclic AMP/Ca-induced ventricular tachycardia in the intact pig heart, *Basic Res. Cardiol.,* 75, 772, 1980.

78. **Tsien, R. W.,** Adrenalin-like effect of intracellular iontophoresis of cyclic AMP in cardiac Purkinje fibers, *Nature New Biol.,* 245, 120, 1973.

79. **Mehegan, J. P., Muir, W. W., Nuvertferth, D. V., Fertel, R. H., and McGuirk, S. M.,** Electrophy-siologic effect of cyclic GMP on canine cardiac Purkinje fibers, *J. Cardiovasc. Pharmacol.,* 7, 30, 1985.

80. **Nawrath, H.,** Does cyclic GMP mediate the negative inotropic effect of acetylcholine in the heart, *Nature (London),* 267, 72, 1977.

81. **Taniguchi, T., Figiwara, M., Lee, J. J., and Hidaka, H.,** Cyclic 3':5' nucleotide phosphodiesterase of rabbit sinoatrial node, *Biochim. Biophys. Acta,* 522, 465, 1978.

82. **Tuganowski, W., Kopec, P., Kopyta, M., and Wezowska, J.,** Iontophoretic application of autonomic mediators and cyclic nucleotides in the sinus node cells, *Naunyn Schmiedebergs Arch. Pharmakol.,* 299, 65, 1979.

83. **Franco-Suarez, R., Somani, T., and Mulrow, P. J.,** Bradycardia after infusions of atrial natriuretic factor, *Ann. Int. Med.,* 107, 594, 1987.

84. **Nicholls, M. C. and Richards, A. M.,** Human studies with atrial natriuretic factor, in *Endocrinology and Metabolism Clinics of North America,* Vol. 16, W. B. Saunders, Philadelphia, 1987, 199.

Chapter 3

ATRIAL NATRIURETIC FACTOR: ITS CIRCULATING FORMS AND PROHORMONE PROCESSING

Gaétan Thibault

TABLE OF CONTENTS

I. INTRODUCTION

Since de Bold's discovery in 1981[1] that heart atria contain a factor which possesses natriuretic and diuretic properties, it now appears that this factor is a new peptidic hormone integral to the well-known renin-angiotensin-aldosterone system. Atrial natriuretic factor (ANF) counterbalances this system by inhibiting aldosterone and renin secretion and by relaxing angiotensin II- or norepinephrine-induced contraction of vascular tissues. Many excellent reviews have detailed the physiological effects of ANF.[2-4]

This chapter will first describe the different forms of ANF which are found in the circulation and will then discuss the possible sites and mechanisms of proANF processing.

II. CIRCULATING FORMS OF ANF

ANF is mainly synthesized in atrial cardiocytes, but specific ANF mRNA can also be detected in other tissues such as ventricles, lungs, and adrenal glands.[5-7] The peptide is stored in the specific granules of atrial cardiocytes as the full prohormone (proANF) which contains 126 amino acids.[8] Earlier investigations have demonstrated that the C-terminal portion of the propeptide exerts biological activity. Among various peptides which have been assays *in vivo* and *in vitro* by different systems, ANF(99—126) and ANF(101—126) have shown the greatest potency.[9]

Considering these facts, it appears logical that the biologically active circulating form of ANF should be a peptide containing 25 to 35 residues and representing the C-terminal portion of proANF. Radioimmunoassay (RIA) of the ANF C-terminal portion confirmed its presence in rat and human plasma at concentrations in the range of 10 to 50 fmol/ml.[10-12] Since amino acid sequencing and analyses require relatively large quantities (50 to 100 pmol) of an unknown peptide to elucidate its structure, and considering the low yield of the purification procedures, concentrations have to be artificially increased to overcome these difficulties.

We have previously observed that morphine sulfate elevates plasma immunoreactive ANF by more than 50-fold.[13] Sprague-Dawley rats were therefore injected with morphine and blood was collected via the aorta. Following extraction of the immunoreactive material and purification by affinity chromatography and reverse-phase HPLC, the peptide was identified by Edman degradation on an amino acid sequencer as ANF(99—126).[14] Schwartz et al. used a similar strategy.[15] Their rats were injected with Arg 8-vasopressin, which increased the plasma ANF concentration tenfold. Following extraction and purification of the material, they also identified ANF(99—126) as the major circulating form.

Experiments with isolated hearts perfused by the Langendorff technique have revealed that a short C-terminal peptide is also released in the effluent.[16] We have identified this peptide — after collection of the perfusates on C_{18} Sep-Pak and purification — as the 28-residue peptide, ANF(99—126).[17] Identical results have recently been obtained with isolated perfused rabbit hearts[18] and neonatal rat hearts.[19] It is interesting to note that, in all these experiments, only a small proportion (less than 10%) of total ANF was detected as proANF.

ANF(99—126) has also been reported to be the circulating form in humans.[20-22] The peptide was isolated from either 10 l of normal human plasma[21] or 1000 l of hemofiltrate of patients with renal insufficiency.[20] Yandle et al. avoided the ethical problem of large blood collections by using blood from the coronary sinus, in which the ANF concentration is much more elevated.[22] In all these cases, ANF(99—126) represented the major peptide in human blood.

However, some other ANF peptides also circulate as minor forms in rat plasma. Schwartz et al.[15] found that about 10% of immunoreactive ANF is ANF(103—126). Yandle et al.[22] also detected a derivative of ANF(99—126) in human plasma. The peptide was hydrolyzed between residues 105 and 106 and it represented about 20% of total plasma ANF. These degraded peptides may be artifacts of purification or partial proteotytic hydrolysis of the original peptide in blood, rather than the directly secreted product. In fact, we have shown that the incubation of ANF(99—126) in rat plasma results in a slow, but progressive appearance of ANF(103—126).[23] Blood does not, therefore, seem to be a major degradation site of the ANF peptide and, as compared to angiotensin, its inactivation is rather slow.

A peculiar peptide has also been found in human blood. Some groups have reported the presence in human plasma of β-ANF, which is an antiparallel dimer of human ANF(99—126).[24-25] In some cases, this peptide accounts for as much as 25% of total ANF. It is believed to originate from the atria and appears to be converted into ANF(99—126) in the blood. The real physiological significance of this phenomenon remains to be elucidated.

During the processing of proANF, leading to the eventual secretion of ANF(99—126), the N-terminal portion, ANF(1—98), should also be generated at an equimolar ratio and released in the bloodstream. Similar events are known to occur with the C-peptide of proinsulin and the neurophysines. Recently, Katsube et al.[26] and Michener et al.,[27] using an antibody against a rat fragment, ANF(48—67), reported the presence in rat plasma of a putative immunoreactive N-terminal fragment. No clear identification was made. Employing antisera against a rat peptide, ANF(11—37), we developed an RIA to measure ANF(1—98) and we characterized it after purification from both human and rat plasma.[28,29] Isolation of ANF N-terminal from rat plasma (320 ml) or from human plasma (1.5 l) was achieved by immunoaffinity chromatography (using a purified N-terminal antibody coupled to CNBr-activated Sepharose 4B) and by reverse-phase HPLC. The purified peptide was characterized by amino acid sequencing and by molecular sieving. In both cases, the first 12 residues were identical to those of ANF(1—98). For the human ANF N-terminal, two sequences were overlapping and corresponded to peptides beginning in positions 1 and 4 of proANF. The total lengths of the peptides were estimated by molecular sieving on a BioSil TSK-125 column. The rat ANF N-terminal possesses a molecular weight of 10.5 kDa, which is identical to that of ANF(1—98). The molecular weight of the human peptide ranges between 8 and 10.5 kDa. These data indicate that, in human plasma, some partial degradation may occur in the circulation either at the N-terminal or C-terminal end of human ANF(1—98).

Concentrations of ANF N-terminal in the plasma have been found to be in the range of 400 to 500 fmol/ml in humans[29] and 200 to 400 fmol/ml in rats.[28] During severe water deprivation in the rat, its concentration decreases to 10% of its original value, as does ANF(99—126).[30] Morphine, which is known to increase ANF(99—126), also elevates the ANF N-terminal.[28] In patients with renal insufficiency, plasma values of ANF N-terminal rise up to 7000 fmol/ml. Katsube et al.[26] have shown that, during bilateral nephrectomy in the rat, there is a tremendous increase of ANF(1—98). These results suggest that the kidneys may be one of the important pathways of elimination of the N-terminal peptide. The half-life of ANF(1—98) in the rat has been found to be 2.5 min, compared to about 20 s for ANF(99—126).[28] This slower disappearance probably explains its higher concentration in the blood.

ProANF has also been detected in human plasma. Following C_{18} extraction and analysis by HPLC, a higher molecular weight form resembling proANF has been found in some plasma.[31,32] The biological significance of this finding is not clear. However, it may suggest that in some pathological situations, such as cardiomyopathy, proANF can be secreted. The precursor may also originate from different tissues, such as ventricles, during cardiac hypertrophy.

In summary, ANF(99—126), which is the biologically active peptide, and ANF(1—98) are the two main circulating forms under normal conditions (Table 1). The other detected peptides probably represent degraded products. The importance of these other peptides in the physiological actions of ANF remains to be determined. The presence of proANF in blood may be important for the clinical evaluation of cardiac function.

TABLE 1
Circulating Forms of ANF

	Human	**Rat**
Stored form	ANF(1—126)	ANF(1—126)
Secreted form	ANF(99—126)?	ANF(99—126)
Circulating forms	ANF(99—126)	ANF(99—126)
	ANF(1—98) and shorter fragments	ANF(1—98)
	β-ANF?	ANF(103—126)
	Open form of ANF(99—126)?	
	ProANF?	
Half-Life		
ANF(99—126)	2.5—5 min	15—30 sec
ANF (1—98)	?	2.5—5 min
Concentrations (fmol/ml)		
ANF (99—126)	5—15	10—25
ANF (1—98)	400—500	200—500

III. PROCESSING OF PROANF

All the data on the circulating forms of ANF suggest that the maturation of proANF involves proteolytic cleavage following the arginyl residue in position 98, which results in the two main circulating forms, ANF(99—126) and ANF(1—98).

Typically, peptidic prohormones are stored in secretory granules in which maturation takes place usually by serine proteases.[33,34] However, the case of proANF appears to be completely different. Analysis of ANF in atrial extracts of many species has shown that proANF is the main component.[16,35-37] Isolation of atrial granules by differential centrifugation and Percoll gradient, and analysis of their content have undoubtedly demonstrated that proANF is the major, if not the only, intracellular stored form.[8] These results, therefore, suggest that maturation does not take place within the atrial granule, as demonstrated for other peptidic hormones.

Bloch et al. have reported that proANF is cleaved into the 3-kDa C-terminal peptide when incubated in serum.[38,39] It has, therefore, been hypothesized that proANF is processed in the blood after its release by cardiocytes to generate the active moiety. To confirm these results, we performed some experiments involving the *in vitro* incubation of proANF in blood, plasma, and serum and the analysis of proANF after its injection *in vivo*.[40] We confirmed that proANF is effectively cleaved by serum proteases into the 3-kDa ANF C-terminal. However, this hydrolysis is 6 times slower in plasma and 12 times slower in whole blood containing EDTA. If the incubation is done in whole blood to which $CaCl_2$ is added to start the coagulation process, proANF hydrolysis almost reaches the values obtained in serum. These results suggest that proANF hydrolysis is due in great part to enzymes involved in the coagulation cascade. Furthermore, intravenous injection of 25 μg of proANF demonstrates a lack of specific processing of the prohormone. Analysis of the blood by molecular-sieving HPLC and specific RIA at different times after injection does not reveal any important generation of the ANF C-terminus.[40]

Because of the minimal activation measured in blood and in the circulation, it is unlikely that the site of processing of the precursor would be the bloodstream. Gibson et al.,[41] using inhibitors of proteases, were unable to block the processing of proANF in isolated perfused rat hearts. Their conclusion was, therefore, the same as ours.

Finally, proANF itself cannot be detected under normal conditions in blood taken from the coronary sinus,[11,12] indicating that this peptide does not appear to be a normal constituent of blood. These facts exclude the possibility of maturation of the propeptide in the circulation even if some blood proteases, such as kallikrein or thrombin, have been reported to cleave it adequately.[41]

Until now, it seems that maturation does not take place either in atrial granules or in the bloodstream, and only speculations can be expressed. Other sites of processing remain possible. (1) During exocytosis of ANF,[42] there is fusion of the granular membrane to the sarcolemma. It is conceivable that a protease located on the plasma membrane or on the granule membrane can be activated during fusion and allow rapid processing of the precursor. (2) When released in the space between cardiocytes and endothelium cells, proANF can be cleaved by an extracellular protease which can be either attached to the external face of the membrane or float in the intercellular medium. (3) ProANF, once secreted, can be picked up by specific sites on capillary endothelial cell membranes, processed in these cells, and released in the blood as the C-terminal peptide. There is actually no experimental evidence supporting any of these hypotheses. Whatever the site, processing must be excessively rapid since the prohormone cannot be measured in the coronary sinus.[11,22]

The facts are even more complicated by studies on ANF secretion by atrial cardiocytes in culture. All the reports indicate that proANF is the main form released in the medium, and ANF(99—126) is a minor form which may or may not be generated if serum is present.[38,39,43,44] On the other hand, all experiments with isolated hearts perfused with physiological buffers have demonstrated that only ANF(99—126) is released.[16-19] It is possible that the tridimensional organization of atrial cardiocytes in tissue in relation to other cells is essential for the maturation of proANF. The disorganization of myocytes, as in culture, may lead to a loss of the ability of the system to cleave adequately the precursor.

Although the site of processing is still unknown, tentative attempts have been made to identify enzymes which may be implicated in that mechanism. Plasma kallikrein and thrombin are capable of generating the ANF C-terminal and are thought to be partly responsible for the cleavage of proANF in serum.[41] Intra-atrial enzymes have also been implicated. Imada et al. reported the presence in bovine atria of a membrane-bound protease which generates ANF(99—126) from proANF.[45,46] The enzyme, which was solubilized and partially purified from bovine atria, possesses a native molecular weight of 200 kDa and is composed of subunits of 30 kDa. This enzyme appears to be associated with microsomal and granular fractions.

We have recently described the presence in rat atria of an enzyme, IRCM serine protease #1, which, upon incubation with proANF, can generate C-terminal peptides.[47,48] This enzyme has a molecular mass of 180 kDa determined by gel filtration, but 96 kDa in the presence of SDS and 44 kDa in the presence of SDS and β-mercaptoethanol by gel electrophoresis. We cannot detect this enzyme in a purified granular fraction. The serine protease can also adequately process different precursors, such as proopiomelanocortin, at the right residues to generate active peptides. Although both the proteases which we have just described possess a similar molecular weight and specificity, it is not yet known if they are identical and if they represent the right processing enzyme for proANF. Coimmunolocalization of proANF and of this enzyme will have to be performed to prove that it is responsible for the transformation of the precursor.

In summary, although the different forms of ANF in the circulation are well characterized, the study of proANF processing has only just begun.

ACKNOWLEDGMENTS

The work presented was supported by a grant from the Medical Research Council of Canada to the Multidisciplinary Research Group on Hypertension and by the Canadian Heart Foundation, the National Research Council of Canada, Bio-Méga, Inc., and Pfizer (England).

REFERENCES

1. **de Bold, A. J., Borenstein, H. B., Veress, A. T., and Sonnenberg, H.,** A rapid and potent natriuretic response to intravenous injection of atrial myocardial extract in rats, *Life Sci.,* 28, 89, 1981.
2. **Cantin, M. and Genest, J.,** The heart and the atrial natriuretic factor, *Endocrine Rev.,* 6, 107, 1985.
3. **Atlas, S. A.,** Atrial natriuretic factor: a new hormone of cardiac origin, in *Recent Progress in Hormone Research,* Vol. 42, Greep, R. O., Ed., Academic Press, Orlando, 1986, 207.
4. **Ballermann, B. J. and Brenner, B. M.,** Role of atrial peptides in body fluid homeostasis, *Circ. Res.,* 58, 619, 1986.
5. **Nemer, M., Lavigne, V. P., Drouin, J., Thibault, G., Gannon, M., and Antakly, T.,** Expression of atrial natriuretic factor gene in heart ventricular tissues, *Peptides,* 7, 1147, 1986.
6. **Gardner, D. G., Descheffer, C. F., Ganong, W. F., Hane, S., Fiddes, J., Baxter, J. D., and Lewicki, J.,** Extra-atrial expression of the gene for atrial natriuretic factor, *Proc. Natl. Acad. Sci. U.S.A.,* 83, 6697, 1986.
7. **Gardner, D. J., Vlasuk, G. P., Baxter, J. D., Fiddes, J. C., and Lewicki, J. A.,** Identification of atrial natriuretic gene transcripts in the central nervous system of the rat, *Proc. Natl. Acad. Sci. U.S.A.,* 84, 2175, 1987.
8. **Thibault, G., Garcia, R., Gutkowska, J., Bilodeau, J., Lazure, C., Seidah, N. G., Chrétien, M., Genest, J., and Cantin, M.,** The propeptide (Asn 1-Tyr 126) is the storage form of rat atrial natriuretic factor, *Biochem. J.,* 241, 265, 1987.
9. **Thibault, G., Garcia, R., Schiffrin, E. L., De Léan, A., Schiller, P. W., Hamet, P., Gutkowska, J., Genest, J., and Cantin, M.,** Structure-activity relationships of atrial natriuretic peptides, in *Atrial Hormones and Other Natriuretic Factors,* Vol. 7, Mulrow, P. J. and Schrier, R., Eds., American Physiological Society, Bethesda, MD, 1987, 77.
10. **Gutkowska, J., Bourassa, M., Roy, D., Thibault, G., Garcia, R., Cantin, M., and Genest, J.,** Immunoreactive atrial natriuretic factor (IR-ANF) in human plasma, *Biochem. Biophys. Res. Commun.,* 128, 1350, 1985.
11. **Yandle, T. G., Espiner, E. A., Nicholls, M. G., and Duff, H.,** Radioimmunoassay and characterization of atrial natriuretic peptide in human plasma, *J. Clin. Endocrinol. Metab.,* 63, 72, 1986.
12. **Miyata, A., Kangawa, K., Toshimore, T., Hatoh, T., and Matsuo, H.,** Molecular forms of atrial natriuretic polypeptides in mammalian tissues and plasma, *Biochem. Biophys. Res. Commun.,* 129, 248, 1985.
13. **Horky, K., Gutkowska, J., Garcia, R., Thibault, G., Genest, J., and Cantin, M.,** Effect of different anesthetics on immunoreactive atrial natriuretic factor concentrations in rat plasma, *Biochem. Biophys. Res. Commun.,* 129, 651, 1985.
14. **Thibault, G., Lazure, C., Schiffrin, E. L., Gutkowska, J., Chartier, L., Garcia, R., Seidah, N. G., Chrétien, M., Genest, J., and Cantin, M.,** Identification of a biologically active circulating form of rat atrial natriuretic factor, *Biochem. Biophys. Res. Commun.,* 130, 981, 1985.
15. **Schwartz, D., Geller, D. M., Manning, P. T., Seigel, N. R., Fok, K. F., Smith, C. F., and Needleman, P.,** Ser-Leu-Arg-Arg-atriopeptin III: the major circulating form of atrial peptide, *Science,* 229, 397, 1985.
16. **Lang, R. E., Tholken, H., Ganten, D., Luft, F. C., Ruskoaho, H., and Unger, Th.,** Atrial natriuretic factor — a circulating hormone stimulated by volume loading, *Nature (London),* 314, 264, 1985.
17. **Thibault, G., Garcia, R., Gutkowska, J., Lazure, C., Seidah, N. G., Chrétien, M., Genest, J., and Cantin, M.,** Identification of the released form of atrial natriuretic factor by the perfused rat heart, *Proc. Soc. Exp. Biol. Med.,* 182, 137, 1986.
18. **Wei, Y., Geller, D., Siegel, N. R., and Needleman, P.,** Identification of the cardiac and circulating form of atriopeptin in rabbit, *Biochem. Biophys. Res. Commun.,* 138, 1263, 1986.
19. **Shields, P. P. and Glembotski, C. C.,** Characterization of the molecular forms of ANP released by perfused neonatal rat hearts, *Biochem. Biophys. Res. Commun.,* 146, 547, 1987.
20. **Forssmann, K., Hock, D., Herbst, F., Schulz-Knappe, P., Talartschik, J., Scheler, F., and Forssmann, W. G.,** Isolation and structural analysis of the circulating human cardiodilatin (alpha ANP), *Klin. Wochenschr.,* 64, 1276, 1986.
21. **Theiss, G., John, A., Morich, F., Neuser, D., Schröder, W., Stasch, J. P., and Wohlfeil, S.,** α-h-ANP is the only form of circulating ANF in humans, *FEBS Lett.,* 218, 159, 1987.
22. **Yandle, T., Crozier, I., Nicholls, G., Espiner, E., Carne, A., Brennan, S.,** Amino acid sequence of atrial natriuretic peptides in human coronary sinus plasma, *Biochem. Biophys. Res. Commun.,* 146, 832, 1987.
23. **Murthy, K. K., Thibault, G., Garcia, R., Gutkowska, J., Genest, J., and Cantin, M.,** Degradation of atrial natriuretic factor in the rat, *Biochem. J.,* 240, 461, 1986.
24. **Miyata, A., Toshimori, T., Hashiguchi, T., Kangawa, K., and Matsuo, H.,** Molecular forms of atrial natriuretic polypeptides circulating in human plasma, *Biochem. Biophys. Res. Commun.,* 142, 461, 1987.

25. **Itoh, H., Nakao, K., Shiono, S., Mukoyama, M., Morii, N., Sugawara, A., Yamada, T., Saito, Y., Arai, H., Kambayashi, Y., Inouye, K., and Imua, H.,** Conversion of β-human atrial natriuretic polypeptide into α-human atrial natriuretic polypeptide in human plasma *in vitro, Biochem. Biophys. Res. Commun.,* 143, 560, 1987.

26. **Katsube, N., Schwartz, D., and Needleman, P.,** Atriopeptin turnover: quantitative relationship between *in vivo* changes in plasma levels and atrial content, *J. Pharmacol. Exp. Ther.,* 239, 474, 1986.

27. **Michener, M. L., Gierse, J. K., Seetharam, R., Fok, K. F., Olins, P. O., Mai, M. S., and Needleman, P.,** Proteolytic processing of atriopeptin prohormone, *Mol. Pharmacol.,* 30, 552, 1986.

28. **Thibault, G., Murthy, K. K., Gutkowska, J., Seidah, N. G., Lazure, C., Chrétien, M., and Cantin, M.,** NH_2-terminal fragment of rat pro-atrial natriuretic factor in the circulation: identification, radioimmunoassay and half-life, *Peptides,* 9, 47, 1988.

29. **Sundsjford, J. A., Thibault, G., Larochelle, P., and Cantin, M.,** Identification and plasma concentrations of the N-terminal fragment of proatrial natriuretic factor in man, *J. Clin. Endocrinol. Metab.,* 66, 605, 1988.

30. **Gauquelin, G., Thibault, G., Cantin, M., Schiffrin, E. L., and Garcia, R.,** Glomerular ANF receptors during rehydration in the rat. Correlation with plasma N- and C-terminal concentrations, *Circulation,* 76 (Suppl. 4), 269, 1987.

31. **Arendt, R. M., Gerbes, A. L., Stangl, E., Glatthor, C., Schimak, M., Ritter, D., Riedel, A., Zähringer, J., Kemkes, B., and Erdmann, E.,** Baseline and stimulated plasma levels: is an impaired stimulus-response coupling diagnostically meaningful?, *Klin. Wochenschr.,* 65, (Suppl. 8), 122, 1987.

32. **Stangl, E., Zähringer, J., and Arendt, R. M.,** The molecular size of circulating atrial natriuretic factor in patients with cardiovascular diseases, *J. Hypertens.,* 4 (Suppl. 6), 5550, 1986.

33. **Lazure, C., Seidah, N. G., Pelaprat, D., and Chrétien, M.,** Proteases and post-translational processing of prohormones: a review, *Can. J. Biochem. Cell. Biol.,* 61, 501, 1983.

34. **Gainer, H., Russel, J. T., and Loh, Y. P.,** The enzymology and intracellular organization of peptide precursor processing: the secretory vesicle hypothesis, *Neuroendocrinology,* 40, 171, 1985.

35. **Vuolteenaho, O., Arganiaa, O., and Ling, N.,** Atrial natriuretic polypeptide (ANF): rat atria store high molecular weight precursor but secrete processed peptides of 25—35 amino acids, *Biochem. Biophys. Res. Commun.,* 129, 82, 1985.

36. **Morii, N., Nakao, K., Kihara, M., Sugawara, A., Sakamoto, M., Yamori, Y., and Imura, H.,** Decreased content in left atrium and increased plasma concentration of atrial natriuretic polypeptide in spontaneously hypertensive rats (SHR) and SHR stroke-prone, *Biochem. Biophys. Res. Commun.,* 135, 74, 1986.

37. **Snajdar, D. M. and Rapp, J. P.,** Elevated atrial natriuretic polypeptide in plasma of hypertensive Dahl salt-sensitive rats, *Biochem. Biophys. Res. Commun.,* 37, 876, 1986.

38. **Bloch, K. D., Scott, J. A., Zisfein, J. B., Fallon, J. T., Margolies, M. N., Seidman, C. E., Matsueda, G. R., Homcy, C. J., Graham, R. M., and Seidman, J. G.,** Biosynthesis and secretion of proatrial natriuretic factor by cultured rat cardiocytes, *Science,* 230, 1168, 1985.

39. **Bloch, K. P., Zisfein, J. B., Margolies, M. N., Homcy, C. V., Seidman, J. G., and Graham, R. M.,** A serum protease cleaves pro-ANF into a 14-kilodalton peptide and ANF, *Am. J. Physiol.,* 252, E147, 1987.

40. **Murthy, K. K., Thibault, G., and Cantin, M.,** Contribution of blood and system circulation to the processing of pro-atrial natriuretic factor, *Biochem. J.,* 250, 665, 1988.

41. **Gibson, T. R., Sheilds, P. P., and Glembotski, C. C.,** The conversion of atrial natriuretic peptide (ANF)-(1—126) to ANF (99—122) by rat serum: contribution to ANF cleavage in isolated perfused rat hearts, *Endocrinology,* 120, 764, 1987.

42. **Page, E., Goings, G. E., Power, B., and Upshaw-Early, J.,** Ultrastructural features of atrial peptide secretion, *Am. J. Physiol.,* 251, H340, 1986.

43. **Glembotski, C. C., and Gibson, T. R.,** Molecular forms of immunoreactive atrial natriuretic peptide released from cultured rat atrial myocytes, *Biochem. Biophys. Res. Commun.,* 132, 1008, 1985.

44. **Zisfein, J. B., Sylvestre, D., Homcy, C. J., and Graham, R. M.,** Analysis of atrial natriuretic factor biosynthesis and secretion in adult and neonatal rat atrial cardiocytes, *Life Sci.,* 41, 1953, 1987.

45. **Imada, T., Takayanagi, R., and Inagami, T.,** Identification of a peptidase which processes atrial natriuretic factor precursor to its active form with 28 amino acid residues in particulate fractions of rat atrial homogenate, *Biochem. Biophys. Res. Commun.,* 143, 587, 1987.

46. **Imada, T. and Inagami, T.,** Purification and characterizaton of pro-ANF processing peptidase from bovine atria, *Circulation,* 76 (Suppl. 4), 318, 1987.

47. **Seidah, N. G., Cromlish, J. A., Hamelin, J., Thibault, G., and Chrétien, M.,** Homologous IRCM-serine protease from pituitary, heart atrium and ventricle: a common pro-hormone maturation enzyme?, *Biosci. Rep.,* 6, 835, 1986.

48. **Thibault, G., Seidah, N. G., Cromlish, J. A., Garcia, R., Gutkowska, J., Chrétien, M., Genest, J., and Cantin, M.,** Intracellular storage form of atrial natriuretic factor, *J. Hypertens.,* 4 (Suppl. 6), S535, 1986.

Chapter 4

PROCESSING OF PROANF: DISCOVERY, PURIFICATION, AND CHARACTERIZATION OF THE SPECIFIC PROANF PROCESSING ENZYME ATRIOACTIVASE

Teruaki Imada and Tadashi Inagami

TABLE OF CONTENTS

I. INTRODUCTION

Atrial natriuretic factor (ANF) is a peptide hormone which is synthesized and secreted mainly from atrial myocytes.[1] In the early stages of the discovery of ANF, many ANFs with varying molecular sizes were identified in atrial extract in several laboratories. These included high molecular weights (15,000 to 12,000), medium molecular weights (~6,000), and low molecular weights (~3,000). Even among the low molecular weight ANFs isolated from the rat atrium, the size of the peptide ranged from 21 to 35 amino acid residues (Table 1). These results indicated that these peptides of varying sizes were derived from a common precursor. Indeed, it was noted that this peptide hormone is labile to the tissue proteases and it has been suspected that most of them were the products of nonspecific proteolysis of the precursor or naturally occurring active peptides.

Rapid inactivation of such proteases in the tissue by boiling before homogenization enabled Miyata et al.[8] to identify the native molecular form. By this method, major molecular forms of atrial ANF were identified as pro-ANF with 126 amino acid residues. Recently, it was confirmed that isolated rat atrial-specific granules contained exclusively proANF (Figure 1).[11]

On the other hand, isolation and structural analysis of ANF in rat plasma showed that ANF(99—126), a 28-amino-acid residue from the carboxy terminal portion of proANF,[12,13] is the circulating form. Thus, contrary to more complex situations where prohormones and active hormones coexist in the storage granules and also in blood, the distinct localization of proANF and mature ANF(99—126) in different spaces was observed.

The amino acid sequence of pro-ANF was deduced from the cDNA of rat and human ANF mRNA by us and other groups.[14-21] It was shown that the signal peptide comprising the amino terminal (24 residues) and Arg-Arg at the carboxyl terminal of pre-proANF was removed before the proANF was packaged in storage granules. The examination of the amino acid sequence of proANF indicates that the conversion of proANF to 28-residue active ANF requires the cleavage of the peptide bond between Arg_{98} and Ser_{99} in the sequence shown in Figure 2.

This is in contrast to the mechanisms of prohormone-to-hormone conversion in many other tissues in which double basic sequences such as -Lys-Arg- and Arg-Arg are the structural features for the site of cleavage. Thus, although proANF contains such a double basic sequence at Arg_{101}-Arg_{102}, interestingly, it is not the cleavage site in the proANF activation of atrial proANF.

These observations suggest the following unique charcteristics of the processing of ANF.

1. The conversion of proANF to ANF(99—126) occurs during or just after the secretion from atria.
2. The enzyme which is responsible for the processing of ANF preferentially cleaves the position of a single Arg sequence rather than a double Arg sequence, which is seen near the atrial processing position.

In this chapter, we will focus on the site of the processing and the purification and characterization of the enzyme, atrioactivase, responsible for this processing, which was recently purified by us.

II. SITE OF PROCESSING OF PROANF

Several model systems have been developed for the investigation of the release mechanism of ANF from rat heart, including isolated perfused heart (Langendorf heart preparation),[22,23] heart-lung preparation,[24] primary cell culture of atrial mycocytes,[25-27] and organ

TABLE 1
Isolated Rat Atrial Natriuretic
Factors of Low Molecular Weight

No. of amino acid residues	Peptides	Ref.
35	ANF I	2
33	ANF(1—33)	4
32	ANF(2—33)	5
31	ANF II	2
	ANF(3—33)	4, 5
28	Cardionatrin	6, 7
	α-rANP	8
26	ANF(8—33)	4
25	ANF IV	2, 3
	Auriculin B	9
	α-rANP(4—28)	8
24	Auriculin A	9
	Atriopeptin III	10
23	Atriopeptin II	10
22	Atriopeptin I	10

culture of atria.[28] Using these systems, the molecular forms of released ANF were determined. As summarized in Table 2, two contradictory observations were made with these systems. Analysis of the effluent from Langendorf heart[22,23] and heart-lung preparation[24] showed that the released form is the processed 28-residue peptide, ANF(99—126). These results suggest that proANF in atrial granules is processed as it is released. It is consistent with the results that extract of human plasma collected from the coronary sinus, where ANF concentration is highest and, hence, considered as the site where freshly secreted ANF is drained, contains exclusively the small form of ANF with 28-amino-acid residues.[29,30]

On the other hand, Bloch et al.[25,27] and Glembotski and Gibson[26] showed that the media of cultured neonatal rat atrial myocytes contain only proANF. They also demonstrated the presence of enzyme(s) which process proANF to ANF(99—126) in rat serum and speculated that the secreted proANF may be processed in the circulation.[25,26,31] We have also observed the conversion of proANF to ANF(99—126) by serum and identified the serum enzyme as thrombin.[52] However, the enzyme in the serum was not detected in plasma and it seemed unlikely that the enzyme works under the physiological condition[32,33] in which the precursors of the proteases were not activated. These observations may be explained by the possible loss of the proANF activating enzyme upon placing atriocytes in certain culture media.

Since the activation occurs during the process of ANF secretion in the heart perfused with media not containing serum, the possibility that the activation occurs in the blood by blood enzyme was eliminated. Such a possibility was also eliminated by demonstrating the lack of activation upon incubation of rat or human blood plasma with proANF.[52] We have also eliminated the alternative possibility that the activation may be mediated by endothelial cells lining the inner surface of the atrium by demonstrating the lack of activation upon treating proANF with cultured endothelial cells or with atria in organ culture.

By this elimination process, the only viable mechanism for the activation of proANF was that the processing occurs at the time of secretion. The eventual proof of this hypothesis had to be provided by the purification of a specific activating enzyme for proANF in the atrium. To facilitate the assay and detection of the enzyme, we designed a specific fluorogenic substrate, Boc-Ala-Gly-Pro-Arg-MCA (AGPR-MCA), which consisted of the amino acid sequence on the amino terminal side of the peptide bond cleaved by the processing enzyme (Figure 2).

```
        -63 AGAGAGAAACCAGAGAGTGAGCCGAGACAGCAAACATCAGATCGTGCCCCGACCCACGCCAGC   -1

  1 ATG GGC TCC TTC TCC ATC ACC AAG GGC TTC TTC CTC TTC CTG GCC TTT TGG CTC CCA GGC   60
    Met Gly Ser Phe Ser Ile Thr Lys Gly Phe Phe Leu Phe Leu Ala Phe Trp Leu Pro Gly
     1                          10                                          20

 61 CAT ATT GGA GCA AAT CCC GTA TAC AGT GCG GTG TCC AAC ACA GAT CTG ATG GAT TTC AAG  120
    His Ile Gly Ala Asn Pro Val Tyr Ser Ala Val Ser Asn Thr Asp Leu Met Asp Phe Lys
                      ↑              30                                      40

121 AAC CTG CTA GAC CAC CTG GAG GAG AAG ATG CCG GTA GAA GAT GAG GTC ATG CCT CCG CAG  180
    Asn Leu Leu Asp His Leu Glu Glu Lys Met Pro Val Glu Asp Glu Val Met Pro Pro Gln
                                  50                                          60

181 GCC CTG AGC GAG CAG ACC GAT GAA GCG GGG GCG GCA CTT AGC TCC CTC TCT GAG GTG CCT  240
    Ala Leu Ser Glu Gln Thr Asp Glu Ala Gly Ala Ala Leu Ser Ser Leu Ser Glu Val Pro
                                  70                                          80

241 CCC TGG ACT GGG GAA GTC AAC CCG TCT CAG AGA GAT GGA GGT GCT CTC GGG CGC GGC CCC  300
    Pro Trp Thr Gly Glu Val Asn Pro Ser Gln Arg Asp Gly Gly Ala Leu Gly Arg Gly Pro
                                  90                                         100

301 TGG GAC CCC TCC GAT AGA TCT GCC CTC TTG AAA AGC AAA CTG AGG GCT CTG CTC GCT GGC  360
    Trp Asp Pro Ser Asp Arg Ser Ala Leu Leu Lys Ser Lys Leu Arg Ala Leu Leu Ala Gly
                                 110                                         120

361 CCT CGG AGC CTG CGA AGG TCA AGC TGC TTC GGG GGT AGG ATT GAC AGG ATT GGA GCC CAG  420
    Pro Arg Ser Leu Arg Arg Ser Ser Cys Phe Gly Gly Arg Ile Asp Arg Ile Gly Ala Gln
                                 130                                         140

421 AGC GGA CTA GGC TGC AAC AGC TTC CGG TAC CGA AGA TAA CAGCCAAATCTGCTCGAGCAGATCGCA  486
    Ser Gly Leu Gly Cys Asn Ser Phe Arg Tyr Arg Arg ***
                                 150

487 AAAGATCCCAAGCCCTTGCGGTGTGTCACACAGCTTGGTCGCATTGCCACTGAGAGGTGGTGAATACCCTCCTGGAGCT  565

566 GCAGCTTCCTGTCTTCATCTATCACGATCGATGTTAAGTGTAGATGAGTGGTTTAGTGAGGCCTTACCTCTCCCACTCT  644

645 GCATATTAAGGTAGATCCTCACCCCTTTCAGAAAGCAGTTGGAAAAAAATAAATCCGAATAAACTTCAGCACCACGGAC  723
```

FIGURE 1.   Nucleotide sequence of rat ANF cDNA. Nucleotides are numbered in the 5′ and 3′ direction, beginning with the first residue of the ATG triplet encoding the translational initiation methionine; nucleotides on the 5′ side of residue 1 are indicated by negative numbers. The deduced amino acid sequence is shown below the nucleotide sequence. A potential cleavage site for the signal peptide is indicated by an arrow between residues 24 and 25. Potential poly (A) addition signals (AATAAA) are underlined. The boxed region shows the amino acid sequence previously determined by automated Edman degradation of the 25-amino-acid ANF peptide. (Data from Maki, M., Takayanagi, R., Misoro, K. S., Pardey, K. N., Tibbetts, C. T., and Inagami, T., *Nature (London)*, 309, 722, 1984. With permission.)

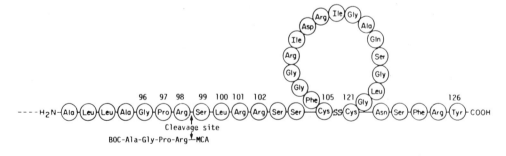

FIGURE 2.   Carboxy terminal portion of rat pro-ANF and the structure of synthetic substrate for the enzyme. BOC indicates *t*-butyloxycarbonyl. MCA indicates the fluorogenic moiety aminomethylcoumarine.

TABLE 2
Forms of Rat ANF in the Atrium, Cultured Atriocytes and Secreted Peptide

	ProANF	ANF(99—126)	Ref.
Atrium	+		8, 11, 28
Plasma		+	12, 13, 28
Krebs-Ringer perfusate of the heart		+	22, 23, a
Blood perfusate of the heart		+	24
ProANF + plasma	+		a
ProANF + serum (thrombin)		+	a
ProANF + cardiac endothelial cells	+		a
Cultured atriocytes	+		25—27
Atriocyte culture medium	+		25—27

Note: a = unpublished results from our laboratory.

TABLE 3
Purification of ProANF Processing Enzyme from Bovine Atria

Step	Protein (mg)	Total activity (U)[a]	Specific activity (U/mg)	Purity (fold)	Yield (%)
1.6 M KCl extract	6000	20.8	0.0035	1.0	100
Heparin-agarose	40	11.7	0.293	83.7	56
Arginine-agarose	2.31	4.58	1.98	565.7	22
Sephacryl S-300	2.00	5.26	2.63	751.4	25
Aprotinin-agarose	0.258	4.08	15.8	4514.3	19
Arginine-agarose	0.097	3.09	31.9	9114.3	15

[a]   μmol of Boc-Ala-Gly-Pro-Arg-MCA hydrolyzed/min.

III. PURIFICATION AND CHARACTERIZATION OF THE ENZYME, ATRIOACTIVASE, FROM BOVINE ATRIA

A. PURIFICATION

The enzyme was found to be bound to the microsomal membrane fraction of rat atrial extract and was solubilized by 1.6 M KCl solution.[34] It was found to possess the general properties compatible with a seryl protease and produced 28-amino-acid ANF by selectively cleaving the peptide bond Arg_{98}-Ser_{99} rather than other arginyl peptide bonds such as those in Arg_{101}-Arg_{102}-Ser_{103}.

For the purification of this enzyme, we used bovine atria as the source tissue. Although the whole sequence of bovine proANF had not yet been determined, we found the substrate for the rat enzyme useful for searching the bovine enzyme. Table 3 shows the summary of the purification of the enzyme. Using these five successive chromatographic steps, the enzyme was purified from bovine atrial extract.

B. CHARACTERIZATION

Atrioactivase had a high affinity to heparin agarose and was stabilized by the addition of heparin. The molecular weight of the enzyme was 580 kDa on gel filtration, whereas on SDS-polyacrylamide gel electrophoresis, a cluster of bands was seen around 30 kDa (Figure 3). Treatment of SDS-treated enzyme with endoglycosidase N reduced it two distinct bands with molecular weights near 28 and 30 kDa, respectively. The activity was inhibited by

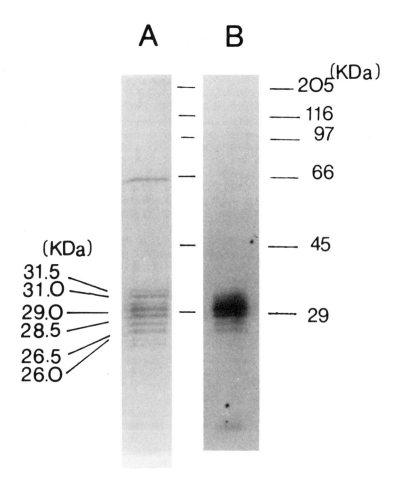

FIGURE 3.   Estimation of molecular weight of atrioactivase of SDS-polyacrylamide gel electrophoresis. (A) Silver staining of 100 ng of purified enzyme; (B) fluorography of 100 ng of the [³H]-DFP-treated enzyme. The 60-kDa band in lane A is an artifact of silver staining. Standards used here are myosin, 205 kDa; β-galactosidase, 116 kDa; phospholylase b, 97 kDa; bovine serum albumin, 65 kDa; egg albumin, 45 kDa; carbonic anhydrase, 29 kDa.

DFP, aprotinin, leupeptin, and benzamidine, but not by alkylating reagent or by chelating reagents. The activity was also inhibited by NaCl dose dependently. The enzyme produced the 28-amino-acid residue peptide ANF(99—126) from partially purified bovine proANF by the selective cleavage of the arginyl peptide bond in the -pro-Arg-Ser- sequence in proANF (Figure 4). The enzyme was localized mainly in the microsomal or plasma membrane fraction, rather than in the granule fraction.

This enzyme seemed to resemble the high molecular weight seryl proteases recently purified from several tissues, including tryptase. Tryptases isolated from human lung[35,36] and human pituitary[37] were shown to have a high affinity to heparin and to be stabilized by heparin. However, their molecular weights were 120 to 130 kDa, which were much smaller than the atrial enzyme. Whereas high ionic concentrations stabilize tryptases, the atrial enzyme rapidly lost the enzyme activity under the same condition.

An enzyme isolated from rat liver was shown to have a 600-kDa molecular mass, which is close to that of the atrial enzyme.[38] However, the liver enzyme exists only in the cytosol fraction and the substrate specificity was completely different from the atrial enzyme.

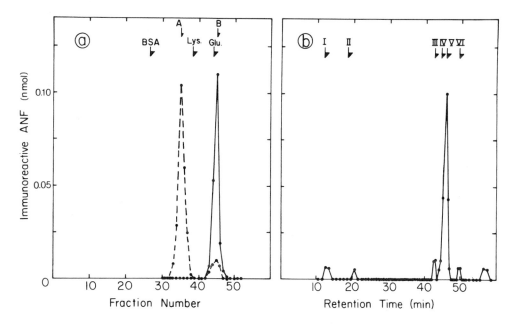

FIGURE 4.   (a) Detection of molecular weight: change of immunoreactive ANF by the atrial enzyme treatment. Fifty μl of the reaction mixtures (proANF incubated with or without the enzyme) were applied to the column and the amount of immunoreactive ANF in the fractions were determined by the method described under Experimental Procedures. Elution positions of standard proteins indicated by arrows were BSA, bovine serum albumin; lys, lysozyme; Glu, glucagon. Elution positions of proANF and ANF(99—126) were indicated by arrows A and B, respectively. (b) Characterization of the atrial enzyme-treated proANF on octadecylcylanyl column. Fifty μl of the reaction mixture (proANF incubated with the enzyme) was applied to the column and the amount of immunoreactive ANF in the fractions were determined by the method described under Experimental Procedures. Synthetic ANFs used here were I, ANF(103—123); II, ANF(105—121); III, ANF(102—126); IV, ANF(96—126); V, ANF(99—126); VI, ANF(103—126).

Atrioactivase seemed to be different from the enzyme reported by Baxter et al.[39] Our enzyme is a seryl protease, whereas the enzyme reported by these authors was a cysteinyl protease.

The localization of the enzyme in the plasma membrane or microsomal fraction rather than the granule fraction agrees with the observation that only proANF exists in the atrial granules. This suggests that it works on proANF during the secretion process of atrial granules. Recently, Page et al.[40] showed the possibility of the involvement of the endoplasmic reticulum and Golgi body in the processing of proANF by histochemical work.

Further investigation of the precise intracellular distribution of atrioactivase may disclose the mechanism of the processing of ANF.

IV. PROANF-PROCESSING SYSTEM IN EXTRA-ATRIAL TISSUES

In previous chapters, we focused on the processing system in atria. Recently, ANF biosynthesis and secretion has been reported in extra-atrial tissues, including the brain,[41-44] ventricle,[45,46] and adrenal.[47] In these tissues, several interesting features of stored ANF distinguishable from those in atria have been reported.

First, the storage forms do not seem to be exclusively proANF, but contain a large amount of processed forms (Table 4). It suggests that the processing site in these tissue cells may be different from that of atria. Furthermore, in rat brain, peptides shorter than ANF(99—126) seem to be produced by some processing enzymes different from that found in the atria.[43,44]

TABLE 4
Storage Form of ANF in Various Tissues

Tissue	Species	Molecular form	Ref.
Atria	Rat, rabbit	ProANF	1, 11
	human	ProANF, (β-form)	48
		ANF(99—126)	
Ventricle	Rat	ProANF, ANF(99—126)	45
Adrenal	Rat	ProANF, ANF(99—126)	51
Brain	Rat	ProANF, ANF(102—125),	43, 44
		ANF(103—126)	
Plasma	Rat, human	ANF(99—126)	12, 13, 29, 30

Another intriguing and yet unresolved problem is the presence in human atria of the β-form of ANF(β-hANP), which is the antiparallel dimer of ANF(99—126), which is not reported in other species.[48]

Recent results indicate that the β-form is increased in certain heart diseases.[49,50] At present, the mechanism of formation of the β-form in human atria is not clear. Since it seems to be present in the ANF secretory granules and the β-form is the antiparallel dimer of the 28-residue ANf(99—126), it is likely that the proteolytic cleavage of Arg_{98}-Ser_{99} may have taken place in the granule. This is in agreement with the observations that human atria contains some ANF(99—126) (α-hANP) as well as proANF.[48] Whether the β-form was produced by the antiparallel dimerization of the 28-residue ANF(99—126) or proANF dimerizes before the proteolytic cleavage is not clear.

REFERENCES

1. **Cantin, M. and Genest, J.,** The heart and the atrial natriuretic factor, *Endocrine Rev.,* 6, 107, 1985.
2. **Misono, K. S., Grammer, R. T., Fukumi, H., and Inagami, T.,** Rat atrial natriuretic factor: isolation, structure and biological activities of four major peptides, *Biochem. Biophys. Res. Commun.,* 123, 444, 1984.
3. **Misono, K. S., Fukumi, H., Grammer, R. T., and Inagami, T.,** Rat atrial natriuretic factor: complete amino acid sequence and disulfide linkage essential for biological activity, *Biochem. Biophys. Res. Commun.,* 119, 524, 1984.
4. **Seidah, N. G., Lazure, C., Chrétien, M., Thibault, G., Garcia, R., Cantin, M., Genest, J., Nutt, R. F., Brady, S. F., Lyle, T. A., Paleveda, W. J., Colton, C. D., Ciccarone, T. M., and Veber, D. F.,** Amino acid sequence of homologous rat atrial peptides: natriuretic activity of native and synthetic forms, *Proc. Natl. Acad. Sci. U.S.A.,* 81, 2640, 1984.
5. **Napier, M. A., Dewey, R. S., Albers-Schönberg, G., Bennett, C. D., Rodkey, J. A., Marsh, E. A., Whinnery, M., Seymour, A. A., and Blaine, E. H.,** Isolation and sequence determination of peptide components of atrial natriuretic factor, *Biochem. Biophys. Res. Commun.,* 120, 981, 1984.
6. **Flynn, T. G., Davies, P. L., Kennedy, B. P., deBold, M. L., and deBold, A. J.,** Alignment of rat cardionatrin sequences with the cDNA derived sequence of preprocardionatrin, *Science,* 228, 323, 1985.
7. **Flynn, T. G., deBold, M. L., and deBold, A. J.,** The amino acid sequence of an atrial peptide with potent diuretic and natriuretic properties, *Biochem. Biophys. Res. Commun.,* 117, 859, 1983.
8. **Miyata, A., Kangawa, K., Tsukasa, T., Hatoh, T., and Matsuo, H.,** Molecular forms of atrial natriuretic polypeptides in mammalian tissues and plasma, *Biochem. Biophys. Res. Commun.,* 129, 248, 1985.
9. **Atlas, S. A., Kleinert, H. D., Camargo, M. J., Januszewicz, A., Sealey, J. E., Laragh, J. H., Schilling, J. W., Lewicki, J. A., Johnson, L. K., and Maack, T.,** Purification, sequencing and synthesis of natriuretic and vasoactive rat atrial peptide, *Nature (London),* 309, 717, 1984.
10. **Currie, M. G., Geller, D. M., Cole, B. R., Siegel, N. R., Fok, K. F., Adams, S. P., Eubanks, S. R., Galluppi, C. R., and Needleman, P.,** Purification and sequence analysis of bioactive atrial peptides (atriopeptins), *Science,* 223, 67, 1984.

11. **Thibault, G., Garcia, R., Gutkowska, J., Bilodeau, J., Lazure, C., Seidah, N. G., Chrétien, M., Genest, J., and Cantin, M.,** The propeptide Asn^1-Tyr^{126} is the storage form of rat atrial natriuretic factor, *Biochem. J.,* 241, 265, 1987.

12. **Schwartz, D., Geller, D. M., Manning, P. T., Siegel, N. R., Fok, K. F., Smith, C. E., and Needleman, P.,** Ser-Leu-Arg-Arg-Atriopeptin III: the major circulating form of atrial peptide, *Science,* 229, 397, 1985.

13. **Thibault, G., Lazure, C., Schiffrin, E. L., Gutkowska, J., Chartier, L., Garcia, R., Seidah, N. G., Chretien, M., Genest, J., and Cantin, M.,** Identification of biologically active circulating form of rat atrial natriuretic factor, *Biochem. Biophys. Res. Commun.,* 130, 981, 1985.

14. **Maki, M., Takayanagi, R., Misono, K. S., Pandey, K. N., Tibbetts, C. T. and Inagami, T.,** Structure of rat atrial natriuretic factor precursor deduced from cDNA sequence, *Nature (London),* 309, 722, 1984.

15. **Yamanaka, M., Greenberg, B., Johnson, L., Seilhamer, J., Brewer, M., Friedmann, T., Miller, J., Atlas, S., Laragh, J., Lewicki, J., and Fiddes, J.,** Cloning and sequence analysis of the cDNA for the rat atrial natriuretic factor precursor, *Nature (London),* 309, 719, 1984.

16. **Seidman, C. E., Duby, A. D., Choi, E., Graham, R. M., Haber, E., Homcy, C., Smith, J. H., and Seidman, J. C.,** The structure of rat preproatrial natriuretic factor as defined by a complementary DNA clone, *Science,* 225, 324, 1984.

17. **Oikawa, S., Imai, M., Ueno, A., Tanaka, S., Noguchi, T., Nakazato, H., Kangawa, K., Fukuda, A., and Matsuo, H.,** Cloning sequence analysis of cDNA encoding a precursor for human atrial natriuretic polypeptide, *Nature (London),* 309, 724, 1984.

18. **Nakayama, K., Ohkubo, H., Hiros, T., Inayama, S., and Nakanishi, S.,** mRNA sequence for human cardiodilatin-atrial natriuretic factor precursor and regulation of precursor mRNA in rat atria, *Nature (London),* 310, 699, 1984.

19. **Nemer, M., Chamberland, M., Sirois, D., Argentin, S., Drouin, J., Dixon, R. A. F., Zivin, R. A., and Condra, J. H.,** Gene structure of human cardiac hormone precursor, pronatriodilatin, *Nature (London),* 312, 654, 1984.

20. **Greenberg, B. D., Bencen, G. H., Seilhamer, J. J., Lewicki, J. A., and Fiddes, J. C.,** Nucleotide sequence of the gene encoding human atrial natriuretic factor precursor, *Nature (London),* 312, 656, 1984.

21. **Kangawa, K., Tawaragi, Y., Oikawa, S., Mizuno, A., Sakuragawa, Y., Nakazato, H., Fukuda, A., Minamino, N., and Matsuo, H.,** Identification of rat atrial natriuretic polypeptide and characterization of the cDNA encoding its precursor, *Nature (London),* 312, 152, 1984.

22. **Thibault, G., Garcia, R., Gutkowska, J., Lazure, C., Seidah, N. G., Chrétien, M., Genest, J., and Cantin, M.,** Identification of the released form of atrial natriuretic factor by the perfused rat heart, *Proc. Soc. Exp. Biol. Med.,* 182, 137, 1986.

23. **Shields, P. P. and Glembotski, C. C.,** Characterization of the molecular forms of ANP released by neonatal perfused rat heart, *Biochem. Biophys. Res. Commun.,* 146, 547, 1987.

24. **Onwochei, M. O., Snajdar, R. M., and Rapp, J. P.,** Release of atrial natriuretic factor from heart-lung preparations of inbred Dahl rats, *Am. J. Physiol.,* 253, H1044, 1987.

25. **Bloch, K. D., Scott, J. A., Zisfein, J. B., Fallon, J. T., Margolies, M. N., Seidman, C. E., Matsueda, G. R., Homcy, C. J., Graham, R. M., and Siedman, J. G.,** Biosynthesis and secretion of proatrial natriuretic factor by cultured rat cardiocytes, *Science,* 230, 1168, 1985.

26. **Glembotski, C. C. and Gibson, T. R.,** Molecular forms of immunoreactive atrial natriuretic peptide released from cultured rat atrial myocytes, *Biochem. Biophys. Res. Commun.,* 132, 1008, 1985.

27. **Bloch, K. D., Seidman, J. G., Naftilan, J. D., Fallon, J. T., and Seidman, C. E.,** Neonatal atria and ventricles secrete atrial natriuretic factor via tissue-specific secretory pathways, *Cell,* 47, 695, 1986.

28. **Vuolteenaho, O., Arjamaa, O., and Ling, N.,** Atrial natriuretic polypeptides (ANP): rat atria store high molecular weight precursor but secrete processed peptides of 25—35 amino acids, *Biochem. Biophys. Res. Commun.,* 129, 82, 1985.

29. **Sugawara, A., Nakao, K., Morii, N., Sakamoto, M., Suda, M., Shimokura, M., Kiso, Y., Kihara, M., Yamori, Y., Nishimura, K., Soneda, J., Ban, T., and Imura, H.,** α-human atrial natriuretic polypeptide is released from the heart and circulates in the body, *Biochem. Biophys. Res. Commun.,* 129, 439, 1985.

30. **Yandle, T., Crozier, I., Nicholls, G., Espiner, E., Caarne, A., and Brennan, S.,** Amino acid sequence of atrial natriuretic peptides in human coronary sinus plasma, *Biochem. Biophys. Res. Commun.,* 146, 832, 1987.

31. **Bloch, K. D., Zisfein, J. B., Margolies, M. N., Homcy, C. J., Seidman, J. G., and Graham, R. M.,** A serum protease cleaves proANF into a 14-kilodalton peptide and ANF, *Am. J. Physiol.,* 252, E147, 1987.

32. **Michener, M. L., Gierge, J. K., Seetharam, R., Fok, K. F., Olins, P. O., Mai, M. S., and Needleman, P.,** Proteolytic processing of atriopeptin prohormone, *Mol. Pharmacol.,* 30, 552, 1987.

33. **Gibson, T. R., Shields, P. P., and Glembotski, C. C.,** The conversion of atrial natriuretic peptide (ANP)-(1—126) to ANF-(99—126) by rat serum: contribution to ANP cleavage in isolated perfused rat hearts, *Endocrinology,* 120, 764, 1987.

34. **Imada, T., Takayanagi, R., and Inagami, T.,** Identification of a peptidase which processes atrial natriuretic factor precursor to its active form with 28 amino acid residues in particulate fractions of rat atrial homogenate, *Biochem. Biophys. Res. Commun.,* 143, 587, 1987.
35. **Smith, T. J., Hougland, M. W., and Johnson, D. A.,** Human lung tryptase: purification and characterization, *J. Biol. Chem.,* 259, 11046, 1984.
36. **Schwartz, L. B., Lewis, R. A., and Austin, K. F.,** Tryptase from human pulmonary must cells: purification and characterization, *J. Biol. Chem.,* 256, 11938, 1981.
37. **Cromlish, J. A., Seidah, N. G., Marcinkiewicz, M., Hamelin, J., Johnson, D. A., and Chréttien, M.,** Human pituitary tryptase: molecular forms, NH_2-terminal sequence, immunocytochemical localization, and specificity with prohormone and fluorogenic substrates, *J. Biol. Chem.,* 262, 1363, 1987.
38. **Tanaka, K., Ii, K., Ichihara, A., Waxman, L., and Goldberg, A. L.,** A high molecular weight protease in the cytosol of rat liver. I. Purification, enzymological properties, and tissue distribution, *J. Biol. Chem.,* 261, 15197, 1988.
39. **Baxter, J. H., Wilson, I. B., and Harris, R. B.,** Identification of an endogenous protease that processes atrial natriuretic peptide at its amino terminus, *Peptides,* 7, 407, 1986.
40. **Page, E., Goings, G. E., Power, B., and Upshaw-Barley, R.,** Ultrastructural features of atrial peptide secretion, *Am. J. Physiol.,* 251, H340, 1986.
41. **Tanaka, I., Misono, K. S., and Inagami, T.,** Atrial natriuretic factor in rat hypothalamus, atria and plasma: determination by specific radioimmunoassay, *Biochem. Biophys. Res. Commun.,* 124, 663, 1984.
42. **Tanaka, I. and Inagami, T.,** Release of immunoreactive atrial natriuretic factor from rat hypothalamus *in vitro, Eur. J. Pharmacol.,* 122, 353, 1986.
43. **Zamir, N., Skofitsh, G., Eskay, R. L., and Jacobowitz, D. M.,** Distribution of immunoreactive atrial natriuretic peptide in the central nervous system of the rat, *Brain Res.,* 365, 105, 1986.
44. **Morii, N., Nakao, K., Morii, N., Sugawara, A., Sakamoto, M., Suda, N., Shimokua, M., Kiso, Y., Itoh, H., Sakamoto, M., Kihara, N., Yamori, Y., and Imura, H.,** The occurrence of atrial natriuretic polypeptide in brain, *Biochem. Biophys. Res. Commun.,* 127, 413, 1985.
45. **Takayanagi, R., Imada, T., and Inagami, T.,** Synthesis and presence of atrial natriuretic factor in rat ventricle, *Biochem. Biophys. Res. Commun.,* 142, 483, 1987.
46. **Gardner, D. G., Deschepper, C. F., Ganong, W. F., Hane, S., Fiddes, J., Baxter, J. D., and Lewicki, J.,** Extra-atrial expression of the gene for atrial natriuretic factor, *Proc. Natl. Acad. Sci. U.S.A.,* 83, 6697, 1986.
47. **McKenzie, J. C., Tanaka, I., Misono, K. S., and Inagami, T.,** Immunocytochemical localization of atrial natriuretic factor in the kidney, adrenal medulla, pituitary and atrium, *J. Histochem. Cytochem.,* 33, 828, 1985.
48. **Kangawa, K., Fukuda, A., and Matsuo, H.,** Structural identification of β- and α-human atrial natriuretic polypeptides, *Nature (London),* 313, 397, 1985.
49. **Song, D. L., Wang, Y.-N., Molina, C. R., Chang, J. K., Cong, Y., Chang, D., and Murad, F.,** β-human atrial natriuretic polypeptides in human plasma, *Circulation,* 76 (Suppl. 4), 134, 1987.
50. **Hiroe, M., Naruse, M., Nagata, M., Naruse, K., Shizume, K., Sekiguchi, M., Hirosawa, K., Hashimoto, A., and Koyanagi, H.,** Increased beta-human atrial natriuretic peptide (ANP) levels in the atria of mitral valvular disease and sick sinus syndrome, *Circulation,* 76 (Suppl. 4), 270, 1987.
51. **Ong, H., Lazure, C., Nguyen, T. T., McNicoll, N., Seidah, N., Chrétien, M., and DeLéan, A.,** Bovine adrenal chromaffin granules are a site of synthesis of atrial natriuretic factor, *Biochem. Biophys. Res. Commun.,* 147, 957, 1987.
52. **Imada, T. and Inagami, T.,** unpublished observation.

Chapter 5

REGULATION OF ANF BIOSYNTHESIS, SECRETION, AND POST-TRANSLATIONAL PROCESSING IN THE HEART

Christopher C. Glembotski and Paul P. Shields

TABLE OF CONTENTS

I. INTRODUCTION

In the adult mammal, the cardiac atrium is the primary tissue that expresses the gene for ANF. Among endocrine cells, atrial myocytes are unique in that they possess not only ANF-containing secretory granules, but also densely arranged myofibril contractile elements. Although ANF in the atria is similar to other endocrine peptides in that it is stored within secretory granules, it is relatively distinctive in that its storage form represents a high molecular weight precursor [15 kDa, ANF(1—126)][1-3] of the circulating form of the peptide [3 kDa, ANF(99—126)].[4,5] With the exception of one other hemostatic hormone, angiotensin, most other peptide hormones are stored within secretory granules, primarily as the final bioactive product peptide.[6,7] While the bioactive form of angiotensin, angiotensin II, is cleaved from its precursor, angiotensinogen, within the circulation, the tissue location and mechanism of ANF processing is presently not known. Because of the potentially important role played by ANF in regulating blood pressure, efforts of many investigators have focused on determining (1) the factors that regulate the expression of the ANF gene, (2) the mechanism of the post-translational processing of ANF, and (3) how ANF secretion is regulated. This review will focus on these topics as they have been studied using various animal, tissue, and cell culture model systems.

II. REGULATION OF ANF GENE EXPRESSION

Recently, biochemical studies have been performed to determine whether various physiological and hormonal manipulations affect ANF levels at either the transcriptional or translational levels. To date, those studies have suggested that the key regulators of atrial ANF mRNA and peptide levels include salt and hydration state, as well as adrenal and thyroid hormones.

A. SALT AND HYDRATION STATE

Early studies demonstrated that a low sodium diet decreased the level of ANF mRNA in the atria of rats by 31%, compared to animals fed a normal sodium diet (Table 1, Section 1).[8] Additionally, it was shown that water deprivation also resulted in decreased atrial ANF mRNA and plasma ANF levels (Table 1, Section 2).[8,9] However, the quantity of the hormone contained in the atria, when expressed per gram of tissue, actually increased.[8] Thus, it seems as if dehydration causes a coordinate drop in ANF gene expression and in atrial secretion rate, which together result in decreased plasma levels of the hormone and increased atrial levels. The response of the ANF system to increased sodium load is likely a complicated physiological process; it seems likely that this response is the result of the direct actions of hormones and/or neurotransmitters at the atrial myocyte level. Further studies will be required to identify such direct effector molecules.

B. HORMONAL REGULATION
1. Adrenal Hormones
a. In Vivo *Studies*

Since various cardiovascular parameters are regulated by gluco- and mineralocorticoids, several studies have focused on evaluating the potential roles of the adrenal hormones in the regulation of the ANF system. The atria of adrenalectomized rats were shown to possesses similar quantities of ANF as control animals. However, under conditions of increased dietary sodium, the atrial ANF levels of the adrenalectomized animals decreased while that of the control group remained similar to levels observed under normal sodium diet (Table 1, Section 3).[10] This may indicate that adrenal hormones are important in the maintenance of the ANF biosynthetic rate during situations of increased salt load, but may have little effect during

TABLE 1
Effectors of ANF mRNA and Peptide Levels

Model	Treatment	mRNA[a]	ANF[b]	Plasma ANF	Other	Ref.
1. Rat[c]	Low Na diet	↓	ND	ND		8
2. Rat	H₂O deprivation	↓	↑	↓	Pulmonary and ven-	8,9
	H₂O deprivation + Dex[e]	↑	ND	ND	tricular ANF mRNA also ↑ with Dex	11
3. Rat	AdX[f]	ND	—	—		10
	AdX + high Na diet	ND	↓	↓		10
	AdX + Dex or DOCA[g]	ND	—	—		10
	AdX + Dex and DOCA	ND	↑	↑		10
4. Rat	AdX + Dex	↑	ND	↑		11
5. Dog[c]	DOCA	↑	ND	↑	DOCA escape	13
6. Cell[d]	Dex	↑	ND	ND	↑ ANF mRNA also in cultured ventricu- lar cells	11, 16
	Dex or hydrocortisone	ND	↑	ND	↑ cellular and se- creted ANF and proper processing in atrial and ventricular cells	17
7. Rat	H₂O deprivation + ThyX[h]	↓	ND	—		22
	H₂O deprivation + ThyX + T₄	—	ND	↑		22
8. Cell	T₃	↑	↑	ND	↑ ANF secretion rates	22—24
9. Rat	AVP, phenylephrine, Ang II	ND	ND	↑		4, 26

Note: ND indicates not determined in this study; — indicates a value similar to those obtained in controls.

[a] ANF mRNA derived from atrial tissue or cultured atrial cells, unless otherwise indicated.
[b] ANF derived from atrial tissue or cultured atrial cells, unless otherwise indicated.
[c] Rat and dog model systems indicate results obtained using intact animal preparations.
[d] Cell model systems indicate results obtained with primary myocytes derived from neonatal rat atria or ventricles.
[e] Dex = dexamethasone, a synthetic glucocorticoid.
[f] AdX = adrenalectomized.
[g] DOCA = deoxycorticosterone acetate, a mineralocorticoid.
[h] ThyX = thyroidectomized.

normal salt intake. Interestingly, in the same study, the coadministration of a glucocorticoid (dexamethasone) and a mineralocorticoid (deoxycorticosterone acetate [DOCA]) to the adrenalectomized animals resulted in a five- to sixfold increase in atrial ANF levels, compared to adrenalectomized animals not receiving replacement therapy. Since neither dexamethasone nor DOCA alone caused the increase in atrial ANF levels, it was hypothesized that glucocorticoids may stimulate atrial ANF biosynthesis, but only in the presence of mineralocorticoids, which may serve a permissive role. In a more recent study, it was shown that in control and adrenalectomized rats, DOCA alone had little effect on the ANF system, but dexamethasone alone produced at least a two- to threefold increase in plasma ANF levels.[11] Additionally, it was shown in the same study that dexamethasone treatment also resulted in an increase in atrial ANF mRNA levels (Table 1, Section 4). Although several aspects of these studies are contradictory, it nevertheless appears as though glucocorticoids function to maintain atrial ANF levels and may be particularly important during times of salt load.

Further studies have evaluated the role of mineralocorticoids in regulating atrial and plasma ANF. When DOCA is administered, the sodium-retaining effect of the mineralocorticoid is observed as an increase in plasma sodium; after several days, plasma sodium levels decrease slowly to normal as a result of increased natriuresis.[12] During such a ''DOCA escape'' phenomenon, it has been shown that plasma ANF concentrations increase approximately two- to threefold with a time course which is coordinate with the role of ANF as a natriuretic hormone.[13] In the same study, left and right atrial ANF mRNA levels were also observed to increase by approximately four- and sevenfold, respectively; atrial levels of ANF itself were not reported (Table 1, Section 5).

b. In Vitro *Cell Culture Studies*

Several studies have utilized primary cultures of atrial myocytes as a model system to assess the potential direct effects of hormones on ANF biosynthesis. The development of complete serum-free media for the maintenance of atrial cultures with high ANF content and secretion rates demonstrated the importance of steroid hormones as medium components.[14] Early studies indicated that glucocorticoids increased culture levels of ANF, while mineralocorticoids had little or no effect.[15] Dexamethasone and hydrocortisone have been shown to increase primary atrial myocyte ANF mRNA and cellular ANF levels, as well as increasing ANF secretion (Table 1, Section 6).[11,16,17] It seems reasonable that glucocorticoids would play a role in the regulation of gene expression since a region of the ANF gene possesses a consensus sequence consistent with its role as a glucocorticoid regulatory element.[18] However, it is still possible that glucocorticoids could affect ANF gene expression at least in part through mineralocorticoid receptors; true mineralocorticoid receptors have recently been identified in the heart in pharmacological[19] and molecular[20] studies.

2. Thyroid Hormone
a. In Vivo *Studies*

The recent findings demonstrating increased plasma ANF levels in hyperthyroid rats and decreased plasma ANF levels in hypothyroid rats[21] have indicated the possible involvement of thyroxine in the regulation of ANF gene expression. The thyroidectomized rat has provided a useful model system for studies of ANF gene expression. When thyroidectomized (ThyX) rats were dehydrated, atrial ANF mRNA levels decreased, while plasma ANF levels remained near the level of ThyX hydrated animals (Table 1, Section 7).[22] Moreover, when ThyX dehydrated rats were given thyroid hormone, atrial ANF mRNA levels returned to approximately those levels observed in ThyX hydrated rats. Interestingly, in this study plasma ANF levels did not always correlate with atrial ANF mRNA levels, indicating that circulating levels of ANF may be in part regulated by mechanisms distinct from ANF gene expression, for example, altered secretion and/or degradation rates. Thus, it appears that basal levels of ANF gene expression in the atria are rather high, and only during times of volume stress (e.g., dehydration), does thyroxine contribute to the modulation of atrial ANF mRNA levels.

b. In Vitro *Cell Culture Studies*

A number of laboratories have shown further that physiological levels of thyroid hormone are capable of increasing the quantity of ANF mRNA and ANF in primary myocytes by two- to threefold, with a comparable increase in the quantity of secreted ANF (Table 1, Section 8).[15,16,22-24] It thus appears as though thyroxine is capable of directly affecting the expression of the ANF gene in atrial and ventricular myocytes. The mechanism through which thyroid hormone regulates ANF gene expression is not clear. However the recent description of DNA sequences capable of specifically binding the thyroid hormone receptor should begin to explain the function of this hormone.[25] Moreover, if both glucocorticoids and thyroid hormone function through ANF gene-associated regulatory elements, it will be of interest to determine whether they interact at the same or different enhancer elements and, thus, whether their effects on ANF gene expression are additive.

III. ANF SECRETION AND POST-TRANSLATIONAL PROCESSING

In addition to regulation at the level of gene expression, it is possible that plasma levels of ANF may also be regulated in part by the rate of cleavage of ANF(99—126) from ANF(1—126) and the rate of secretion of ANF from myocytes. Many studies have been directed at trying to understand the factors that regulate ANF secretion and the mechanism of the post-translational processing of ANF.

A. SECRETION

1. *In Vivo* Studies

Several model systems have been utilized with the goal of identifying substances that can affect the secretion of ANF. In rats, it has been shown that various pressor substances (e.g., phenylephrine, angiotensin II, and vasopressin) are capable of producing a robust increase in plasma levels of ANF(99—126).[4,26] From such studies, it is clear that the plasma ANF levels are responsive to various substances; however, it is not apparent whether such compounds are acting directly on the ANF-secreting myocytes or indirectly via atrial stretch, neuronal reflexes, or alterations of ANF degradation and/or clearance rates. With the use of *in vitro* model systems, several investigators have attempted to clarify such questions.

2. *In Vitro* Tissue Studies

Using the isolated perfused heart preparation, it has been shown that increased right atrial perfusion pressures resulted in increased ANF appearance in the perfusate.[28] This suggests that stretch alone can in some way stimulate ANF release and that complete neural reflexes are not required. This notion has been supported by other studies utilizing vagotemized rats to show that increased volume is capable of increasing plasma ANF levels regardless of whether neural reflexes are intact.[29] Additionally, it has been shown that the active phorbol ester, phorbol 12-myristate 13-acetate (TPA), along with the calcium ionophore, A23187, are capable of stimulating the release of ANF into the perfusate.[30] TPA stimulates protein kinase C (PKC) in a manner similar to diacylglycerol and A23187 increases cytosolic free calcium levels, as does inositol triphosphate (IP3). These results suggest that receptors linked to the phosphoinositide second messenger system would facilitate the stimulation of ANF secretion. The involvement of PKC and intracellular calcium in stimulated ANF secretion is supported further by studies demonstrating that TPA and BAY K8644, a calcium agonist, also behave synergistically to stimulate ANF release from isolated perfused hearts.[31]

3. *In Vitro* Cell Culture Studies

Primary myocyte cultures potentially provide a powerful tool with which to study the regulation of ANF secretion. In part, efforts of our laboratory have concentrated on utilizing this model system in order to identify compounds capable of acutely affecting ANF secretion. The compounds we have tested can be divided into two general categories: (1) hormones, neurotransmitters, and second messengers, and (2) effectors of ion flux or cytosolic calcium levels. Early experiments in our laboratory using various Category 1 compounds indicated that, with regard to ANF secretion, primary atrial myocytes were not responsive. However, in more recent studies, we have shown that culture conditions have a major effect on whether the cells respond to various potential secretagogues. As with the isolated perfused heart,[30,31] TPA and A23187 stimulated ANF secretion by five- to sevenfold from primary atrial myocytes that had been maintained in a glucocorticoid-containing medium; essentially, no stimulation of secretion was observed when cells had been maintained in glucocorticoid-free medium (Figure 1). The PKC-inactive phorbol ester, 4-α-phorbol-12,13-didecanoate,

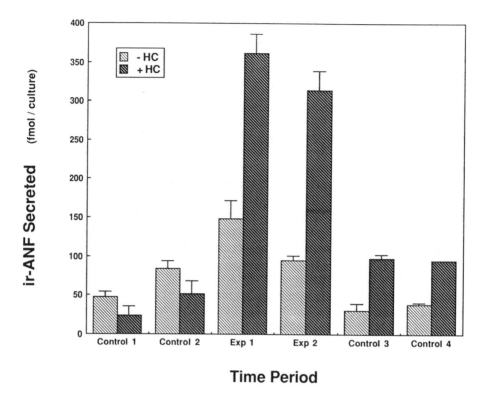

FIGURE 1.   Stimulation of ANF secretion from primary atrial myocytes by TPA and A23187. Primary cultures of atrial myocytes were prepared as previously described[32] and maintained for 7 d in serum-free medium in the presence or absence of 138 nM hydrocortisone. Triplicate cultures were then incubated for two $^1/_2$ h time periods in control medium (Control Periods 1 and 2), followed by two $^1/_2$ h periods in medium containing 0.1 μM TPA/ 1 μM A23187 (Experimental Periods 1 and 2). After the experimental incubations, the cultures were incubated for two $^1/_2$ h time periods in control medium to assess the reversibility of effects. The quantity of ANF secreted into the medium after each incubation was determined by RIA. Error bars represent standard errors of the mean of the values obtained from the three cultures.

was incapable of stimulating ANF secretion from either group of cells. Interestingly, we have also shown that cAMP analogs (e.g., dibutyryl-cAMP) are capable of inhibiting ANF secretion. This result also compares with similar experiments performed with the isolated perfused heart model.[31] Further studies will be required to determine which receptors are involved with the regulation of ANF secretion from myocytes. The primary cell model system should be of particular interest since it enables the evaluation of the long-term effects of agonist stimulation on ANF secretion and biosynthetic rates, as well as allowing the investigation of potential interactions between activators of ANF gene expression (e.g., glucocorticoids) and secretagogues.

Several compounds from Category 2 were found to affect ANF secretion. Depolarizing levels of potassium produced a three- to fourfold increase in ANF secretion, with an EC_{50} of approximately 35 mM (Figure 2). Interestingly, the stimulatory effect of potassium occurred only during the initial 30 min of exposure to the ion; beyond this time period, the cells became refractory with regard to the potassium level (Figure 2, inset). This refractory period is not observed when depolarizing levels of KCl have been used to stimulate the secretion of other peptide hormones, thus further emphasizing the distinction between other endocrine cells and atrial myocytes. Also in contrast to other endocrine peptides, the release of ANF from cultured atrial myocytes was actually inhibited by physiological levels of calcium. When primary atrial myocytes were maintained in calcium-free medium, the rate

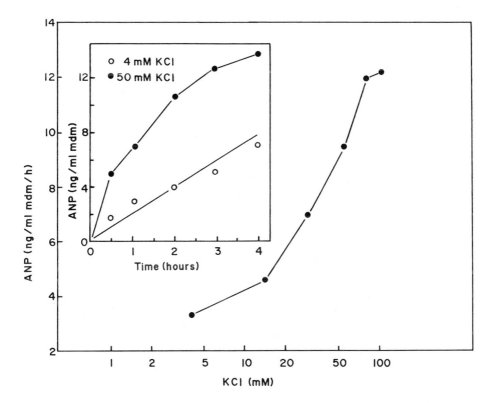

FIGURE 2. Stimulation of ANF secretion from primary atrial myocytes by potassium chloride. Cultures of primary atrial myocytes were prepared and maintained in serum-free medium without glucocorticoids, as described in Figure 1. Cultures were then incubated for 1 h with serum-free medium containing varied concentrations of KCl and the secreted ANF was determined by RIA. Each point represents the average of determinations from three different cultures; the triplicate cultures varied from one another by less than 5%. A time course (inset) was performed by incubating parallel cultures with 4 or 50 mM KCl for various times, followed by ANF RIA analysis of the spent medium. Again, each point is the average value determined from triplicate cultures.

of ANF secretion increased two- to threefold, compared to cells maintained in physiological levels of calcium (Figure 3). When depolarizing levels of potassium were added to calcium-free medium, the stimulation of ANF secretion remained at about twofold. This suggested that both ionic manipulations may be altering the membrane potential in similar ways to affect ANF secretion. Both calcium-free and potassium-mediated stimulation of ANF secretion were reversible. Although the inhibitory effect of calcium on ANF secretion is relatively unique among peptide endocrine systems, several other secretory systems behave similarly. It is possible that ANF secretion is coupled to cytosolic calcium very differently than other hormones since the contractile cycle in the same cardiac myocyte is regulated by transient changes in cytosolic-free calcium levels.

B. ANF BIOSYNTHESIS AND POST-TRANSLATIONAL PROCESSING

One of the most intriguing features of the heart ANF system is the biosynthetic mechanism. In the rat, the ANF gene encodes a translation product that possesses an NH_2-terminal signal sequence, which is likely cotranslationally cleaved from the nascent polypeptide, and results in a 128-amino-acid precursor peptide, proANF(1—128).[18] The arginine residues at positions 127 and 128 are presumed to be cleaved from the peptide very soon after translation since the primary storage form of the hormone in the heart is ANF(1—126) (Figure 4).[1—3,32] Interestingly, the primary form of the hormone in the circulation and in the perfusate from the isolated heart preparations is ANF(99—126). Thus, there is no apparent location for the

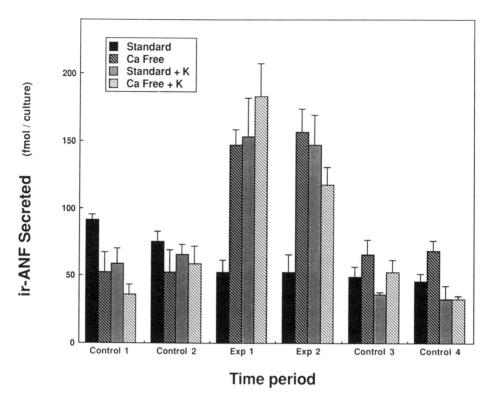

FIGURE 3. The effect of calcium on ANF secretion from primary atrial myocytes. This experiment was performed similarly to that described in Figure 1, except the media used during the experimental time periods were either identical to the control media (i.e., Standard), calcium-free with 1 μM EGTA (Ca Free), supplemented with KCl to 35 mM (Standard + K), or calcium-free and KCl supplemented (Ca Free + K).

storage of the circulating peptide, nor is it clear where the proteolytic cleavage of ANF(1—126) to form ANF(99—126) occurs.

1. Primary Atrial Myocytes as a Model System

Several laboratories have utilized the primary myocyte preparation as a model system for studies of the biosynthesis, processing, and release of ANF-related peptides. In early studies, it was demonstrated that primary cultures of atrial myocytes could be maintained in serum-free medium such that the cells contained and secreted ANF(1—126).[14,33,34] Interestingly, since the cultured cells secreted ANF(1—126) instead of ANF(99—126), it was hypothesized that the cleavage to form the circulating hormone in fact took place in the circulation. In the same studies it was shown that rat serum was capable of cleaving ANF(1—126) to form ANF(99—126). This cleavage was apparently performed by kallikrein- and/or thrombin-like activities since chloromethylketone (CMK) inhibitors of these enzymes were able to inhibit the serum-mediated cleavage of ANF(1—126).[3] Moreover, the serum-mediated cleavage was shown to be nonphysiological since plasma was incapable of performing the cleavage to any large extent and since isolated hearts could be perfused with CMK inhibitors, yet the primary form of ANF found in the perfusate was ANF(99—126). The last finding indicated further that the cleavage occurs either in the myocytes just prior to secretion or on the surface of the tissue as ANF(1—126) is diffusing from the cells of origin, perhaps within the enthothelial spaces.

2. Primary Atrial Myocytes that Process ANF

In our laboratory, recent interest has focused on the apparent paradoxical finding that

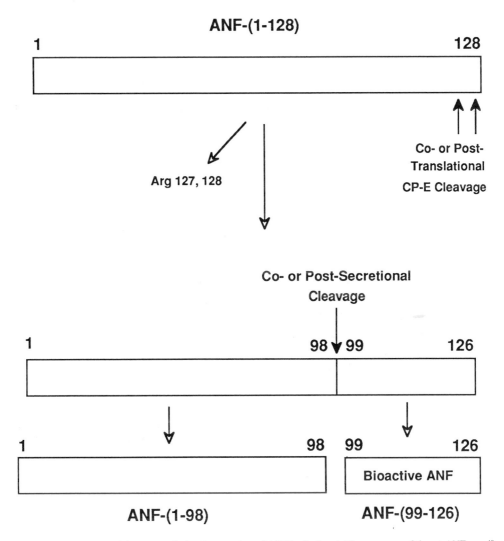

ANF-(1-128)

1   128

Arg 127, 128

Co- or Post-Translational CP-E Cleavage

Co- or Post-Secretional Cleavage

1   98   99   126

1   98   99   126

Bioactive ANF

ANF-(1-98)   **ANF-(99-126)**

FIGURE 4. Diagram of the postranslational processing of ANF in the heart. The sequence of the rat ANF gene[18] indicates that the primary translation product possesses 128 amino acids. This peptide [ANF(1—128)] is presumably rapidly converted to ANF(1—126) by the carboxypeptidase E that has been localized to many endocrine tissues.[32] Since ANF(1—128) has not been positively identified in cells, its existence is presently hypothetical. ANF(1—126) is then co- or postsecretionally cleaved between Arg_{98} and Ser_{99} to form the two product peptides, ANF(1—98) and ANF(99-126).

the isolated perfused heart contains ANF(1—126) and apparently releases ANF(99—126), while the cultured cells both contain and release ANF(1—126). Efforts have been undertaken to describe a defined complete serum-free medium (CSFM) that results in the long-term maintenance of primary myocytes that possess and secrete ANF in relatively large quantities and that mimic the processing events observed *in vivo*.

    We have found that one of several formulations tested (CSFM-2), which was modified from that of Freersken et al.,[35] resulted in long-term cultures with a morphology quite different from that observed when the cells were maintained in our previously described medium (CSFM-1).[14,34] In CSFM-1, the ANF-containing myocytes, as viewed by immunocytochemistry, were defined, individual spindle-shaped cells; however, in CSFM-2, the ANF-containing cells are much larger and form multicellular "colonies" with other ANF-containing cells. Although both medium formulations supported the relatively long-term

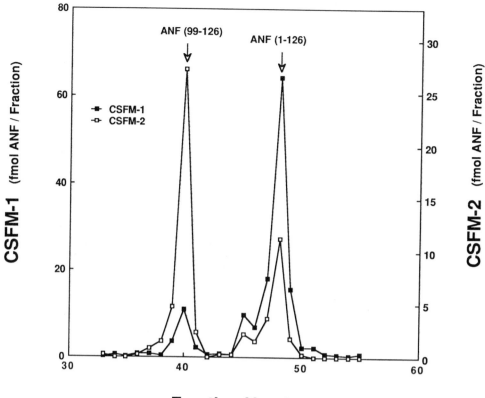

Fraction Number

FIGURE 5.   Reversed-phase HPLC analysis of the molecular forms of immunoactive ANF secreted by primary atrial myocytes. Cultures of atrial myocytes were maintained in either CSFM-1[32] or CSFM-2[33], as described in Figure 1. Spent media derived from $^1/_2$ h secretion periods were collected and analyzed by RP-HPLC and RIA, as previously described.[3] Further experiments indicated that the hydroxycorticosterone in CSFM-2 was responsible for conferring processing ability to the cultures. The elution positions of synthetic ANF(99—126) and purified ANF(1—126)[3] were determined in parallel analyses.

maintenance of ANF-containing cultures, those cultures maintained in CSFM-2 were much longer lived and were found to contain and secrete large quantities of ANF after as long as 45 days.

The molecular forms of ANF contained and secreted by the cultures were assessed utilizing RIA or biosynthetic labeling coupled with HPLC. Interestingly, the cells maintained in either medium contain only ANF(1—126), while the form of ANF secreted by the cells differed, depending on the medium conditions. Those cultures maintained in CSFM-1 released primarily ANF(1—126)-like material, as previously observed,[14,33] whereas cultures maintained in CSFM-2 secreted large quantities of ANF(99—126)-like material (Figure 5). Biosynthetically labeled ANF(99—126)-like material was isolated by quantitative immunoprecipitation from the medium of cells maintained in CSFM-2. Using reversed-phase, size exclusion, and ion exchange HPLC, the labeled ANF(99—126)-like material could be distinguished from other forms of ANF, such as ANF(92—126), (96—126), (101—126), (103—126), and (103—123). Thus, it appears as if the primary atrial cells maintained in CSFM-2 are capable of releasing ANF(99—126) while they contain ANF(1—126), similar to what has been observed in rats and in the isolated perfused heart model system.

In further preliminary studies, we have found that the addition of various glucocorticoids to CSFM-1 results in a medium like CSFM-2 that supports processing (Table 1, Section 6).

Mineralocorticoids do not appear to have the same effect. Further studies will be required to establish whether glucocorticoids confer processing ability to the cultures by regulating the expression of the responsible enzyme or some other, perhaps indirect, mechanism.

Several experiments utilizing protease inhibitors have been focused on determining the location and nature of the ANF processing protease. The addition of the thrombin inhibitor, D-Phe-Pro-Arg-chloromethyl ketone, to the medium did not alter the processing capability of the cultures. This was also true for leupeptin and phenylmethylsulfonyl fluoride (PMSF). It is thus apparent that either these inhibitors cannot gain access to the responsible protease or the enzyme is not susceptible to these compounds.

3. Primary Ventricular Myocytes as a Model System

Recently, it has been shown that in prenatal and early neonatal rat, both atria and ventricles express the gene for ANF.[36-38] However, the tissues diverge as a function of development such that the concentration of ANF in the atria increases with age, whereas the level of ANF in the ventricles decreases with age.[37] An interesting contrast between the two tissues with regard to the expression of ANF is that the atria store the peptide in secretory granules, while it appears as if the ventricles do not possess large numbers of secretory granules. Moreover, recent studies have demonstrated that in cultures derived from neonatal animals, the rate of ANF secretion from ventricular myocytes is much greater than that from atrial myocytes; it has been suggested that atrial cells possess the "regulated" pathway of secretion, while ventricular cells possess only the constitutive pathway and thus release the hormone as quickly as it is synthesized.[37]

Considering these differences between neonatal atrial and ventricular cells, it was of interest to evaluate whether there are also differences between the cells with regard to the post-translational processing of ANF. We found that when ventricular cells were maintained in CSFM-2, they contained ANF(1—126), while ANF(99—126) was the major form of the peptide that accumulated in the medium. Moreover, ANF processing in the ventricular cultures was also shown to depend on the presence of glucocorticoids. Thus, it appears as if both atrial and ventricular cells are capable of converting ANF(1—126) to the circulating form of the hormone, ANF(99-126), in an essentially cosecretional fashion. This implies that processing is not dependent on the presence of granules and, therefore, it seems likely that the responsible protease(s) are located either in organelles common to both the constitutive and regulated pathways (i.e., RER, Golgi apparatus) or on the surface of the myocyte.

IV. CONCLUSIONS

The combination of animal, isolated heart, and cell culture model systems have proven useful in determining various features of ANF biosynthesis and secretion. Physiological studies have demonstrated that salt and water balance play an important role in regulating ANF gene expression and plasma levels of ANF. Using both physiological manipulations and cell culture techniques, it has been shown that thyroid hormone and glucocorticoids increase ANF gene expression. Observations made using all three model systems have indicated that the post-translational cleavage of ANF(1—126) to form ANF(99—126) must occur essentially cosecretionally at the level of the heart. The fact that primary myocytes maintained in serum-free medium are capable of secreting ANF(99—126) indicates that the processing event is associated with the myocyte itself and that both atrial and ventricular cells are capable of performing the cleavage. Thus, processing occurs regardless of whether ANF is secreted by the constitutive or regulated pathway.

It is of interest to note that glucocorticoids both enhance the expression of the ANF gene and support the proper post-translational processing. It is not yet clear whether the expression of the responsible processing enzyme is also regulated by glucocorticoids, nor is it known whether the enzyme is intra- or extracellular. The ability of cultured atrial myocytes to differentially respond to potential secretagogues, depending on the presence of glucocorticoids, is also noteworthy; it is possible that processing and the receptor-regulated release of ANF are obligately coupled events. Interestingly, primary cells maintained in the presence of glucocorticoids possess a different morphology and beat more consistently and rapidly than those maintained without glucocorticoids. Since the beat rate of cultured cells has been associated with their metabolic health,[39] it seems as if glucocorticoids may be responsible for increasing the survival of myocytes in culture.

Many questions regarding the biosynthesis, secretion, and processing of ANF remain to be answered. The use of various serum-free media and the primary myocyte model system will be of great value in studies designed to describe the mechanism of ANF processing and secretion. Such studies will also begin to delineate the key regulated points of the ANF system and will contribute to our understanding of the factors involved in the regulation of plasma levels of this hormone.

ACKNOWLEDGMENTS

This work was supported by NIH Grant NS-25037 and NIH Predoctoral Training Grant GM-07229. Christopher C. Glembotsky is an Established Investigator of the American Heart Association, Grant No. 860173. We thank Tom Gibson for enlightening scientific discussion and critical review of the manuscript.

REFERENCES

1. **Flynn, T. G., Davies, P. L., Kennedy, B. P., deBold, M. L., and deBold, A. J.,** Alignment of rat cardionatrin sequences with the preprocardionatrin sequence from complementary DNA, *Science,* 228, 323, 1985.
2. **Thibault, G., Garcia, R., Gutkowska, J., Bilodeau, J., Lazure, C., Seidah, N. G., Chretien, M., Genest, J., and Cantin, J.,** The propeptide Asn^1-Tyr^{126} is the storage form of rat atrial natriuretic factor, *Biochem. J.,* 241, 256, 1987.
3. **Gibson, T. R., Shields, P. P., and Glembotski, C. C.,** The conversion of atrial natriuretic peptide (ANF)-(1—126) to ANF-(99—126) by rat serum: contribution to ANP cleavage in isolated perfused rat hearts, *Endocrinology,* 120, 764, 1987.
4. **Schwartz, D., Geller, D. M., Manning, P. T., Siegel, N. R., Fok, K. F., Smith, C. E., and Needleman, P.,** Ser-Leu-Arg-Arg-atriopeptide III: the major circulating form of atrial peptide, *Science,* 229, 397, 1985.
5. **Thibault, G., Lazure, C., Shiffrin, E. L., Gutkowska, J., and Cantin, M.,** Identification of a biologically active circulating form of rat atrial natriuretic factor, *Biochem. Biophys. Res. Commun.,* 130, 981, 1985.
6. **Mains, R. E., Eipper, B. A., Glembotski, C. C., and Dores, R. J.,** Strategies for the biosynthesis of bioactive peptides, *Trends Neurosci.,* 6, 229, 1983.
7. **Lynch, D. R. and Snyder, S. H.,** Neuropeptides: multiple molecular forms, metabolic pathways, and receptors, *Annu. Rev. Biochem.,* 55, 773, 1986.
8. **Takayanagi, R., Tanaka, I., Maki, M., and Inagami, T.,** Effects of changes in water-sodium balance on levels of atrial natriuretic factor messenger RNA and peptide in rats, *Life Sci.,* 36, 1843, 1985.
9. **Nakayama, K., Ohkubo, H., Hirose, T., Inayama, S., and Nakanishi, S.,** Sequence for human cardiodilatin-atrial natriuretic factor precursor and regulation of precursor mRNA in rat atria, *Nature (London),* 310, 699, 1984.
10. **Garcia, R., Debinski, W., Gutkowska, J., Kuchel, O., Thibault, G., Genest, J., and Cantin, M.,** Gluco- and mineralocorticoids may regulate the natriuretic effect and the synthesis and release of atrial natriuretic factor by the rat atria in vivo, *Biochem. Biophys. Res. Commun.,* 131, 806, 1985.
11. **Gardner, D. G., Hane, S., Trachewsky, D., Schenk, D., and Baxter, J. D.,** Atrial natriuretic peptide mRNA is regulated by glucocorticoids in vivo, *Biochem. Biophys. Res. Commun.,* 139, 1047, 1986.
12. **Knox, F. G., Burnett, J. C., Kohan, D. E., Spielman, W. S., and Strand, J. C.,** Escape from the sodium-retaining effects of mineralocorticoids, *Kidney Int.,* 17, 263, 1980.

13. **Metzler, C. H., Gardner, D. G., Keil, L. C., Baxter, J. D., and Ramsay, D. J.,** Increased synthesis and release of atrial peptide during DOCA escape in conscious dogs, *Am. J. Physiol.,* R188, 1987.

14. **Glembotski, C. C. and Gibson, T. R.,** Molecular forms of immunoactive atrial natriuretic peptide released from cultured rat atrial myocytes, *Biochem. Biophys. Res. Commun.,* 132, 1008, 1985.

15. **Glembotski, C. C. and Gibson, T. R.,** Rat atrial myocytes synthesize, store, and secrete atrial natriuretic peptide (1—126), *Endocrinology,* 118 (Suppl.), 257, 1986.

16. **Gardner, D. G., Gertz, B. J., Baxter, J. D., Vlasuk, G., Fiddes, J. C., and Lewicki, J. A.,** Molecular biology of the gene for atrial natriuretic factor (ANF), in 2nd World Congr. Biologically Active Atrial Peptides, New York, May 20 to 21, 1987, 183.

17. **Shields, P. P. and Glembotski, C. C.,** *J. Biol. Chem.,* 263, 8091, 1988.

18. **Argentin, S., Nemer, M., Drouin, J., Scott, G. K., Kennedy, B. P., and Davies, P. L.,** The gene for rat atrial natriuretic factor, *J. Biol. Chem.,* 260, 4568, 1985.

19. **Barnett, C. A. and Pritchett, E. L.,** Detection of corticosteroid type I binding sites in heart, *Mol. Cell Endocrinol.,* 56, 191, 1988.

20. **Arriza, J. L., Weinberger, C., Cerelli, G., Glaser, T. J., Handlein, B. L., Housman, D. E., and Evans, R.,** Cloning of human mineralocorticoid receptor complementary DNA: structural and functional kinship with the glucocorticoid receptor, *Science,* 237, 268, 1987.

21. **Kohno, M., Takaori, K., Matasuura, T., Marakawa, K., Kanayama, Y., and Takeda, T.,** Atrial natriuretic polypeptide in atria and plasma in experimental hyperthyroidism and hypothyroidism, *Biochem. Biophys. Res. Commun.,* 134, 178, 1986.

22. **Gardner, D. G., Bertz, B. J., and Hane, S.,** Thyroid hormone increases rat atrial natriuretic peptide messenger ribonucleic acid accumulation *in vivo* and *in vitro, Mol. Endocrinol.,* 1, 260, 1987.

23. **Matsubara, H., Hirata, Y., Yoshimi, H., Takata, S., Takagi, Y., Iida, T., Yamane, Y., Umeda, Y., Nishikawa, M., and Inada, M.,** Effects of steroid and thyroid hormones on synthesis of atrial natriuretic peptide by cultured atrial myocytes of rat, *Biochem. Biophys. Res. Commun.,* 145, 336, 1987.

24. **Argentin, S., Drouin, J., and Nemer, M.,** Thyroid hormone stimulates rat pro-natriodilatin mRNA levels in primary cardiocyte cultures, *Biochem. Biophys. Res. Commun.,* 146, 1336, 1987.

25. **Glass, C. K., Franco, R., Weinberg, C., Albert, V. R., Evans, R. E., and Rosenfeld, M. G.,** A c-erb-A binding site in rat growth hormone gene mediates trans-activation by thyroid hormone, *Nature (London),* 329, 738, 1987.

26. **Manning, P. T., Schwartz, D., Katsube, N. C., Holmberg, S. W., and Needleman, P.,** Vassopressin-stimulated release of atriopeptin: endocrine antagonists in fluid homeostasis, *Science,* 229, 395, 1985.

27. **Baranowska, B., Gutkowska, J., and Cantin, M.,** Effects of α_1- and α_2-adrenergic agonists on plasma immunoreactive atrial natriuretic factor (IR-ANF) in conscious rats, in 2nd World Congr. Biologically Active Atrial Peptides, New York, May 20 to 21, 1987, 219.

28. **Lang, R. E., Tholken, H., Ganten, D., Luft, F. C., Ruskoaho, H., and Unger, Th.,** Atrial natriuretic factor — a circulating hormone stimulated by volume loading, *Nature (London),* 314, 264, 1985.

29. **Eskay, R., Zukowska-Grojec, Z., Haass, M., Dave, J. R., and Zamir, N.,** Circulating atrial natriuretic peptides in conscious rats: regulation of release by multiple factors, *Science,* 232, 636, 1986.

30. **Ruskoaho, H., Toth, M., and Lang, R. E.,** Atrial natriuretic peptide secretion: synergistic effect of phorbol ester and A23187, *Biochem. Biophys. Res. Commun.,* 133, 581, 1985.

31. **Ruskoaho, H., Toth, M., Ganten, D., Unger, Th., and Lang, R. E.,** The phorbol ester induced atrial natriuretic peptide secretion is stimulated by forskolin and BAY K8644 and inhibited by 8-bromo-cyclicGMP, *Biochem. Biophys. Res. Commun.,* 139, 266, 1986.

32. **Fricker, L. D. and Snyder, S. H.,** Purification and characterization of enkephaline convertase, an enkephalin-synthesizing carboxypeptidase, *J. Biol. Chem.,* 258, 10950, 1983.

33. **Bloch, K. D., Scott, J. A., Zisfein, J. B., Fallon, J. T., Margolies, M. N., Seidman, C. E., Matsueda, G. R., Homcy, C. J., and Graham, R. M.,** Biosynthesis and secretion of proatrial natriuretic factor by cultured rat cardiocytes, *Science,* 230, 1168, 1985.

34. **Glembotski, C. C., Oronzi, M. E., Li, X., Shields, P. P., Johnston, J. F., Kallen, R. G., and Gibson, T. R.,** The characterization of atrial natriuretic peptide (ANP) expression by primary cultures of atrial myocytes using an ANP-specific monoclonal antibody and an ANP messenger ribonucleic acid probe, *Endocrinology,* 121, 843, 1987.

35. **Freerksen, D. L., Schroedl, N. A., and Hartzell, C. R.,** Control of enzyme activity levels by serum and hydrocortisone in neonatal rat heart cells cultured in serum-free medium, *J. Cell Physiol.,* 120, 126, 1984.

36. **Takayanagi, R., Imada, T., and Inagami, T.,** Synthesis and presence of atrial natriuretic factor in rat ventricle, *Biochem. Biophys. Res. Commun.,* 142, 483, 1987.

37. **Bloch, K. D., Seidman, J. G., Naftilan, J. D., Fallon, J. T., and Seidman, C. E.,** Neonatal atria and ventricles secrete atrial natriuretic factor via tissue-specific pathways, *Cell,* 47, 695, 1986.

38. **Gardner, D. G., Deschepper, C. R., Ganong, W. F., Hane, S., Fiddes, J., Baxter, J. D., and Lewicki, J.,** Extra-atrial expression of the gene for atrial natriuretic factor, *Proc. Natl. Acad. Sci. U.S.A.*, 83, 6697, 1986.
39. **Mohammed, S. N. W., Holmes, R., and Hartzell, C. R.,** A serum-free, chemically defined medium for function and growth of primary neonatal rat heart cell cultures, *In Vitro*, 19, 471, 1983.

Chapter 6

REGULATION OF ANF RELEASE

Rüdiger von Harsdorf, Jing Ru Hu, and Rudolf E. Lang

TABLE OF CONTENTS

I. INTRODUCTION

The hypothesis of a natriuretic factor — originally an intriguing possibility and now an experimentally documented reality — has occupied the minds of scientists for more than 30 years. The idea of its existence was originally based on the observation that blood volume expansion induces natriuresis, even when glomerular filtration does not change, and that stretching of the cardiac atria is associated with an increase in urinary sodium excretion. Nevertheless, the question of whether humoral regulation of salt-water homeostases relies only on the action of vasopressin and the renin angiotensin system or depends on still another hormone continued to be a subject of controversy and intense research until it was found that the heart atria contain a natriuretic and diuretic peptide.[1] This peptide, now termed ANF, fulfills the classic characteristics of a hormone: it is stored in secretory granule-like vesicles of atrial cardiocytes, is released from the heart in response to certain stimuli such as atrial distension, and is transported in the blood to various end organs endowed with specific receptors which mediate its effects.[2-4] As with many other endocrine systems, there may be a variety of ways by which the release of ANF is controlled. It has been found that increased blood volume or high salt intake are potent stimuli for ANF secretion.[5-9] A large number of studies have suggested that changes in atrial size play an important role in the regulation of ANF release from the heart. It was found that distension of the left atrium, achieved by inflating a balloon, increases plasma ANF levels in dogs.[10] High plasma ANF levels were observed in patients with cardiac failure or pulmonary diseases.[11-15] Water immersion, which shifts blood to the thorax and increases right atrial stretch, was reported to be associated with high plasma ANF levels in humans and in rats.[16,17] Elevated concentrations of circulating ANF were also measured during chronic hypoxia or mineralocorticoid excess.[18,19] All these observations are consistent with the idea that atrial stretch is the principal stimulus for ANF release. Whether other factors, such as the autonomic nervous system or humoral substances, are also involved in the regulation of ANF release will be the subject of the first section of this chapter. The second part will deal with the possible role of calcium and other intracellular signals in the mediation of ANF secretion.

II. THE AUTONOMIC NERVOUS SYSTEM AND ANF RELEASE

Neural pathways influence the release of quite a number of hormones. One example is insulin, whose secretion in response to glucose is amplified by beta adrenergic stimulation. In the case of vasopressin, it has been shown that activation of stretch receptors in the left atrium inhibits the release of this hormone by a vagally mediated reflex.[20] The dense innervation of the heart and particularly of the cardiac atria with adrenergic and cholinergic nerve fibers raises the possibility that the autonomic nervous system is directly involved in the control of ANF release. Indeed, it has been reported that in conscious dogs the natriuresis observed in response to left atrial distension is abolished by cardiac denervation.[21] This is in conflict with other studies, however, in which expansion of the blood volume in anesthetized rats produced a natriuretic response independent of whether the vagal afferents were intact or severed.[22]

More to the point, recent studies in dogs, demonstrating that atrial stretch may increase sodium excretion independently of the release of ANF, raised some doubts as to whether natriuresis is even a good indicator of circulating ANF.[23] Studies in animals with cervical vagotomy, autonomic blockade, or electrical nerve stimulation, in which plasma ANF levels were measured radioimmunologically, do not support a major role of nervous pathways in ANF secretion.[10,17,24] In one investigation, mitral obstruction was used to provide atrial wall stretch and stimulation of atrial receptors.[10] This resulted in a marked rise in plasma ANF concentration which was not significantly affected by bilateral cervical vagotomy or beta blockade. In another study in rabbits, the possible contribution of cardiac afferents to the release of ANF was tested by electrical nerve stimulation. Hormone levels did not change during moderate sympathetic or vagal nerve stimulation unless atrial pressure was affected, despite the expected responses in heart rate.[25] This again reinforces the view that distension of atrial cardiocytes is the primary stimulus of ANF release and that this effect does not require mediation by cardiac nerves.

The most convincing evidence comes from experiments using the isolated heart. A rise in cardiac preload or afterload was reported to produce a several-fold increase in ANF release from a rat heart-lung preparation.[26,27] In our own studies in the isolated perfused rat heart, a marked elevation of ANF in the perfusate was obtained in response to a graded volume load to the right atrium which showed a strong positive correlation with right atrial pressure.[5,28] A 1 mmHg rise in right atrial pressure was found to increase the concentration of ANF in the perfusate by about 30 to 40%. This is in good accordance with observations in human subjects.[15] Additional evidence that mechanical stretch of the atria is the primary stimulus of ANF release has been provided by experiments in conscious rats with ganglionic blockade. which showed an unimpaired response of ANF release to volume or salt loading.[24] Similarly, the rise in ANF following pharmacologically induced blood pressure elevations was still observed after elimination of control reflexes by pithing, although the responses were markedly attenuated, compared with those in intact control rats. That mechanical stretch alone can elicit ANF release is further supported by studies in which isolated rat atria were superfused *in vitro* and exposed to resting tensions of various degrees.[29] An increase in tension caused a marked rise in peptide secretion, an effect probably not mediated by the release of neurotransmitters from endogenous nerve endings since it was also obtained in the presence of neurotransmitter antagonists.

Although the above results suggest that neuronal pathways are not required for stretch-induced ANF release, they do not entirely exclude a role for autonomic nerves in the control of ANF release. In this regard, it should be noted that both epinephrine and acetylcholine have been reported to stimulate the secretion of ANF from isolated atria.[30,31] A dose-dependent rise of ANF release was observed upon infusion of the alpha$_1$-receptor agonist phenylephrine into isolated hearts at concentrations between 10^{-7} and 10^{-4} M, whereas the beta-agonist isoproterenal failed to affect hormone release.[32] These results are somewhat in conflict with those of another study performed in atrial slices, in which neither alpha- nor beta-adrenergic agonists nor cholinergic agonists showed an effect.[33] The reasons for these discrepancies are not well understood. The possibility of receptor down-regulation or autoinhibition of hormone release in the latter study cannot be ruled out since the tissue was incubated for a relatively long period in a static incubation system. In a more recent study, a beta adrenoceptor mechanism was implicated in the regulation of ANF release.[34] It was demonstrated that dispersed superfused rat atrial myocytes liberate high amounts of ANF in response to very low concentrations of beta-adrenoreceptor agonists. Further support for a role of beta receptors in the mediation of ANF release comes from experiments using isolated left rat atria which were kept in a superfusion chamber and stimulated electrically.[35] In this model, ANF release was obtained with both alpha- and beta-andrenoceptor agonists. The response to noradrenaline was blocked by metacholine, indicating that the parasympathetic nervous system also plays a part in the regulation of ANF release.

There is no doubt that the autonomic nervous system affects ANF release in an indirect manner. Alterations in sympathetic nerve activity are known to be associated with changes in venous and arterial tone which, in turn, might cause alterations in ANF release through changes in atrial pressure. Indeed, it has been shown that infusion of pressor doses of phenylephrine increased plasma ANF levels in rats.[36] This is in keeping with the observation that patients with severe hypertension present higher ANF plasma levels than do normotensives.[37,38] It is further conceivable that changes in the inotropic state due to alterations in autonomic nerve activity might have some influence on ANF release since atrial filling pressure and cardiac performance are intimately connected.

III. HUMORAL FACTORS AND ANF RELEASE

Considering the natriuretic potency of ANF, it appears reasonable to speculate that, by analogy, the secretion of this hormone is regulated by the plasma sodium concentration. There is, indeed, a wealth of literature reporting a strong positive correlation between sodium intake and ANF plasma levels.[8,39] Similarly, infusion of high sodium salt solutions stimulate ANF release.[9] However, the most likely explanation for these observations may be that osmotically induced changes in plasma volume affected ANF release by altering atrial pressure. Some authors have suggested that high sodium concentration or an increased extracellular osmolality elicit ANF secretion on their own by acting directly on the heart.[40,41] This was concluded from experiments using isolated atria or atrial cardiocytes bathed in high salt solutions. However, the changes in sodium chloride concentration and osmolality necessary to produce an ANF response were very large in these studies or else the hormone release failed to show calcium dependency, which raises some doubts as to the specificity of the effects. Other authors, using a rat heart-lung preparation, have been unable to detect any changes in ANF secretion following administration of media with sodium concentrations over a range of 132 to 166 meq/l.[27]

Plasma ANF levels have been reported to change in response to a number of other peptides known to circulate in the blood. Thus, it has been shown that intravenous administration of pressor doses of vasopressin or angiotensin results in a dose-dependent increase in plasma ANF concentration in both rat and man.[36,42] Vasopressin has been demonstrated to stimulate ANF secretion by acting directly on the heart.[31] The physiological significance of this observation, however, is uncertain since the effects were obtained at doses far exceeding vasopressin concentrations found in plasma. It appears more likely that ANF responses to vasopressin are due to the hemodynamic effects of this hormone. This is suggested by the observation that there is a strong correlation between ANF plasma levels and right atrial pressure, which increases following administration of vasopressin due to a decrease in venous capacitance and the ensuing augmentation of venous return to the heart.[36] A similar mechanism may underlie the effects on ANF release of other peptides such as neuropeptide Y, a strong vasoconstrictor peptide found in sympathetic nerve fibers, as well as dynorphin, which has also recently been reported to increase plasma ANF levels following systemic administration.[43,44] Neither vasopressin nor the renin angiotensin system appear to play a major role in mediating the effect of acute volume expansion or salt loading on ANF release. This was shown by experiments in rats in which both captopril and vasopressin antagonists failed to alter the ANF response to these stimuli.[24]

The control of the release of one hormone by another hormone is a well-known phenomenon in endocrinology. Typical examples are the anterior pituitary hormones, which control a number of endocrine glands, while their own secretion is regulated by hypothalamic releasing factors. It is intriguing to speculate that the release of ANF from the heart may similarly depend on the action of an ANF-releasing hormone. Although such a substance has not been identified as yet, there might exist a factor having at least a permissive effect on ANF secretion. According to a recent report, both the basal and stimulated release of ANF is reduced in rats with hypophysectomy, but is completely restored when the anterior pituitary gland is reimplanted under the kidney capsule.[45] This points to a possible role of a pituitary factor in the regulation of ANF secretion. Although differences in mean arterial blood pressure were excluded as a possible cause for this phenomenon, the role of other hemodynamic factors, such as changes in blood volume or venous capacitance, was not adequately controlled in these experiments. Thus, the question of whether the observed effects were indirect or direct remains unanswered.

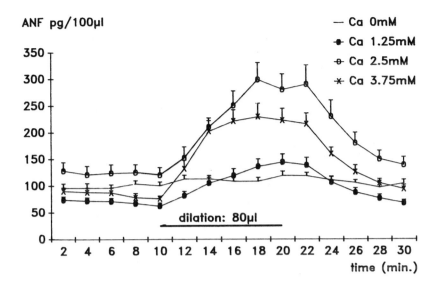

FIGURE 1. Effect of calcium concentration in the perfusion medium on ANF release from isolated perfused rat hearts. Hearts were perfused at a constant rate of 5 ml/min and paced electrically (4 Hz). ANF release was stimulated by inflating a small latex balloon inserted into the right atria.

IV. CALCIUM AND THE CONTROL OF ANF SECRETION

It is now generally agreed that atrial stretch is the principal stimulus of ANF release. However, it is not clear precisely how stretch per se induces the secretion of this cardiac hormone. Since the original discovery that extracellular calcium is a prerequisite for stimulation of insulin release by glucose, numerous studies have emphasized the fundamental role of calcium in stimulus-secretion coupling.[46] With a few exceptions, the weight of experimental evidence is consistent with the concept that a rise in free calcium inside the endocrine cell triggers hormonal exocytosis. The most important sources of cytosolic free calcium are the extracellular fluid, from which calcium entry is controlled by voltage and agonist-gated channels, and internal stores, of which the endoplasmic reticulum seems to be the most important for calcium mobilization. Since the morphology of the extrusion of ANF from the heart resembles very closely that of other hormones and since distension of heart muscle may be accompanied by an increase in free cytosolic calcium concentration in cardiac myocytes, it is intriguing to speculate that ANF secretion in response to atria stretch is a calcium-dependent process.[47,48] To address this question, we have performed a number of experiments in which ANF release from the isolated perfused rat heart or isolated atria was studied under various experimental conditions known to affect intracellular calcium levels.

In the first series of experiments, the effect of atrial stretch on ANF release was examined in isolated rat hearts perfused with Krebs-Henseleit buffer containing either a 1.25, 2.5, or 3.75 mM calcium concentration, or else no calcium. The hearts, which had been prepared according to the Langendorff technique, were perfused at a constant rate of 5 ml/min and paced electrically at a frequency of 4 Hz. For distension of the right atria, a small latex balloon was inserted into the right atrium via the inferior vena cava. The balloon was attached via a catheter to a 1-ml syringe filled with water. After an equilibrium period of 1 h and a 10-min control period, during which basal secretion of ANF was determined, the balloon was inflated to a volume of 80 µl for 10 min. This caused a gradually developing rise in ANF concentration of the perfusate to a maximum of about 250% of basal secretion after 10 min (Figure 1). Upon deflation, ANF levels slowly returned to basal levels. Raising the calcium concentration in the perfusion buffer to 3.75 mM markedly enhanced the ANF response to atrial stretch, yielding peak concentrations of ANF in the perfusate of about 300% above control levels. This was independent of whether the increase in osmotic pressure obtained by raising the calcium concentration was compensated for by reducing sodium concentration. The force of contraction developed at high calcium concentrations was slightly higher than that of hearts perfused with physiological calcium concentrations. Absence of calcium from the perfusion buffer almost completely prevented the increase in ANF release obtained during atrial dilatation in the presence of calcium.

These data clearly demonstrate that extracellular calcium is an absolute prerequisite for stretch-induced ANF release. Extracellular calcium may equilibrate with an intracellular stimulatory calcium pool through the mediation of voltage-regulated calcium channels in the cell membrane.[49] This possibility was tested in another set of experiments in which balloon dilatation of the right atria of electrically paced isolated rat hearts was performed in the presence and absence of the calcium channel blockers verapamil and diltiazem. Infusion of each drug was started 10 min before balloon inflation and maintained through the whole dilatation period. At concentrations between 10^{-7} to 10^{-6} M of verapamil and diltiazem, the ventricular force of contraction decreased by about 50%. At higher concentrations, the hearts stopped contracting. The dilatation-induced rise in ANF release decreased in a dose-dependent manner. A half-maximal reduction was observed at a concentration of 10^{-6} M verapamil or diltiazem (Figure 2).

Basal ANF secretion was not altered much by the calcium channel blockers. This gives rise to the speculation that calcium channel activation occurred in parallel with the changes in muscle length. Distension-operated calcium channels have recently been described in rabbit vein preparations and in vascular endothelial cells.[50,51] As for the heart, it has been reported that stretch reduces not only the resting membrane potential, but also stimulates ^{45}Ca uptake in isolated rat atria.[52] This would be consistent with the contention that stretching of cardiac muscle fibers is accompanied by a gradually developing increase in the amplitude of calcium transients, as measured by injection of the calcium-sensitive photoprotein aequorin.[48] Thus, it may be the stretch-induced increase in intracellular free calcium concentration which mediates the secretion of ANF. If so, ANF should also be released from the heart in response to other stimuli known to increase intracellular free calcium. One of those stimuli may be depolarization of the cell membrane during each action potential.

This possibility was tested in experiments using isolated left or right atria kept in a perfusion chamber. ANF release from nonbeating left atria was about one fifth of that from spontaneously beating right atria. Upon electrical stimulation at 3 Hz, ANF concentration in the perfusion medium of left atria gradually increased, reaching half the level of ANF measured in the bathing fluid of right atria. The rise in electrically stimulated ANF release was entirely prevented by addition of the calcium channel blocker verapamil or by omission of calcium from the perifusion medium (Figure 3). Endogenous neurotransmitter substances in the media are unlikely to mediate this effect since the ANF response was not influenced by adrenergic or cholinergic blockade. Thus, electrical stimulation by mediating calcium entry may have augmented the concentration of calcium in intracellular stores. This, in turn, might have led to a slowly developing increase in free cytosolic calcium in response to depolarization, paralleled by a graded rise in ANF release.

Intracellular calcium has also been shown to increase following inhibition of sodium/potassium ATPase.[53] When electrically paced left atria are exposed to oubain, ANF release is stimulated in a dose-dependent manner (Figure 4). Although the changes in cytoplasmic free calcium evoked by this treatment may sufficiently explain this response, other mechanisms, such as a direct action of oubain on the secretory granule membrane, must also be considered.

Cytosolic free calcium may promote exocytosis in at least two ways. It may bind to

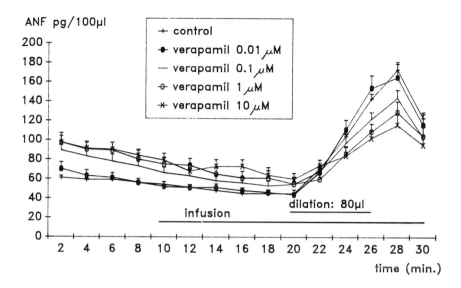

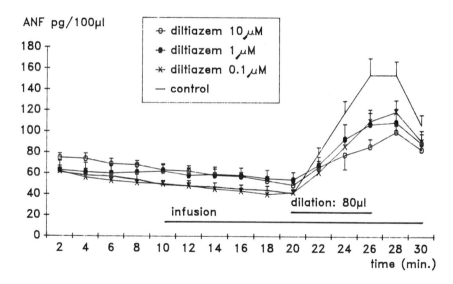

FIGURE 2. Effect of verapamil and diltiazem on stretch-induced ANF release from isolated per-fused rat hearts. Drug infusion was started 10 min before balloon dilatation of the right atria.

calmodulin, whose possible importance in the regulation of hormone secretion is suggested by a number of studies, or serve as a cofactor in the activation of protein kinase C. Protein kinase C may be an important target for calcium in the control of ANF release since this enzyme has been shown to be involved in many secretory processes, including hormone and neurotransmitter release.[54] This prompted us to investigate its possible role in the control of ANF secretion in the isolated perfused rat heart preparation. Since diacylglycerol, the natural activator of protein kinase C, does not penetrate the cell membrane, we used the structurally related and more lipophilic phorbol-ester, 12-*O*-tetradecanoyl-phorbol-13-acetate (TPA), to stimulate the enzyme.[55] The hearts were perfused at a constant flow of 10 ml/min. After an equilibrium period of 20 min, the substances to be tested were administered for 30 min and ANF measured in the perfusate. While hormone release over time was fairly

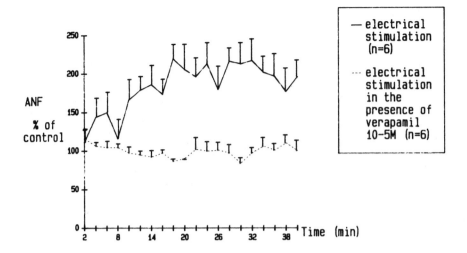

FIGURE 3.   Release of ANF from electrically paced left atria: effect of verapamil. Left atria were superfused in an organ bath chamber; field stimulation was started after a 1-h equilibrium period. ANF concentrations are expressed as percent of average concentration measured before electrical stimulation (4 Hz).

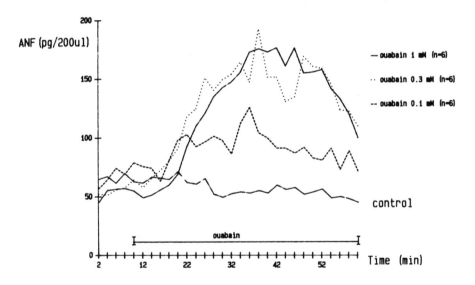

FIGURE 4.   Effect of ouabain on electrically stimulated ANF release from superfused left atria (4 Hz).

stable under basal conditions, it increased gradually during infusion of 10^{-7} M TPA. To control the specificity of this effect, we also infused the biologically inactive phorbolester 4 d PDD, which did not alter the ANF levels.[56]

If the activity of protein kinase C depends on the presence of calcium, the biological effects produced by this enzyme should vary in parallel with changes in the cytosolic free calcium concentration. This seems, indeed, to be the case. When we infused the calcium channel agonist Bay K 8644, which is believed to increase the number of calcium channels opening in response to an electric stimulus, a slowly developing increase in ANF secretion was observed. We found a greater than additive effect when we infused TPA in addition to Bay K 8644.[57] This is consistent with the proposed sensitization of protein kinase C to calcium by the phorbolester.[55] A very similar picture was obtained when the calcium channel agonist was replaced by the calcium ionophore A23187.[56] Due to the different mode of action, the latter provokes an instant rise in ANF release following administration. This again argues for a specific role of calcium in the regulation of this hormone. As in the previous experiment, the effect of TPA appears to be potentiated by the calcium activating agent.

These observations suggest that the phosphatidyl-inositol-phosphate system with inositol phosphate and diacylglycerol as intracellular signals may be involved in the mediation of ANF release. The existence of this signal system in the heart is well documented and its activation by a number of substances, including alpha-adrenoceptor and muscarinic receptor agonists, has recently been reported.[58,59] If the phosphatidyl-inositol-phosphate system plays a role in the control of ANF, it should be possible to release the hormone by infusing such substances. To test this hypothesis, we infused the muscarinic receptor agonist carbachol, the alpha-adrenoceptor agonist phenylephrine, and the beta-adrenoceptor agonist isoproterenol at concentrations of 10^{-5} M into the isolated rat heart, which was electrically paced and perfused at a constant flow rate. Phenylephrine and carbachol, which are both known to act through the activation of the phosphoinositol system, increased the ANF concentration in the perfusate. The response to carbachol was biphasic, showing first a transient decrease, followed by a rapidly developing increase. ANF release was only transiently elevated by isoproterenol and then tended to decrease, although the force of contraction was largely enhanced. This demonstrates that ANF release is not simply a function of the inotropic state of the heart. Although the stimulation of hormone secretion by phenylephrine and carbachol suggests a mediator role of phosphoinositols, it is presently not clear whether this system is activated by atrial wall stress.

V. CONCLUSION

The regulation of ANF release has been the subject of intense research during the past few years since the discovery of this hormone. The most effective stimulus for ANF release appears to be atrial distension. A number of studies strongly suggest that calcium plays a crucial role in this process. The role of other intracellular signals is not completely understood, although there is some indirect evidence that the phosphatidylinositol system might be involved. Stretch-induced ANF secretion does not require intact innervation of the heart, but this does not necessarily exclude a modulatory effect of the nervous system. Since neurotransmitters have been shown to alter markedly the rate of ANF release, a role of autonomic nerves in the control of secretion of this hormone is very likely.

REFERENCES

1. **deBold, A. J., Borenstein, H. B., Veress, A. T., and Sonnenberg, H.,** A rapid and potent natriuretic response to intravenous injection of atrial myocardial extract in rats, *Life Sci.,* 28, 89, 1981.
2. **Cantin, M. and Genest, J.,** The heart and the atrial natriuretic factor, *Endocrine Rev.,* 6, 107, 1985.
3. **Needleman, P., Adams, S. P., Cole, B. R., Currie, M. G., Geller, D. M., Michener, M. L., Saper, C. B., Schwartz, D., and Standaert, D. G.,** Atriopeptins as cardiac hormones, *Hypertension,* 87, 469, 1985.
4. **Lang, R. E., Unger, Th., and Ganten, D.,** Atrial natriuretic peptide: a new factor in blood pressure control, *Hypertension,* 5, 255, 1987.
5. **Lang, R. E., Tholken, H., Ganten, D., Luft, F. C., Ruskoaho, H., and Unger, Th.,** Atrial natriuretic factor — a circulating hormone stimulated by colume loading, *Nature (London),* 314, 264, 1985.
6. **Rascher, W., Tulassay, T., and Lang, R. E.,** Atrial natriuretic peptide in plasma of volume-overloaded children with chronic renal failure, *Lancet,* 2, 303, 1985.

7. **Yamaji, T., Ishibashi, M., and Takaku, F.,** Atrial natriuretic factor in human blood, *J. Clin. Invest.,* 76, 1705, 1985.
8. **Sagnella, G. A., Markandu, N. D., Shorf, A. C., and MacGregor, G. A.,** Effects of changes in dietary sodium intake and saline infusion on immunoreactive atrial natriuretic peptide in human plasma, *Lancet,* 2, 1208, 1985.
9. **Eskay, R., Zukowska-Grojec, Z., Haass, M., Jitendra, R. D., and Zamir, N.,** Circulating atrial natriuretic peptides in conscious rats: regulation of release by multiple factors, *Science,* 232, 636, 1985.
10. **Ledsome, J. R., Wilson, N., Courneya, C. A., and Rankin, A. J.,** Release of atrial natriuretic peptide by atrial distension, *Can. J. Physiol. Pharmacol.,* 63, 739, 1985.
11. **Lang, R. E., Unger, Th., Ganten, D., Wil, J., Bidlingmaier, F., and Doglemann, D.,** Alpha-atrial natriuretic peptide concentrations in plasma of children with congenital heart and pulmonary diseases, *Br. Med. J.,* 291, 1241, 1985.
12. **Tikkanen, I., Fyhrquist, F., Metsarinne, K., and Leidenius, R.,** Plasma atrial natriuretic peptide in cardiac disease and during infusion in healthy volunteers, *Lancet,* 2, 66, 1985.
13. **Shenker, Y., Sider, R. S., Ostafin, E. A., and Grekin, R. J.,** Plasma levels of immunoreactive atrial natriuretic factor in healthy subjects and in patients with edema, *J. Clin. Invest.,* 76, 1684, 1985.
14. **Lang, R. E., Dietz, R., Merkel, A., Unger, T., Ruskoaho, H., and Ganten, D.,** Plasma atrial natriuretic peptide values in cardiac disease, *J. Hypertens.,* 4 (Suppl.), S119, 1986.
15. **Raine, A. E. G., Erne, P., Burgisser, E., Muller, F. B., Bolli, P., Burkhart, F., and Buhler, F. R.,** Atrial natriuretic peptide and atrial pressure in patients with congestive heart failure, *N. Engl. J. Med.,* 315, 533, 1986.
16. **Epstein, M., Loutzenhiser, R., Friedland, E., Aceto, R. M., Camargo, M. J. F., and Atlas, S. A.,** Relationship of increased plasma atrial natriuretic factor and renal sodium handling during immersion-induced central hypervolemia in normal humans, *J. Clin. Invest.,* 79, 738, 1987.
17. **Katsube, N., Schwaryz, D., and Needleman, P.,** Release of atriopeptin in the rat by vasoconstrictors or water immersion correlates with changes in right atrial pressure, *Biochem. Biophys. Res. Commun.,* 133, 937, 1985.
18. **Baertschi, A. J., Hausmaninger, C., Walsh, R. S., Mentzer, R. M., Jr., Wyatt, D. A., and Pence, R. A.,** Hypoxia-induced release of atrial natriuretic factor (ANF) from the isolated rat and rabbit heart, *Biochem. Biophys. Res. Commun.,* 140, 427, 1986.
19. **Ballermann, B. J., Bloch, K. D., Seidman, J. G., and Brenner, B. M.,** Atrial natriuretic peptide transcription, secretion, and glomerular receptor activity during mineralocorticoid escape in the rat, *J. Clin. Invest.,* 78, 840, 1986.
20. **Henry, J. P., Gauer, O. H., and Reeves, J. L.,** Evidence of the atrial location of receptors influencing urine flow, *Circ. Res.,* 4, 85, 1956.
21. **Kaczmarczyk, G., Drake, A., Eisele, R., Mognhaupt, R., Noble, M. I. M., Simgen, B., Stubbs, J., and Reinhardt, H. W.,** The role of the cardiac nerves in the regulation of sodium excretion in conscious dogs, *Pfluegers Arch.,* 390, 125, 1981.
22. **Achermann, U.,** Control of renal function in isovolemic hemodilution or in vagotomized, infused rats, *Pfluegers Arch.,* 386, 111, 1980.
23. **Goetz, K. L., Wang, B. C., Geer, P. G., Leadly, R. J., and Reinhardt, H. W.,** Atrial stretch increases sodium excretion independently of releases of atrial peptides, *Am. J. Physiol.,* 250, R946, 1986.
24. **Haass, M., Zukowska-Grojec, Z., Kopin, I. J., and Zamir, N.,** Role of autonomic nervous system and vasoactive hormones in the release of atrial natriuretic peptides in conscious rats, *J. Cardiovasc. Pharmacol.,* 10, 424, 1987.
25. **Rankin, A. J., Wilson, N., and Lesome, J. R.,** Effects of autonomic stimulation on plasma immunoreactive atrial natriuretic peptide in the anesthetized rabbit, *Can. J. Physiol. Pharmacol.,* 65, 532, 1986.
26. **Dietz, J. R.,** Release of natriuretic factor from rat heart-lung preparation by atrial distension, *Am. J. Physiol.,* 247, R1093, 1984.
27. **Dietz, J. R.,** Control of atrial natriuretic factor release from a rat heart-lung preparation, *Am. J. Physiol.,* 252, R498, 1987.
28. **Ruskoaho, H., Tholken, H., and Lang, R. E.,** Increase in atrial pressure releases atrial natriuretic peptide from isolated perfused rat hearts, *Eur. J. Physiol.,* 407, 170, 1986.
29. **Schiebinger, R. J. and Linden, J.,** The influence of resting tension on immunoreactive atrial natriuretic peptide secretion by rat atria superfused in vitro, *Circ. Res.,* 59, 105, 1986.
30. **Sonnenberg, H., Krebs, R. F., and Veress, A. T.,** Release of atrial natriuretic factor from incubated rat heart atria, *IRCS Med. Sci.,* 12, 783, 1984.
31. **Sonnenberg, H. and Veress, A. T.,** Cellular mechanism of release of atrial natriuretic factor, *Biochem. Biophys. Res. Commun.,* 124, 443, 1984.
32. **Currie, M. G. and Newman, W. H.,** Evidence for alpha-1 adrenergic receptor regulation of atriopeptic release from the isolated rat heart, *Biochem. Biophys. Res. Commun.,* 137, 94, 1986.

33. **Garcia, R., Lachance, D., Thibarlt, G., Gutkowska, J., and Cantin, M.,** *Biological Action of Arterial Peptides,* Vol. 1, Brenner, B. M. and Laragh, J. H., Eds., Raven Press, New York, 1987, 35.

34. **Gibbs, D. M.,** Beta-adrenergic control of atrial natriuretic factor secretion from dispersed rat atrial myocytes, *Regul. Peptides,* 19, 73, 1987.

35. **Schiebinger, R. J., Baker, M. Z., and Linden, J.,** Effect of adrenergic and muscarinic cholinergic agonists on atrial natriuretic peptide secretion by isolated rat atria, *J. Clin. Invest.,* 80, 1687, 1987.

36. **Mannign, P. T., Schwartz, D., Katsube, N. C., Holmberg, S. W., and Needleman, P.,** Vasopressin-stimulated release of atriopeptin: endocrine antagonists in fluid homeostasis, *Science,* 229, 395, 1985.

37. **Sugawara, A., Nakao, K., Sakamoto, M., Morii, N., Yamada, T., Itoh, H., Shiono, S., and Imura, H.,** Plasma concentration of atrial natriuretic polypeptide in essential hypertension, *Lancet,* 2, 1426, 1985.

38. **Sagnella, G. A., Markandu, N. D., Shore, A. C., and MacGregor, G. A.,** Raised circulating levels of atrial natriuretic peptides in essential hypertension, *Lancet,* 1, 179, 1986.

39. **Yandle, T. G., Espiner, E. A., Nicholls, M. G., and Duff, H.,** Radioimmunoassay and characterization of atrial natriuretic peptide in human plasma, *J. Clin. Endocrinol. Metab.,* 63, 72, 1986.

40. **Arjamaa, I. and Vuolteenaho, O.,** Sodium ion stimulates the release of atrial natriuretic polypeptides (ANP) from rat atria, *Biochem. Biophys. Res. Commun.,* 132, 375, 1985.

41. **Gibbs, D. M.,** Noncalcium-dependent modulation of in vitro atrial natriuretic factor release by extracellular osmolality, *Endocrinology,* 120, 194, 1987.

42. **Ueglinger, D. E., Weidmann, P., Gnadinger, M. P., Shaw, S., and Lang, R. E.,** Depressor effects and release of atrial natriuretic peptide during norepinephrine or angiotensin II infusion in man, *J. Clin. Endocrinol. Metab.,* 63, 669, 1986.

43. **Baranowska, B. and Gutkowska, J.,** Opposite effects of neuropeptide Y (NPY) and polypeptide YY (PYY) on plasma immunoreactive atrial natriuretic factor (IR-ANF) in rats, *Biochem. Biophys. Res. Commun.,* 145, 680, 1987.

44. **Tang, J., Xie, C. W., Gao, X. M., and Chang, J. K.,** Dynorphin A(1-10) amide stimulates the release of atrial natriuretic polypeptide (ANP) from rat atrium, *Eur. J. Pharmacol.,* 136, 449, 1987.

45. **Zamir, N., Haass, M., Dave, J. R., and Zudowska-Grojec, Z.,** Anterior pituitary gland modulates the release of atrial natriuretic peptides from cardiac atria, *Proc. Natl. Acad. Sci. U.S.A.,* 84, 541, 1987.

46. **Wollheim, C. B. and Sharp, G. W. G.,** Regulation of insulin release by calcium, *Physiol. Rev.,* 61, 914, 1981.

47. **Page, E., Gings, G. E., Power, B., and Upshaw-Earley, J.,** Ultrastructural features of atrial peptide secretion, *Am. J. Physiol.,* 251, H340, 1986.

48. **Allen, D. G. and Kurihara, S.,** The effects of muscle length on intracellular calcium transients in mammalian cardiac muscle, *J. Physiol.,* 327, 79, 1982.

49. **Reuter, H.,** Ion channels in cardiac cell membranes, *Annu. Rev. Physiol.,* 46, 473, 1984.

50. **Winquist, R. J. and Baskin, E. P.,** Calcium channels resistant to organic calcium entry blockers in a rabbit vein, *Am. J. Physiol.,* 345, H1024, 1983.

51. **Lansman, J. B., Hallam, T. J., and Rink, T. J.,** Single stretch-activated ion channels in vascular endothelial cells as mechanotransducers, *Nature (London),* 325, 811, 1987.

52. **Macchia, D. D. and Page, E.,** Stretch activated net plasmalemmal ion fluxes and depolarization in rat atria, *Biophys. J.,* 51, 255a, 1987.

53. **Allen, D. G. and Blinks, J. R.,** Calcium transients in aequorin-injected frog cardiac muscle, *Nature (London),* 273, 509, 1978.

54. **Berridge, M. J.,** Inositol trisphoysphate and diacylglycerol: two interacting second messengers, *Annu. Rev. Biochem.,* 56, 159, 1987.

55. **Nishizuka, Y.,** The role of protein kinase C in cell surface signal transduction and tumor promotion, *Nature (London),* 308, 693, 1984.

56. **Ruskoaho, H., Toth, M., and Lang, R. E.,** Atrial natriuretic peptide secretion: synergistic effect of phorbol ester and A23187, *Biochem. Biophys. Res. Commun.,* 133, 581, 1985.

57. **Ruskoaho, H., Toth, M., Ganten, D., Unger, Th., and Lang, R. E.,** The phorbol ester induced atrial natriuretic peptide secretion is stimulated by forskolin and bay K8644 and inhibited b 8-bromo-cyclic GMP, *Biochem. Biophys. Res. Commun.,* 139, 266, 1986.

58. **Brown, J. H., Buxton, I. L. and Brunton, L. L.,** Alpha-1-adrenergic and muscarinic cholinergic stimulation of phosphoinositide hydrolysis in adult rat cardiomyocytes, *Circ. Res.,* 57, 532, 1985.

59. **Brown, J. H. and Brown Masters, S.,** Muscarinic regulation of phosphatidylinositol turnover and cyclic nucleotide metabolism in the heart, *Fed. Proc.,* 43, 2613, 1984.

Chapter 7

STRUCTURE AND FUNCTION OF ATRIAL NATRIURETIC RECEPTOR SUBTYPES

Dale C. Leitman and Ferid Murad

TABLE OF CONTENTS

I. INTRODUCTION

Shortly after its identification and synthesis, it became clear that atrial natriuretic peptide (ANP) had unique and unanticipated biological actions. In addition to producing natriuresis and diuresis,[1] ANP was shown to produce relaxation of smooth muscle[2,3] and inhibit the secretion of aldosterone,[4,5] renin,[6,7] and vasopressin.[8] ANP has also been reported to inhibit water and sodium intake after central administration[9] and stimulate testosterone synthesis in Leydig cells.[10,11] While it has become clear that ANP exhibits more than just natriuretic and diuretic properties, the cellular actions that mediate the diverse biological actions of ANP are not known. Two general experimental approaches have been used to elucidate the mechanism of action of ANP. ANP has been tested to determine if it can regulate any of the previously discovered second messenger systems in a variety of tissues and cultured cells. In addition, the pharmacological and biochemical properties of the membrane receptors for ANP have been characterized in a number of tissues and cells.

Peptide hormones, such as ANP, initiate their biological actions by binding to specific glycoprotein receptors in the plasma membrane. The binding of the hormone to its receptor results in the formation of an intracellular second messenger which mediates the effects of the hormone. The process whereby peptide hormones transmit their information into the cell to produce its biological action is known as signal transduction. An understanding of the mechanism of signal transduction for ANP is essential for the development of therapeutic agents that mimic the remarkable properties of ANP. In this chapter, we will focus on the pharmacological and biochemical properties of ANP receptors and the coupling of one of the ANP receptors to the guanylate cyclase-cyclic GMP system. In previous articles, we have discussed possible functions of cyclic GMP and intracellular sites where cyclic GMP may interact to elicit its biological effects.[12-15]

II. IDENTIFICATION AND BINDING PROPERTIES OF ANP RECEPTORS

The initial step in the mechanism of action of ANP is the binding of ANP to specific membrane receptors. ANP receptors have been identified in tissues by two methods: radioligand binding and radioautography localization studies. In both methods, ANP receptors have been characterized using a radioactive iodinated form of ANP. Table 1 summarizes the identification of ANP receptors in a variety of tissues and cultured cells by radioligand binding studies. Several general conclusions can be ascertained from these studies. In most studies, a single class of ANP receptors was identified in tissues and cells with equilibrium dissociation constants that ranged from 0.025 to 2 nM. However, analysis of competition binding curves by computer programs has revealed that two classes of ANP binding sites exist in bovine adrenal glomerulosa,[16] rabbit kidney cortex,[17] and rat glomeruli.[18] The low-affinity ANP binding sites detected in these studies may not be physiologically relevant since plasma ANP levels are normally lower (range 1 to 100 pM) than the K_d for the low-affinity site (Table 1). It can also be appreciated that ANP binding sites are present in a wide variety of tissues and cells, including many cell types that are not directly involved in blood pressure and vascular volume homeostasis. For example, high-affinity ANP binding sites have been identified in human platelets,[19,20] brain,[21,22] Leydig cells,[23] cardiac messenchymal cells,[24] lung fibroblasts,[23,25] osteoblasts,[26] granulosa-lutein cells,[27] and thymocytes.[28]

In a revealing study by De Lean et al.,[29] the abundance of ANP receptors was compared in various segments of the dog kidney. These investigators discovered that the highest ANP receptor density was present in the glomeruli, followed by the collecting ducts and thick ascending loop of Henle (Table 1). In contrast, no ANP receptors were detected in the proximal tubule. The greater density of receptors in the glomeruli and collecting duct,

TABLE 1
ANP Receptors in Tissues and Cell Types

ANP receptor source	Equilibrium dissociation	Binding capacity	Ref.
Tissue	nM	fmol/mg protein	
Bovine adrenal cortex	1.8	2,500	37
Bovine adrenal glomerulosa	0.0.25, 3.2	1,300	16
Bovine brain microvessels	0.11	58	86
Rabbit aorta	0.13	96	17
Rabbit kidney cortex	0.052, 490	35	17
Dog glomeruli	0.12	200	29
Dog collecting ducts	0.4	150	29
Dog thick ascending loop of Henle	0.4	3	29
Renal adrenal capsule	0.064	90	87
Rat glomeruli	0.027	390	42
	0.46	484	65
	0.057, 8.0	73	18
Rat renal artery	0.18	23	87
Rat lung	0.28	120	41
Rat thymocytes	0.17	218	28
Guinea pig thalamus/hypothalamus	0.02	4	21
Guinea pig cerebellum	0.06	4.7	21
Human placenta	2.5	96	35
Human kidney cortex	0.4	16	88
Human pheochromocytoma	1.0	400	89
Cells		**ANP receptors/cell**	
Bovine aortic smooth muscle	2.1	550,000	90
	0.82	310,000	23
Bovine endothelial	0.3	10,000—50,000	90
	0.1	16,000	49
Bovine adrenal cortical	0.12	50,000	23
Rat mesenchymal heart	0.2—0.3	190,000—300,000	24
Rat messangial	0.22	12,000	65
Rat lung fibroblasts	0.66	130,000	25
Rat Leydig	0.11	3,000	23
Rat osteoblasts	0.12	42,000	26
Rat aortic smooth muscle	1—2	200,000—300,000	90
Human lung fibroblasts	0.32	80,000	23
Human granulosa-lutein	0.18	160,000—190,000	27
Human platelets	0.025	9.8	19
	0.008	12	20
LLC-PK$_1$	110	240,000	30

compared to the tubular segments, suggested that these are the major sites where ANP acts in the kidney. Table 1 also shows that the most abundant tissue sources of ANP binding sites are the adrenal cortex and glomeruli, whereas the cultured cell type with the greatest number of ANP receptors is vascular aortic smooth muscle cells. Porcine kidney cells, LLC-PK$_1$, have also been reported to have a large population of ANP receptors,[30] but these have extremely low affinity for ANP (110 nM) and, therefore, are not likely to be physiologically relevant.

In addition to radioligand binding studies, radioautography studies indicate that ANP receptors are also located in the cillary process of the eye, hepatocytes, chromaffin cells of the adrenal medulla, epithelial cells of intestinal villi, and the smooth muscle layer of the colon.[31,32] These studies demonstrate that ANP receptors are present in many diverse cell

TABLE 2
Photoaffinity and Chemical Cross-Linking of ANP Receptors in Tissues and Cells

ANP receptor source	Molecular size (kDa)	Type of cross-linking	Ref.
Rat kidney cortex	140	Photoaffinity	33
Rat liver	140	Photoaffinity	33
Rat adrenal	126	Photoaffinity	34
Bovine adrenal cortex	70	DDS	37
Bovine glomerulosa	68, 114	DSS	38
Rabbit aorta	60, 70, 120	Photoaffinity	36
Human placenta	140—160	DSS	35
Human pheocytochromocytoma	70	DSS	89
Cultured cells			
Bovine aortic smooth muscle	66, 180	DSS	92
	66, 130	DSS	23
Bovine aortic endothelial	66, 180	DSS	92
	66, 130	DSS	39
Bovine adrenal cortical	66, 130	DSS	23
Rat lung fibroblasts	66, 130	DSS	25
Rat aortic smooth muscle	60	Photoaffinity	60
Human lung fibroblasts	66, 130	DSS	23
Mouse Leydig tumor	135	Photoaffinity	27

Note: The values in this table for the molecular size of the ANP receptors are from SDS-poly-acrylamide gel analysis performed under reducing conditions.

types. In fact, only a very few cell types have been reported to be devoid of ANP receptors. These include some kidney epithelial cell lines[23] and red and white blood cells.[20] Although the function of ANP receptors in many of these cell types, such as endothelial cells and fibroblasts, is not known, we believe ANP may regulate generalized cellular processes that may include metabolism, proliferation, and differentiation.

III. MOLECULAR CHARACTERISTICS OF ANP RECEPTORS

The characterization of the molecular properties of ANP receptors is a major step toward identifying the signal transduction mechanisms of ANP and also will provide a more rational approach to designing ANP analogs useful for clinical purposes. Most investigators have used photoaffinity or chemical cross-linking techniques to define the molecular properties of ANP receptors. In photoaffinity labeling, membranes or intact cells are incubated with ^{125}I-labeled ANP that contains a photoactivable group. Once the labeled ANP is bound to its receptors, it is covalently cross-linked by ultraviolet irradiation. ^{125}I-labeled ANP has also been irreversibly cross-linked to cells using chemical cross-linking techniques. In this case, the ^{125}I-ANP, which is not derivatized with a photoactive agent, is incubated with membranes or intact cells and then is cross-linked with the bifunctional reagent disuccinimidyl suberate (DSS). In both of these cross-linking methods, the molecular size of the ANP receptor protein is determined by autoradiography after the proteins are separated by sodium dodecyl sulfate (SDS)-polyacrylamide gel electrophoresis. The results with either technique have been generally similar.

Table 2 summarizes the studies that have used cross-linking techniques to identify the molecular size of ANP receptors. Using photoaffinity cross-linking methods, one protein with a molecular size of 120 to 140 kDa has been identified in rat kidney cortex,[33] liver,[33] adrenal gland,[34] and human granulosa-lutein cells[27] under reducing conditions. A single 140-

to 160-kDa ANP binding protein has been found in human placental membranes.[35] In rabbit aorta, three distinct proteins with molecular sizes of 60, 70, and 120 kDa, respectively, have been described.[36] Hirose et al.[37] have reported that bovine adrenal cortex has one ANP binding site with a molecular size of 130 kDa under nonreducing conditions. However, when the proteins were separated under reducing conditions, all of the 130-kDa protein band was converted into a 70-kDa protein band.[37] In another study, a 68- and 114-kDa ANP binding protein has been found in bovine adrenal zona glomerulosa.[38] The structural basis for the differences in molecular size of ANP binding sites may be due to the presence of multiple ANP receptor subtypes, cellular heterogeneity of the tissue, proteolysis of ANP receptors, or differences in cross-linking techniques.

In order to exclude the uncertainty of identifying receptors in tissues containing multiple cell types, we and other investigators have cross-linked ANP to homogeneous populations of cultured cells. We have found that cultured bovine adrenal cortical, aortic endothelial, and aortic smooth muscle and human and rat lung fibroblasts have two ANP binding sites.[23,25,39,40] Under nonreducing conditions, 40 to 60% of the ANP binding sites have a molecular size of 130 kDa, whereas the remaining sites have a molecular size of 66 kDa. When the cellular proteins are separated using reducing conditions, only 1 to 6% of the ANP binding sites are 130 kDa, and the remaining sites have a molecular size of 66 kDa.[23,25,39,40] From these results, we proposed that at least three molecular forms of ANP binding sites exist in intact cells:[23] (1) a nonreducible, single protein with a molecular size of 130 kDa, (2) an ANP binding site that also has a molecular size of 130 kDa, but is made up of two proteins with a molecular size of 66 kDa that are joined by a disulfide bond, and (3) a 66-kDa monomer.

IV. PURIFICATION OF ANP RECEPTOR SUBTYPES

A second approach taken to characterize the ANP receptor has utilized chromatographic methods to purify the receptor proteins. The first step in the purification of membrane receptors involves the solubilization of the protein in a state that retains ligand binding. Fortunately, it was found that ANP binding activity could be readily extracted from membranes after solubilization with a variety of nonionic detergents, including lubrol-PX, Triton X-100, CHAPS, and octyl-glucoside.[41-43] Kuno et al.[41] were the first to purify a nonreducible ANP binding site with a molecular size of 120 to 140 kDa from rat lung. In their purification procedure, lung membranes were solubilized with the nonionic detergent lubrol-PX, and the ANP receptor was purified by sequential column chromatography using GTP-agarose, DEAE-sephacel, phenyl-agarose, and WGA-agarose. Silver staining of the SDS-polyacrylamide gel revealed the presence of one major band with a molecular size of 120 to 140 kDa. Furthermore, only this band was labeled after cross-linking with ^{125}I-ANP. The purified ANP receptor bound ANP with a similar affinity and atrial peptide analog specificity as in lung membranes, and the specific binding activity was increased by 19,000-fold. The mobility on SDS-polyacrylamide gel of the purified 120- to 140-kDa ANP receptor from rat lung was not altered by reducing agents.[41] The nonreducible 120- to 140-kDa ANP protein was also recently purified from bovine adrenal cortex.[44]

A second 130- to 140-kDa ANP protein that is converted into a 60- to 70-kDa protein by reducing agents has been purified from cultured bovine aortic smooth muscle cells,[45] bovine lung,[46] and bovine adrenal cortex.[44] The successful purification of this receptor from these tissues was accomplished using an ANP affinity column. The binding properties and analog specificity of the purified ANP receptor from smooth muscle cells and adrenal cortex after elution from the affinity column at pH 5.0 to 5.5 were similar to those found with intact cultures or membranes.[44,45] The purification of two distinct ANP binding sites confirms the cross-linking studies, which indicated the existence of at least two binding sites for ANP.

The observation that both ANP binding proteins have a similar molecular size (120 to 140 kDa) suggests that these two proteins may have a close structural relationship and may even be interconvertible. However, Takayangi et al.[44] have shown that peptide maps of both the purified nonreducible and reducible 130- to 140-kDa ANP binding sites from bovine adrenal cortex have only a 10% homology, which indicates that the primary structures of these two proteins are distinct. This study and the difference in functional properties (see below) of these two ANP binding sites suggest that these two proteins are encoded by separate genes and are not interconvertible or structurally related.

A major issue raised by the cross-linking and purification studies is whether the reducible 130-kDa ANP binding protein consists of two distinct or identical 60- to 70-kDa subunits. Recent evidence indicates that this protein is a homodimer that consists of the two identical subunits. Shimonaka et al.[46] have purified the reducible 130-kDa ANP binding protein from bovine lung. When the N-terminal portion of the protein was sequenced, only one amino acid sequence was obtained, which suggests that the two subunits were identical or, alternatively, one of the subunits had a blocked N terminus.

V. CLONING OF THE ANP RECEPTOR

Additional evidence that indicates that the reducible 130-kDa ANP receptor consists of two identical subunits is derived from the molecular cloning of the cDNA for this ANP receptor subtype. Fuller et al.[47] have purified the reducible 130-kDa ANP binding site from cultured bovine aortic smooth muscle cells, sequenced the N terminus, and eventually isolated a cDNA to this protein. The predicted molecular size of the primary translation product from the cDNA was 56 kDa. However, when the cDNA was translated in *Xenopus* oocytes, a 65-kDa protein was synthesized that bound ANP with high affinity. Uchida et al.[48] reported that the mRNA for the 60- to 70-kDa ANP receptor subunits is translated into a 58-kDa protein in a reticulolysate *in vitro* translational system. These studies provide evidence that indicates that this ANP receptor subtype is synthesized as a 56-kDa protein, which then is glycosylated to form the mature 60- to 70-kDa protein. The observation that the 60- to 70-kDa ANP binding site binds to a lectin column also indicates that this ANP binding site is a glycoprotein. After translation and glycosylation, apparently two identical subunits are joined by a disulfide bridge to form a 130- to 140-kDa ANP binding site. The successful cloning of the nonreducible 130-kDa ANP receptor subtype has not been reported.

From cross-linking and purification studies, it can be concluded that there are two major ANP receptors. Both of these ANP receptors have a molecular size of 120 to 140 kDa. However, one receptor consists of a single 120- to 140-kDa protein, whereas the other receptor is comprised of two identical 60- to 70-kDa subunits joined by a disulfide bond. In our cross-linking studies, we have found that 40 to 60% of the ANP binding sites in cultured cells may be present as the 60- to 70-kDa monomer. However, it is possible that in the native membrane only the 120- to 140-kDa dimer exists, but the two subunits separate during the solubilization of the cells with SDS, even in the absence of reducing agents. Although it is clear that there are two major ANP binding sites, it remains possible that additional ANP receptor subtypes are present. Furthermore, there may be other proteins associated with these two ANP receptors that do not contain an ANP binding site, but are involved in the coupling or regulation of the ANP receptor signal transduction pathways.

VI. FUNCTIONAL ANP RECEPTOR HETEROGENEITY

The structural properties of the ANP receptors suggest that there are at least two physical forms of ANP receptors. Our laboratory was the first to provide pharmacological evidence to suggest that these two ANP binding sites also have different functional properties.[49] In

ANP binding studies with cultured bovine aortic endothelial[49] and smooth muscle cells,[50] a linear Scatchard plot was found, which indicated that these cell types contain a single class of ANP receptors. However, when comparing the effects of the 26-amino-acid atrial peptide ANP and the 21-amino-acid peptide atriopeptin I on cyclic GMP accumulation in these cultured cells, we found that atriopeptin I is 100- to 1000-fold weaker than ANP at increasing cyclic GMP accumulation.[49,50] Furthermore, at a concentration of 100 nM, ANP increased cyclic GMP by 500-fold in endothelial cells, whereas atriopeptin I stimulated cyclic GMP by only sevenfold.[49] We first suspected that atriopeptin I was a much weaker agonist than ANP because the ANP receptors had a greater affinity for ANP, compared to atriopeptin I. However, when competition binding studies were performed with these two atrial peptides, we found that the ANP receptors exhibited a similar affinity for both ANP and atriopeptin I. These results ruled out the possibility that atriopeptin I was a much weaker agonist than ANP because it did not bind to ANP receptors. Because of the linear Scatchard plot, we next suspected that atriopeptin I was ineffective at activating guanylate cyclase after it became bound to the ANP receptor. In this case, one would expect atriopeptin I to act as an antagonist for the more potent agonist, ANP. However, under a variety of different conditions, atriopeptin I was unable to antagonize the stimulation of cyclic GMP accumulation by ANP.[39,49] In fact, when endothelial cells were treated with less than maximally effective concentrations of both ANP and atriopeptin I, an additive increase in cyclic GMP was observed.[39] From these studies, we proposed that two functionally distinct ANP binding sites exist in endothelial cells.[39] Our results indicated that most of the ANP receptors were not functionally coupled to guanylate cyclase since atriopeptin I could bind to over 80% of the ANP receptors without increasing cyclic GMP levels. Furthermore, we suggested that endothelial cells also contained a small population of a second, distinct ANP receptor that was coupled to guanylate cyclase. Our results also suggested that the guanylate cyclase-coupled ANP binding site must have a much lower affinity for atriopeptin I, compared to ANP, since it was ineffective at increasing cyclic GMP and antagonizing the stimulation of cyclic GMP by ANP. Scarborough et al.[51] have confirmed these results by demonstrating that a marked dissociation in the potency of various ANP analogs to bind to ANP receptors and stimulate cyclic GMP accumulation also occurs in cultured bovine aortic smooth muscle cells. From these studies, they also concluded that functionally distinct ANP receptors were responsible for the marked discrepancy between the potency of ANP analogs to compete for ANP binding sites and increase cyclic GMP.[51]

The identification of multiple ANP binding sites is typically accomplished with specific receptor agonists and antagonists. Unfortunately, no selective ANP agonists and antagonists are available. In order to further explore the existence of ANP receptor heterogeneity, we compared the number and affinity of ANP receptors with the ability of ANP to stimulate particulate guanylate cyclase activity and increase cyclic GMP accumulation in eight different cultured cell types. We reasoned that if only one class of ANP receptors exists in cells, as suggested by Scatchard analysis, there should be a reasonable correlation between the biological potency of ANP and the number of ANP receptors. Table 3 shows that, in general, the cells having the greatest number of ANP binding sites (BAC, HLF, and BASM cells) actually exhibit the weakest stimulation of cyclic GMP accumulation and particulate guanylate cyclase activity. In contrast, ANP produced the greatest increase in the cell types that contained few or no detectable ANP receptors.[23] Remarkably, no ANP binding sites were detected in MDBK cells, despite that ANP increased cyclic GMP accumulation by 300-fold and guanylate cyclase activity by 7.8-fold. These results clearly demonstrate that the number of ANP receptors does not adequately reflect the biological potency of ANP in different cell types. The differences in biological potency also could not be attributed to differences in ANP receptor affinity in the eight cell types. For example, the K_d in the BAC and BAE were very similar, but ANP was 10,000-fold more potent at increasing cyclic GMP in BAE cells, compared to BAC cells.[23] It is highly unlikely that these results could be interpreted

TABLE 3
ANP Receptor Binding and Effects of ANP on Cyclic GMP and Particulate Guanylate Cyclase Activity in Cultured Cells

Cell type	Fold stimulation		Receptors/cell	K_d (nM)
	Cyclic GMP	Guanylate cyclase		
BAC	13	1.5	50,000	0.12
HLF	35	3.1	80,000	0.32
MDCK	58	3.2	N.D.	
BASM	60	2.5	310,000	0.82
RME	120	5.0	N.D.	
RL	260	7.0	3,000	0.11
MDBK	300	7.8	N.D.	
BAE	475	8.0	14,000	0.09

Note: Confluent cells were used to measure cyclic GMP responses, particulate guanylate cyclase activity, and ANP receptors, as previously described.[23] BAC, bovine adrenal cortical cells; HLF, human lung fibroblasts; MDCK, canine kidney epithelial cells; BASM, bovine aortic smooth muscle cells; RME, rat mammary epithelial cells; RL, rat Leydig; MDBK, bovine kidney epithelial cells; BAE, bovine aortic endothelial cells; N.D. = none detectable.

to support a one ANP receptor model. Instead, these results provide additional evidence that supports our hypothesis that multiple, functionally distinct ANP binding sites exist in cells. These results also clearly demonstrate that the number of ANP receptors may not be a valid prediction of the biological response to ANP. For example, if one finds that a tissue or cell type has no or few ANP receptors, it would be unfortunate to assume that this is not an important target tissue for ANP. In future studies, it will be important to measure both ANP binding and the biological response (i.e., cyclic GMP, smooth muscle relaxation, and natriuresis) to ANP, particularly during changes in physiological or pathological states.

The above studies indicated that cells contain two structurally and functionally distinct ANP binding sites and that only one ANP receptor is linked to guanylate cyclase. In order to determine which one of these ANP binding sites was coupled to guanylate cyclase, we cross-linked intact endothelial cells with ^{125}I-labeled ANP in the presence of increasing concentrations of ANP or atriopeptin I. In endothelial cells, 6% of the total ANP binding sites are the nonreducible 130-kDa protein, whereas 94% of the ANP sites have a molecular size of 66 kDa under reducing conditions.[39,40] Our results demonstrated that both atriopeptin I and ANP effectively bind to the 66-kDa ANP binding sites. At a concentration of 100 nM, both ANP and atriopeptin I occupy nearly all of the 66-kDa ANP binding sites. However, at this concentration, ANP produced over a 400-fold increase in cyclic GMP, whereas atriopeptin I produced only a fourfold increase in cyclic GMP. Atriopetin I was much weaker at binding to the nonreducible 130-kDa ANP protein, compared to the 66-kDa protein. In contrast, ANP was equally effective at binding to both the 66- and 130-kDa binding proteins. Because the EC_{50} for cyclic GMP accumulation was closer to the K_I of the 130-kDa ANP binding protein for both ANP and atriopeptin I, we concluded that the 130-kDa ANP binding site is the ANP receptor coupled to guanylate cyclase and the 66-kDa site is not functionally linked to guanylate cyclase. We have previously suggested that the nonreducible 130-kDa ANP receptor (R) coupled to guanylate cyclase be designated ANP-R1 and the uncoupled, reducible 130-kDa ANP binding protein that consists of two 66-kDa subunits be designated ANP-R2.[39,40] Our studies also demonstrated that the C-terminal phenylalanine-arginine-tyrosine residues are not important for binding to ANP-R2 receptor, whereas these three tandem amino acids are critical for binding to the ANP-R1 receptor and activating particulate guanylate cyclase. These results have been confirmed with both purified ANP receptor subtypes from bovine adrenal cortex.[44] Furthermore, Scarborough et al.[51] also found that the disulfide ring is essential for binding to the guanylate cyclase-coupled ANP receptor, but is not required to bind to the uncoupled ANP binding site. It should be emphasized that the two ANP binding sites do not represent a high- and a low-affinity binding site. Both of these sites have nearly equal affinity for ANP when measured with intact cells[39,40] or purified preparations[44] of each ANP receptor subtype. The presence of two receptors that have a similar affinity for ANP and the preponderance of the uncoupled ANP receptors can explain the linear Scatchard plot with many cell types.

Additional support for functional heterogeneity of ANP receptors has come from the purification of the two ANP receptor subtypes. Unexpectedly, our laboratory discovered that the nonreducible 120- to 140-kDa ANP binding site copurified with particulate guanylate cyclase activity.[41] These results suggested that a single transmembrane glycoprotein with a molecular size of 120 to 140 kDa contained at least two functional domains, an ANP binding domain and guanylate cyclase domain. Apparently, the ANP binding domain extends from the outer cell membrane, whereas the region that possesses guanylate cyclase activity is located in the inner portion of the membrane, where it catalyzes the conversion of GTP to cyclic GMP. Other investigators have also shown that particulate guanylate cyclase copuries with the nonreducible 120- to 140-kDa ANP receptor subtype in bovine adrenal gland.[44] In contrast to the nonreducible ANP binding protein (ANP-R1), the reducible ANP binding protein (ANP-R2) does not contain a GTP binding site[23,41] or possess intrinsic guanylate cyclase activity.[44,45]

VII. ANP ACTIVATION OF PARTICULATE GUANYLATE CYCLASE

After binding to the ANP-R1 receptor, ANP activates guanylate cyclase and increases cyclic GMP accumulation. Hamet and co-workers reported that ANP increased cyclic GMP accumulation in kidney minces and cells.[52] Waldman and co-workers showed that ANP increased cyclic GMP by selectively activating the particulate isoenzyme of guanylate cyclase.[3,53,54] ANP increases particulate guanylate cyclase by two- to tenfold in membranes prepared from rabbit aorta and rat kidney, lung, liver, intestine, testes, and adrenal cortex.[3,53,54] The activation of particulate guanylate cyclase was dose-dependent, with an EC_{50} that ranged from 2 to 10 nM. ANP had no effect on soluble guanylate cyclase in all of these preparations. These studies were the first demonstration that a hormone could directly activate the particulate guanylate cyclase-cyclic GMP signal transduction system and suggested that cyclic GMP was the second messenger that mediated the cellular actions of ANP. Following these original studies, ANP has been shown to increase particulate guanylate cyclase activity and cyclic GMP accumulation in many different tissues and cell types.[14] At the present time, the only cell type that contains ANP receptors in which ANP does not increase cyclic GMP is human platelets.[55]

The studies by Waldman and co-workers established that ANP can raise intracellular levels of cyclic GMP by activating the particulate or membrane-associated isoenzyme form of guanylate cyclase. However, these studies could not exclude the possibility that ANP may also indirectly activate the soluble isoenzyme in intact cells since it has not been possible to demonstrate hormonal activation of the soluble isoenzyme in a broken cell preparation which was used in their studies. Other studies have provided compelling evidence that suggests that ANP raises cyclic GMP levels by exclusively activating the particulate isoenzyme. It has been reported that the distribution of particulate guanylate cyclase in different kidney fractions correlates with the magnitude of stimulation of cyclic GMP accumulation by ANP.[56] Table 2 shows that the cell types that exhibited the greatest activation of particulate guanylate cyclase also had the greatest increase in cyclic GMP accumulation. We also demonstrated that an additive increase in cyclic GMP accumulation resulted when rat lung fibroblasts were exposed to both ANP and sodium nitroprusside, which activated only the particulate and soluble guanylate cyclase isoenzymes, respectively.[25] Finally, we found that the increase in cyclic GMP accumulation by ANP in the eight cell types shown in Table 2 is not inhibited by methylene blue, which is a relatively selective inhibitor of soluble guanylate cyclase.[23] These findings demonstrating that ANP does not activate the soluble isoenzyme also indicate that the mechanisms whereby ANP activates the particular isoenzyme are different from the mechanism which other hormones utilize to activate the soluble isoenzyme. For example, we recently found that other natriuretic peptide hormones (e.g., oxytocin) increase cyclic GMP by activating the soluble isoenzyme in cultured LLC-PK$_1$ kidney epithelial cells.[57] When these cells are treated with both ANP and oxytocin, an additive increase in cyclic GMP is observed.[57] These results suggest that agents that increase cyclic GMP by selectively activating the soluble isoenzyme may potentiate the biological effects (e.g., natriuresis) of ANP, which activates only the particulate isoenzyme.

VIII. REGULATION OF ANP RECEPTORS

One site for altering the biological response to ANP during physiological and pathological states is the ANP receptor. The properties of the ANP receptor system can be altered by changes in the affinity or number of ANP receptors and possibly the ratio of the two ANP receptor subtypes.

A. ANP RECEPTORS AND DRUGS

De Lean[58] has reported that amiloride and guanabenz produce a two- to threefold increase in ANP binding to bovine adrenal glomerulosa membranes. The increased ANP binding was attributed to a recruitment in the number of high affinity ANP receptors and was associated with a more pronounced inhibition of aldosterone synthesis.

B. HOMOLOGOUS DOWN-REGULATION OF ANP RECEPTORS

Internalization and down-regulation of membrane receptors is characteristically observed with hormones and other agents that interact with cell surface receptors. The down-regulation of ANP receptors have been most extensively investigated with cultured vascular smooth muscle cells.[59-64] For these studies, smooth muscle cells were exposed to unlabeled ANP for various times and then the remaining number of ANP receptors were determined by radioligand binding studies. After exposing smooth muscle cells to ANP for 16 to 24 h, there is a 40 to 80% decrease in the number of ANP receptors.[57-62] The magnitude of ANP receptor down-regulation was dependent on the time of exposure to ANP and the pretreatment concentration of ANP. The maximal down-regulation of receptors occurred after 4 h of pretreatment[63] and little or no down-regulation occurred when the cells were exposed to concentrations of ANP less than 10 nM.[62] In all studies, the down-regulation of ANP receptors in cultured vascular smooth muscle cells occurred in the absence of any change in ANP receptor affinity.

C. ANP RECEPTORS AND SODIUM AND WATER INTAKE

The number of ANP receptors has also been examined in several different physiological states. Schiffrin et al.[19] have reported that the number of ANP receptors are 1.4-fold higher in platelets from normal men on a low sodium intake, compared to men with a higher sodium intake. Ballermann et al.[65] have reported that there is an approximate four-fold higher ANP receptor density in glomerular membranes from rats that were fed a low sodium diet for 2 weeks, compared to rats on a high sodium diet. In contrast, sodium loading results in a decreased number of ANP receptors in vascular tissue[66] and adrenal zona glomerulosa.[67]

The number of ANP receptors are higher in the adrenal glomerulosa[67] and subfornical organ[68] in rats deprived of water.

D. ANP RECEPTORS IN HYPERTENSION

The number of ANP receptors are lower in tissues from spontaneously hypertensive rats (SHR), compared to Wistar-Kyoto rats (WKY), which are normotensive, age-matched control rats. In the SHR, the number of ANP receptors are decreased in the adrenal gland,[69] glomeruli,[69] sympathetic ganglia,[70] renal basolateral membranes,[71] thymocytes,[72] and localized regions of the brain, including the subfornical organ and choroid plexus.[22,73] In DOCA salt-induced hypertensive rats, a decrease in ANP receptor density occurs in the glomeruli, mesenteric artery, and aorta.[74,75] The down-regulation of ANP receptors with hypertension in SHR may be secondary to elevated plasma ANP levels, which accompanies hypertension in SHR. These studies also suggest that the plasma levels of ANP may be one of the factors that control the number of ANP receptors in cells by altering the rate of down-regulation. It also remains possible that the decline in ANP binding in SHR results from a genetic defect in ANP receptors.

IX. REGULATION OF ANP RECEPTOR SUBTYPES AND STIMULATION OF CYCLIC GMP

Another possible mechanism to alter the ANP receptor system is by changing the ratio of the uncoupled (ANP-R2) and guanylate cyclase-coupled (ANP-R1) ANP receptor subtypes. The importance of the ratio of the two ANP receptor subtypes in determining the biological response to ANP is obvious from our studies that showed that a cell type with few or no detectable ANP receptors can exhibit a much greater increase in cyclic GMP by ANP, compared to cell types rich in ANP receptors.[23] From our cross-linking studies, it is clear that the proportion of ANP-R1 receptors to ANP-R2 receptors is much greater in endothelial cells, compared to smooth muscle cells.[39] The higher ratio of ANP-R1 to ANP-R2 receptors in endothelial cells is associated with a 1000-fold lower EC_{50} and a much greater maximal stimulation of cyclic GMP in endothelial cells.[23,50] We also found that ANP produced a several hundred-fold increase in cyclic GMP accumulation in cell types that contained fewer ANP receptors than could be measured with conventional binding assays.[23] We suspect that ANP is able to produce a marked increase in cyclic GMP in these cells because they have a high ANP-R1 to ANP-R2 receptor ratio, despite the very low total number of ANP receptors in these cells.

Although the possibility that the ANP-R1 to ANP-R2 receptor ratio changes during physiological and pathological conditions has not been directly investigated, studies correlating the number of ANP receptors with the ANP stimulation of cyclic GMP suggest that in some instances a change in the ANP receptor subtype ratio may occur. For example, it may be expected that if only the uncoupled ANP receptor is decreased during homologous down-regulation, high-sodium intake, or SHR, there may not be a diminished increase in cyclic GMP accumulation. In contrast, if the guanylate cyclase-coupled ANP receptor is down-regulated, then a marked decrease in cyclic GMP would be anticipated. Hirata et al.[64] reported that in cultured vascular smooth muscle cells pretreated with ANP, there was no change in the ANP-induced stimulation of cyclic GMP accumulation, despite an 80% decrease in the number of ANP receptors. The magnitude of increase in cyclic GMP accumulation by ANP is also not changed in glomeruli[65] and sympathetic ganglion,[70] despite a marked down-regulation of ANP receptors produced by low sodium intake and SHR, respectively. These studies indicate that in these cases only the uncoupled ANP receptor (ANP-R2) is subject to down-regulation. In contrast, other investigators have reported that the down-regulation of ANP receptors in vascular smooth muscle cells is associated with a marked reduction in the ANP-induced increase in cyclic GMP formation.[62] Although further studies are needed to determine the precise changes in ANP receptor subtypes that accompany changes in physiological states and vascular diseases, these studies suggest that the ratio of coupled to uncoupled ANP receptors may be more important than total receptor number in determining the biological response to ANP. For example, a two- to fivefold greater increase in cyclic GMP accumulation occurs in various regions of the brain from SHR rats,[76] compared to WKY rats, despite a decreased number of ANP binding sites in the brain of SHR rats.[22] Whether the apparent enhanced activation of particulate guanylate cyclase in the brain of SHR rats is due to a shift in the proportion of ANP receptor subtypes to more ANP-R1 receptors remains to be resolved.

X. PHYSIOLOGICAL ROLE OF ANP RECEPTOR SUBTYPES

Whereas it is clear that ANP increases cyclic GMP in every cell type that has ANP receptors, with few exceptions such as platelets,[55] the role of cyclic GMP in mediating the diverse biological actions of ANP is not known. The increase in cyclic GMP in these cells is mediated by the guanylate cyclase-coupled ANP-R1 receptor. It seems clear that the ANP-R1 receptor mediates vascular smooth muscle relaxation since two other classes of vasodilators, the nitrovasodilators and endothelium-dependent vasodilators, also increase cyclic GMP accumulation and cyclic GMP-dependent protein-kinase activity, and relax vascular smooth muscle.[12,13,15] The role of cyclic GMP in other tissues is more obscure. There is evidence that suggests that cyclic GMP may mediate the natriuretic and diuretic action of ANP. Hamet et al.[51] have demonstrated that ANP produces a marked increase in urinary cyclic GMP excretion. Huang et al.[77] have shown that the infusion of dibutyryl cyclic GMP into isolated kidney results in an increase in glomerular filtration rate, which is thought to mediate the natriuretic and diuretic action of ANP. In acute hypovolemia, it has also been reported that monoclonal antibodies to ANP prevents the rise in both plasma ANP levels and urinary cyclic GMP excretion.[78] The finding by Sonnenberg et al.[79] that ANP inhibits sodium transport in the collecting duct suggests that at least part of the natriuresis of ANP may be due to an effect of ANP on sodium transport in the kidney epithelial cells. In the kidney cell line LLC-PK$_1$, it has reported that ANP inhibits sodium transport, and the inhibition can be mimicked by 8-bromocyclic GMP and sodium nitroprusside.[80,81] ANP and 8-bromo cyclic GMP have also been reported to inhibit oxygen consumption in kidney papillary collecting tubule cells.[82] The inhibition of renin[83] secretion in isolated juxtoglomerular cells and the stimulation of testosterone[11] synthesis in Leydig cells also are mimicked by 8-bromo-cyclic GMP. The findings that 8-bromo-cyclic GMP and/or sodium nitroprusside increase glomerular filtration rate and testosterone synthesis and inhibit renin secretion and sodium transport suggest that the ANP-R1 receptor may mediate these biological actions of ANP.

One biological action of ANP that is not mimicked by 8-bromo-cyclic GMP or sodium nitroprusside is the ANP-induced inhibition of aldosterone synthesis.[84] These results suggest that the inhibition of aldosterone synthesis is not mediated by the ANP-R1 receptor, but instead is mediated by a nonguanylate cyclase-coupled receptor. It is also possible that an unidentified third ANP receptor may mediate the inhibition of aldosterone synthesis. As stated previously, we have found that ANP produces a marked increase in cyclic GMP in cell types that have no detectable ANP receptors (Table 3).[23] Therefore, it remains possible that the inhibition of aldosterone is mediated by an unidentified ANP receptor that is present in adrenal cells in such a low abundance that they cannot be measured with current radioligand and cross-linking techniques. In a recent study, Maack et al.[85] have provided evidence that ANP-R2 receptors (called C-receptor by the authors) may be involved in the degradation and clearance of ANP. In this study, a linear ANP analog was synthesized that specifically

TABLE 4
Characteristics of ANP Receptor Subtypes

	ANP-R1	ANP-R2
Molecular size		
Non-reduced	120—140 kDa	130—140 kDa
Reduced	120—140 kDa	60—70 kDa
Affinity for C-terminal truncated analogs	Low	High
Guanylate cyclase activity	Yes	No
Second messenger	Cyclic GMP	?
Possible functions	Smooth muscle relaxation, natriuresis and diuresis, inhibition of renin, stimulation of testosterone	Clearance of ANP, inhibition of aldosterone

binds only to the ANP-R2 receptor. The linear analog was devoid of physiological activity and unable to antagonize the renal effects of native ANP. However, after the administration of the linear ANP analog, the endogenous level of ANP was increased in rats and this was associated with an increase in natriuresis. From these results, it was suggested that by binding to the ANP-R2 receptor, the linear ANP analog prevented the degradation of endogenous ANP since it could not interact act with the ANP-R2 receptor.[85] Although this study indicates that the ANP-R2 receptor may be involved in the clearance of ANP, it does not rule out the possibility that this site may also mediate some of the biological effects of ANP.

XI. SUMMARY

Atrial natriuretic peptide exhibits remarkable and diverse physiological activities. The biological actions of ANP are mediated by specific ANP receptors in the cell membrane. Two ANP receptor subtypes have been characterized pharmacologically and with cross-linking and purification techniques. Table 4 summarizes the characteristics of the two ANP receptor subtypes. The ANP-R1 receptor is a bifunctional, single transmembrane glycoprotein with a molecular size of 120 to 140 kDa that has both an ANP binding site and guanylate cyclase activity. This receptor has a much greater affinity for ANP than the C-terminal truncated analogs and is pharmacologically coupled to increased guanylate cyclase activity and cyclic GMP formation. This ANP receptor promotes physiological processes that are mediated by the second messenger cyclic GMP. The ANP-R2 receptor is 130- to 140-kDa glycoprotein that is composed of two identical 60- to 70-kDa ANP binding proteins that are joined by a disulfide bridge. This ANP binding site does not contain guanylate cyclase activity and has high affinity for C-terminal truncated analogs and linear analogs that lack a disulfide bridge. It is not known if this binding site is associated with a second messenger system. A more complete understanding of the physiological roles and signal transduction pathways for both ANP receptor subtypes will be greatly facilitated with the development of specific agonists and antagonists for each receptor subtype.

REFERENCES

1. **de Bold, A.,** Atrial natriuretic factor: a hormone produced by the heart, *Science,* 230, 767, 1985.
2. **Winquist, R. J., Faison, E. P., Waldman, S. A., Schwartz, K., Murad, F., and Rapoport, R. M.,** Atrial natriuretic factor elicits an endothelium-independent relaxation and activates particulate guanylate cyclase in vascular smooth muscle, *Proc. Natl. Acad. Sci. U.S.A.,* 81, 7661, 1984.
3. **Fiscus, R. R., Rapoport, R. M., Waldman, S. A., and Murad, F.,** Atriopeptin II elevates cyclic GMP, activates cyclic GMP-dependent protein kinase and causes relaxation in rat thoracic aorta, *Biochim. Biophys. Acta,* 846, 179, 1985.
4. **De Lean, A., Racz, K., Gutkowska, J., Nguyen, T.-T., Cantin, M., and Genest, J.,** Specific receptor-mediated inhibition by synthetic atrial natriuretic factor of hormone-stimulated steroidogenesis in cultured bovine adrenal cells, *Endocrinology,* 115, 1636, 1984.
5. **Kudo, T. and Baird, A.,** Inhibition of aldosterone production in the adrenal glomerulosa by atrial natriuretic factor, *Nature (London),* 312, 756, 1984.
6. **Burnett, J. C., Jr., Granger, J. P., and Opgenorth, T. J.,** Effects of synthetic atrial natriuretic factor on renal function and renin release, *Am. J. Physiol.,* 247, F863, 1984.
7. **Maack, T., Marion, D. N., Camargo, M. J. F., Kleinert, H. D., Laragh, J. H., Vaughan, E. D., and Atlas, S. A.,** Effects of auriculin (atrial natriuretic factor) on blood pressure, renal function, and the renin-aldosterone system in dogs, *Am. J. Med.,* 77, 1069, 1984.
8. **Samson, W. K.,** Atrial natriuretic factor inhibits dehydration and hemorrhage-induced vasopressin release, *Neuroendocrinology,* 40, 277, 1985.
9. **Antunes-Rodrigues, J., McCann, S. M., and Samson, W. K.,** Central administration of atrial natriuretic factor inhibits saline preference in the rat, *Endocrinology,* 118, 1726, 1986.
10. **Bex, F. and Corbin, A.,** Atrial natriuretic factor stimulates testosterone production by mouse interstitial cells, *Eur. J. Pharmacol.,* 115, 125, 1985.
11. **Mukhopadhyay, A. K., Schumacher, M., and Leidenberger, F. A.,** Steroidogenic effect of atrial natriuretic factor in mouse Leydig cells is mediated by cyclic GMP, *Biochem. J.,* 239, 463, 1986.
12. **Rapoport, R. M. and Murad, F.,** Endothelium-dependent and nitrovasodilator-induced relaxation of vascular smooth muscle: role of cyclic GMP, *J. Cyclic. Nucleotide Protein Phosphor. Res.,* 9, 281, 1983.
13. **Murad, F.,** Cyclic guanosine monophosphate as a mediator of vasodilation, *J. Clin. Invest.,* 78, 1, 1986.
14. **Leitman, D. C. and Murad, F.,** Atrial natriuretic factor receptor heterogeneity and stimulation of particulate guanylate cyclase and cyclic GMP, *Endocr. Metab. Clin. N. Am.,* 16, 79, 1987.
15. **Waldman, S. A. and Murad, F.,** Cyclic GMP synthesis and function, *Pharmacol. Rev.,* 39, 163, 1987.
16. **De Lean, A., Gutkowska, J., McNicoll, N., Schiller, P. W., Cantin, M., and Genest, J.,** Characterization of specific receptors for atrial natriuretic factor in bovine adrenal zona glomerulosa, *Life Sci.,* 35, 2311, 1984.
17. **Napier, M. A., Vandlen, R. L., Albers-Schonberg, G., Nutt, R. F., Lyle, T., Winquist, R., Faison, E. P., Heinel, L. A., and Blaine, E. H.,** Specific membrane receptors for atrial natriuretic factor in renal and vascular tissues, *Proc. Natl. Acad. Sci. U.S.A.,* 81, 5946, 1984.
18. **Hamada, M., Burmester, H. A., Graci, K. A., Frolich, E. D., and Cole, F. E.,** Atrial natriuretic peptide binding properties of purified rat glomerular membranes, *Life Sci.,* 40, 1731, 1987.
19. **Schiffrin, E. L., Deslongchamps, M., and Thibault, G.,** Platelet binding sites for atrial natriuretic factor in humans: characterization and effects of sodium intake, *Hypertension,* 8 (Suppl. 2), 6, 1986.
20. **Strom, T. M., Weil, J., and Bidlingamaier, F.,** Platelet receptors for atrial natriuretic peptide in man, *Life Sci.,* 40, 769, 1986.
21. **Quiron, R., Dalpe, M., and Dam, T. V.,** Characterization and distribution of receptors for atrial natriuretic peptides in mammalian brain, *Proc. Natl. Acad. Sci. U.S.A.,* 83, 174, 1986.
22. **Saavedra, J. M., Correa, F. M. A., Plunkett, L. M., Israel, A., Kurihara, M., and Shigematsu, K.,** Binding of angiotensin and atrial natriuretic peptide in brain hypertensive rats, *Nature (London),* 320, 758, 1986.
23. **Leitman, D. C., Andresen, J. W., Catalano, R. M., Waldman, S. A., Tuan, J. J., and Murad, F.,** Atrial natriuretic peptide binding, cross-linking and stimulation of cyclic GMP accumulation and particulate guanylate cyclase activity in cultured cells, *J. Biol. Chem.,* 263, 3720, 1988.
24. **Hirata, Y., Tomita, M., Takata, S., and Inoue, I.,** Specific binding sites for atrial natriuretic peptide (ANP) in cultured mesenchymal nonmyocardial cells from rat heart, *Biochem. Biophys. Res. Commun.,* 131, 222, 1985.
25. **Leitman, D. C., Agnost, V. L., Tuan, J., Andresen, J. W., and Murad, F.,** Atrial natriuretic factor and sodium nitroprusside increase cyclic GMP in cultured rat lung fibroblasts by activating different forms of guanylate cyclase, *Biochem. J.,* 244, 66, 1987.
26. **Fletcher, A. E., Allan, E. H., Casley, D. J., and Martin, T. J.,** Atrial natriuretic factor receptors and stimulation of cyclic GMP formation in normal and malignant osteoblasts, *FEBS Lett.,* 208, 263, 1986.

27. **Pandey, K. N., Osteen, K., and Inagami, T.,** Specific receptor-mediated stimulation of progesterone secretion and cGMP accumulation by rat atrial natriuretic factor in cultured human granulosa-lutein (G-L) cells, *Endocrinology,* 121, 1195, 1987.

28. **Kurihara, M., Katamine, S., and Saavedra, J. M.,** Atrial natriuretic peptide, ANP (99-126), receptors in thymocytes and spleen cells, *Biochem. Biophys. Res. Commun.,* 145, 789, 1987.

29. **De Lean, A., Vinay, P., and Cantin, M.,** Distribution of atrial natriuretic factor receptors in dog kidney fractions, *FEBS Lett.,* 193, 239, 1985.

30. **Inui, K.-I., Saito, H., Matsukawa, Y., Nakao, N., Imura, H., Shimokura, M., Kiso, Y., and Hori, R.,** Specific binding activities and cyclic GMP responses by atrial natriuretic polypeptide in kidney epithelial cell line (LLC-PK$_1$), *Biochem. Biophys. Res. Commun.,* 132, 253, 1985.

31. **Bianchi, C., Gutkowska, J., Thibault, G., Garcia, R., Genest, J., and Cantin, M.,** Radioautographic localization of ^{125}I-atrial natriuretic factor (ANF) in rat tissues, *Histochemistry,* 82, 441, 1985.

32. **Bianchi, C., Anand-Srivastava, M. B., De Lean, A., Gutkowska, J., Forthomme, D., Genest, J., and Cantin, M.,** Localization and characterization of specific receptors for atrial natriuretic factor in the ciliary processes of the eye, *Curr. Eye Res.,* 5, 282, 1986.

33. **Yip, C. C., Laing, L. P., and Flynn, T. G.,** Photoaffinity labeling of atrial natriuretic factor receptors of rat kidney cortex plasma membranes, *J. Biol. Chem.,* 260, 8229, 1985.

34. **Misono, K. S., Grammer, R. T., Rigby, J. W., and Inagami, T.,** Photoaffinity labeling of atrial natriuretic factor receptor in bovine and rat adrenal cortical membranes, *Biochem. Biophys. Res. Commun.,* 130, 994, 1985.

35. **Sen, I.,** Identification and solubilization of atrial natriuretic factor receptors in human placenta, *Biochem. Biophys. Res. Commun.,* 135, 480, 1986.

36. **Vandlen, R. L., Arcuri, K. E., and Napier, M. A.,** Identification of a receptor for atrial natriuretic factor in rabbit aorta membranes by affinity cross-linking, *J. Biol. Chem.,* 260, 10889, 1985.

37. **Hirose, S., Akiyama, F., Shinjo, M., Ohno, H., and Murakami, K.,** Solubilization and molecular weight estimation of atrial natriuretic factor receptor from bovine adrenal cortex, *Biochem. Biophys. Res. Commun.,* 130, 574, 1985.

38. **Meloche, S., Ong, H., Cantin, M., and De Lean, A.,** Affinity cross-linking of atrial natriuretic factor to its receptor in bovine adrenal zona glomerulosa, *J. Biol. Chem.,* 261, 1525, 1986.

39. **Leitman, D. C., Andresen, J. W., Kuno, T., Kamisaki, Y., Chang, J.-K., and Murad, F.,** Identification of multiple binding sites for atrial natriuretic factor by affinity cross-linking in cultured endothelial cells, *J. Biol. Chem.,* 261, 11155, 1986.

40. **Leitman, D. C., Andresen, J. W., Kuno, T., Kamisaki, Y., Chang, J.-K., and Murad, F.,** Identification of two binding sites for atrial natriuretic factor in endothelial cells: evidence for a receptor subtype coupled to guanylate cyclase, *Trans. Am. Assoc. Physicians,* 99, 103, 1986.

41. **Kuno, T., Andresen, J. W., Kamisaki, Y., Waldman, S. A., Chang, L. Y., Saheki, S., Leitman, D. C., Nakane, M., and Murad, F.,** Co-purification of an atrial natriuretic factor receptor and particulate guanylate cyclase from rat lung, *J. Biol. Chem.,* 261, 5817, 1986.

42. **Carrier, F., Thibault, G., Schiffrin, E. L., Garcia, R., Gutkowska, J., Cantin, M., and Genest, J.,** Partial characterization and solubilization of receptors for atrial natriuretic factor in rat glomeruli, *Biochem. Biophys. Res. Commun.,* 132, 666, 1985.

43. **Meloche, S., Ong, H., Cantin, M., and De Lean, A.,** Molecular characterization of solubilized atrial natriuretic factor receptor from bovine adrenal zona glomerulosa, *Mol. Pharmacol.,* 30, 537, 1986.

44. **Takayangi, R., Inagami, T., Snajdar, R. M., Imada, T., Tamura, M., and Misono, K. S.,** Two distinct forms of receptors for atrial natriuretic factor in bovine adrenocortical cells: purification, ligand binding, and peptide mapping, *J. Biol. Chem.,* 262, 12104, 1987.

45. **Schenk, D. B., Phelps, M. N., Porter, J. G., Fuller, F., Cordell, B., and Lewicki, J. A.,** Purification and subunit composition of atrial natriuretic peptide receptor, *Proc. Natl. Acad. Sci. U.S.A.,* 84, 1521, 1987.

46. **Shimonaka, M., Saheki, T., Hagiwara, H., Ishido, M., Nogi, A., Fujita, T., Wakita, K., Inada, Y., Kondo, J., and Hirose, S.,** Purification of atrial natriuretic peptide receptor from bovine lung: evidence for a disulfide-linked structure, *J. Biol. Chem.,* 262, 5510, 1987.

47. **Fuller, F., Porter, J. G., Arfsten, A., Miller, J., Schilling, J., Scarborough, R. M., Lewicki, J. A., and Schenk, D. B.,** Atrial natriuretic peptide C-receptor complete sequence and functional expression of cDNA clones, *J. Biol. Chem.,* 263, 9395, 1988.

48. **Uchida, K., Shimonaka, M., Saheki, T., Ito, T., and Hirose, S.,** Identification of the primary translational product of the atrial natriuretic peptide receptor mRNA in a cell-free system using anti-receptor antiserum, *J. Biol. Chem.,* 262, 12401, 1987.

49. **Leitman, D. C. and Murad, F.,** Comparison of binding and cyclic GMP accumulation by atrial natriuretic peptides in endothelial cells, *Biochim. Biophys. Acta,* 885, 74, 1986.

50. **Leitman, D. C., Waldman, S. A., Rapoport, R. M., and Murad, F.,** Specific atrial natriuretic factor receptors mediate increased cyclic GMP accumulation in cultured bovine aortic endothelial and smooth muscle cells, *Trans. Am. Assoc. Physicians,* 98, 243, 1985.

51. **Scarborough, R. M., Schenk, D. B., McEnroe, G. A., Arfsten, A., Kang, L.-L., Schwartz, K., and Lewicki, J. A.**, Truncated atrial natriuretic peptide analogs: comparison between receptor binding and stimulation of cyclic GMP accumulation in cultured vascular smooth muscle cells, *J. Biol. Chem.*, 261, 12960, 1986.

52. **Hamet, P., Tremblay, J., Pang, S. C., Garcia, R., Thibault, G., Gutkowska, J., Cantin, M., and Genest, J.**, Effect of native and synthetic atrial natriuretic factor on cyclic GMP, *Biochem. Biophys. Res. Commun.*, 123, 515, 1984.

53. **Waldman, S. A., Rapoport, R. M., and Murad, F.**, Atrial natriuretic factor selectively activates particulate guanylate cyclase and elevates cyclic GMP in rat tissues, *J. Biol. Chem.*, 259, 14332, 1984.

54. **Waldman, S. A., Rapoport, R. M., Fiscus, R. R., and Murad, F.**, Effects of atriopeptin on particulate guanylate cyclase from rat adrenal, *Biochim. Biophys. Acta*, 845, 298, 1985.

55. **Hamet, P., Tremblay, J., Pang, S. C., Skuherska, R., Schiffrin, E., Garcia, R., Cantin, M., Genest, J., Palmour, R., Ervin, F. R., Martin, S., and Goldwater, R.**, Cyclic GMP as mediator and biological marker of atrial natriuretic factor, *J. Hypertens.*, 4, S49, 1986.

56. **Tremblay, J., Gerzer, R., Vinay, P., Pang, S. C., Beliveau, R., and Hamet, P.**, The increase of cGMP by atrial natriuretic factor correlates with distribution of particulate guanylate cyclase, *FEBS Lett.*, 181, 17, 1985.

57. **Leitman, D. C., Agonst, V. A., Catalano, R. M., Schroder, H., Waldman, S. A., Bennett, B. M., Tuan, J. J., and Murad, F.**, Atrial natriuretic peptide, oxytocin and vasopressin increase cyclic GMP in LLC-PK$_1$ kidney epithelial cells, *Endocrinology*, 122, 1478, 1988.

58. **De Lean, A.**, Amiloride potentiates atrial natriuretic factor inhibitory action by increasing receptor binding in bovine adrenal glomerulosa, *Life Sci.*, 39, 1109, 1986.

59. **Hirata, Y., Tomita, M., Takada, S., and Yoshimi, H.**, Vascular receptor binding activities and cyclic GMP responses by synthetic human and rat atrial natriuretic peptides (ANP) and receptor down-regulation by ANP, *Biochem. Biophys. Res. Commun.*, 128, 538, 1985.

60. **Napier, M. A., Arcuri, K. E., and Vandlen, R. L.**, Binding and internalization of atrial natriuretic factor by high-affinity receptors in A10 smooth muscle cells, *Arch. Biochem. Biophys.*, 248, 516, 1986.

61. **Neuser, D. and Bellermann, P.**, Receptor binding, cGMP stimulation and receptor desensitization by atrial natriuretic peptides in cultured A10 vascular smooth muscle cells, *FEBS Lett.*, 209, 347, 1986.

62. **Roubert, P., Lonchampt, M. O., Chabrier, P. E., Plas, P., Goulin, J., and Braquet, P.**, Down-regulation of atrial natriuretic factor receptors and correlation with cGMP stimulation in rat cultured vascular smooth muscle cells, *Biochem. Biophys. Res. Commun.*, 148, 61, 1987.

63. **Hirata, Y., Takata, S., Takagi, Y., Matsubara, H., and Omae, T.**, Regulation of atrial natriuretic peptide receptors in cultured vascular smooth muscle cells of rat, *Biochem. Biophys. Res. Commun.*, 138, 405, 1986.

64. **Hirata, Y., Hirose, S., Takata, S., Takagi, Y., and Matsubara, H.**, Down-regulation of atrial natriuretic peptide and cyclic GMP response in cultured rat vascular smooth muscle cells, *Eur. J. Pharmacol.*, 135, 439, 1987.

65. **Ballermann, B. J., Hoover, R. L., Karnovsky, M. J., and Brenner, B. M.**, Physiological regulation of atrial natriuretic peptide receptors in rat renal glomeruli, *J. Clin. Invest.*, 76, 2049, 1985.

66. **Schiffrin, E. L., St.-Louis, J., Garcia, R., Thibault, G., Cantin, M., and Genest, J.**, Vascular and adrenal binding sites for atrial natriuretic factor: effects of sodium and hypertension, *Hypertension*, 8 (Suppl. 1), 141, 1986.

67. **Lynch, D. R., Braas, K. M., and Snyder, S. H.**, Atrial natriuretic factor receptors in rat kidney, adrenal gland and brain: autoradiographic localization and fluid balance dependent changes, *Proc. Natl. Acad. Sci. U.S.A.*, 83, 3357, 1986.

68. **Saavedra, J. M., Israel, A., and Kurihara, M.**, Increased atrial natriuretic peptide binding sites in rat subfornical organ after water deprivation, *Endocrinology*, 120, 426, 1987.

69. **Swithers, S. E., Stewart, R. E., and McCarty, R.**, Binding sites for atrial natriuretic factor (ANF) in kidneys and adrenal glands of spontaneous hypertensive (SHR) rats, *Life Sci.*, 40, 1673, 1987.

70. **Gutkind, J. S., Kurihara, M., Castren, E., and Saavedra, J. M.**, Atrial natriuretic peptide receptors in sympathetic ganglia: biochemical response and alterations in genetically hypertensive rats, *Biochem. Biophys. Res. Commun.*, 149, 65, 1987.

71. **Saito, H., Inui, K., Matsukawa, Y., Okano, T., Maegawa, H., Nakao, K., Morii, N., Imura, H., Makino, S., and Hori, R.**, Specific binding of atrial natriuretic polypeptide to renal basolateral membranes in spontaneously hypertensive rats (SHR) and stroke-prone SHR, *Biochem. Biophys. Res. Commun.*, 137, 1079, 1986.

72. **Kurihara, M., Castren, E., Gutkind, J. S., and Saavedra, J. M.**, Lower number of atrial natriuretic peptide receptors in thymocytes and spleen cells of spontaneously hypertensive rats, *Biochem. Biophys. Res. Commun.*, 149, 1132, 1987.

73. **Saavedra, J. M., Israel, A., Kurihara, M., and Fuchs, E.**, Decreased number and affinity of rat atrial natriuretic peptide (6-33) binding sites in the subfornical organ of spontaneously hypertensive rats, *Circ. Res.*, 58, 389, 1986.

74. **Schiffrin, E. L. and St.-Louis, J.**, Decreased density of vascular receptors for atrial natriuretic peptide in DOCA-salt hypertensive rats, *Hypertension*, 9, 504, 1987.

75. **Gauquelin, G., Schiffrin, E. L., Cantin, M., and Garcia, R.**, Specific binding of atrial natriuretic factor to renal glomeruli in DOCA- and DOCA-salt-treated rats correlation with atrial and plasma levels, *Biochem. Biophys. Res. Commun.*, 145, 522, 1987.

76. **Takayanagi, R., Grammer, R. T., and Inagami, T.**, Regional increase of cyclic GMP by atrial natriuretic factor in rat brain: markedly elevated response in spontaneously hypertensive rats, *Life Sci.*, 39, 573, 1986.

77. **Huang, C.-L., Ives, H. E., and Cogan, M. G.**, *In vivo* evidence that cGMP is the second messenger for atrial natriuretic factor, *Proc. Natl. Acad. Sci. U.S.A.*, 83, 8015, 1986.

78. **Stasch, J.-P., Hirth, C., Kazda, S., and Wohlfeil, S.**, The elevation of cyclic GMP as a response to acute hypervolemia is blocked by a monoclonal antibody directed against atrial natriuretic peptides, *Eur. J. Pharmacol.*, 129, 165, 1986.

79. **Sonnenberg, H., Honrath, U., Chong, C. K., and Wilson, D. R.**, Atrial natriuretic factor inhibits sodium transport in medullary collecting duct, *Am. J. Physiol.*, 250, F963, 1986.

80. **Cantiello, H. F. and Ausiello, D. A.**, Atrial natriuretic factor and cGMP inhibit amiloride-sensitive Na^+ transport in the cultured renal epithelial cell line, LLC-PK$_1$, *Biochem. Biophys. Res. Commun.*, 134, 852, 1986.

81. **Mohrmann, M., Cantiello, H. F., Ausiello, D. A.**, Inhibition of epithelial Na^+ transport by atriopeptin, protein kinase c, and pertussis toxin, *Am. J. Physiol.*, 253, F372, 1987.

82. **Zeidel, M. L., Silva, P., Brenner, B. M., and Seifter, J. L.**, cGMP mediates effects of atrial peptides on medullary collecting duct cells, *Am. J. Physiol.*, 252, F559, 1987.

83. **Kurtz, A., Bruna, R. D., Pfeilschifter, J., Taugner, R., and Bauer, C.**, Atrial natriuretic peptide inhibits renin release from juxtaglomerlular cells by a cGMP-mediated process, *Proc. Natl. Acad. Sci. U.S.A.*, 83, 4769, 1986.

84. **Matsuoka, H., Ishii, M., Hirata, Y., Atarashi, K., Sugimoto, T., Kangawa, K., and Matsuo, H.**, Evidence for lack of a role for cGMP in effect of -hANP on aldosterone inhibition, *Am. J. Physiol.*, 252, E643, 1987.

85. **Maack, T., Suzuki, M., Almeida, F. A., Nussenzvieg, D., Scarborough, R. M., McEnroe, G. A., and Lewicki, J. A.**, Physiological role of silent receptors of atrial natriuretic factor, *Science*, 238, 675, 1987.

86. **Chabrier, P. E., Roubert, P., and Braquet, P.**, Specific binding of atrial natriuretic factor in brain microvessels, *Proc. Natl. Acad. Sci. U.S.A.*, 84, 2078, 1987.

87. **Shiffrin, E. L., Chartier, L., Thibault, G., St.-Louis, J., Cantin, M., and Genest, J.**, Vascular and adrenal receptors for atrial natriuretic factor in rat, *Circ. Res.*, 52, 801, 1985.

88. **Ishikawa, Y., Unemura, S., Yasuda, G., Uchino, K., Shindou, T., Minanmizawa, K., Toya, Y., and Kaneko, Y.**, Identification of an atrial natriuretic peptide specific receptor in human kidney, *Biochem. Biophys. Res. Commun.*, 147, 135, 1987.

89. **Shionoiri, H., Hirawa, N., Takasakai, I., Ishikawa, Y., Minamissawa, K., Miyajima, E., Kinoshita, Y., Shimoyama, K., Shimonaka, M., Ishido, M., and Hirose, S.**, Presence of functional receptors for atrial natriuretic peptide in human pheochromocytoma, *Biochem. Biophys. Res. Commun.*, 148, 286, 1987.

90. **Hirata, Y., Tomita, M., Yoshimi, H., Ikeda, M.**, Specific receptors for atrial natriuretic factor (ANF) in cultured vascular smooth muscle cells of rat aorta, *Biochem. Biophys. Res. Commun.*, 125, 562, 1984.

91. **Schenk, D. B., Johnson, L. K., Schwartz, K., Sista, H., Scarborough, R. M., and Lewicki, J. A.**, Distinct atrial natriuretic factor receptor sites on cultured bovine aortic smooth muscle and endothelial cells, *Biochem. Biophys. Res. Commun.*, 127, 433, 1985.

92. **Schenk, D. B., Phelps, M. N., Porter, J. G., Scarborough, R. M., McEnroe, G. A., and Lewicki, J. A.**, Identification of the receptor for atrial natriuretic factor on cultured vascular cells, *J. Biol. Chem.*, 260, 14887, 1985.

Chapter 8

ANP AND SECOND MESSENGER SYSTEMS

Pavel Hamet and Johanne Tremblay

TABLE OF CONTENTS

I. SECOND MESSENGER SYSTEMS

The concept of the second messenger system, originally proposed by Sutherland and colleagues,[1] has mostly been confirmed and enlarged, and almost all of its biochemical components are now well determined. The original description focused on hormone-receptor interactions, information transmission to membrane-bound adenylate cyclase, and cyclic AMP (cAMP) generation as the second messenger. It was also recognized earlier that cAMP levels are not only regulated by its synthesis by adenylate cyclase,[2] but also by its catabolism via phosphodiesterase[3] and by extracellular egression.[4] The effector arm of this system is represented by cAMP-dependent protein kinase, to which cAMP is bound, leading to dissociation of the catalytic subunit which, in turn, is responsible for the phosphorylation of specific substrates, resulting in modification of cellular activity.[5]

One of the potent characteristics of this second messenger system of hormonal information transmission is the amplification of the hormonal response.[6] This amplification may be of several orders of magnitude, i.e., 1 mol of hormone leading to several hundred moles of phosphorylation-regulated product.[2] Although cAMP-related studies have generated a large amount of knowledge on the transmission of hormonal information, electrical stimulation, and cell growth, it was apparent almost from the outset that this cyclic nucleotide cannot explain the transmission of information of many types of stimulants,[7] particularly those related to calcium signals, whose effects are either concurrent or opposed to those of cAMP.[8]

Berridge[9] proposed a useful concept of monodirectional and bidirectional systems. In monodirectional systems, such as secretion, signals to calcium and cAMP either run parallel or potentiate each other. In bidirectional systems such as vascular contraction-relaxation and platelet aggregation-inhibition of aggregation, signals related to calcium and cAMP appear to move in opposite directions. However, understanding of the calcium-regulated pathways became more complete only recently after the discovery of its effector arm, protein kinase C by Nishizuka and colleagues[10-12] and the identification of its second messengers, diacylglycerol and inositol trisphosphate.[13,14] Although the enzymatic cascade in response to hormonal stimulation leading to generation of the second messengers, i.e., the turnover of phosphoinositides, has been known for a long time,[15] its involvement in the cellular transmission of hormonal information has been recognized only in the last few years.[11] At present, the modification of free cytosolic calcium levels and calcium-dependent phosphorylation indeed appears to be a major cellular regulatory system. Nishizuka et al.[12,16] proposed a concept which confines the calcium-related events (with diacylglycerol and inositol trisphosphates as second messengers) to positive pathways, i.e., leading to bidirectional systems to contraction, while the cAMP-related system represents negative pathways, i.e., resulting in vasodilation.

Cyclic GMP (cGMP) is another cyclic nucleotide which participates in the regulation of negative pathways. This nucleotide was first discovered as an organic high-energy phosphate compound in urine.[17] Its role remained unclarified for a long time.[18,19] cGMP generation in several organs has been known to require the presence of extracellular calcium[20] and, misleadingly, cGMP increases were found to occur simultaneously to stimulation of the positive pathways, as in epinephrine-induced platelet aggregation. It was only recognized later that cGMP generation concomitant with stimulation of the positive pathways actually serves as a negative feedback.[21-26] Indeed, during stimulation of the positive pathway, arachidonic acid is released in a calcium-dependent manner by phospholipase-C activation and culminates in the direct stimulation of one of the cGMP-generating enzymes, soluble guanylate cyclase.[27] However, when this cGMP increase is prevented (by omitting extracellular calcium), the positive response is even potentiated.[28] It is now well recognized that cGMP levels can be stimulated directly, without receptor interaction, by nitrovasodilators, including sodium nitroprusside (SNP) and nitroglycerin (NG) or endothelium-derived relaxing factor (EDRF).[23,29-31] These agents directly stimulate soluble guanylate cyclase and increase cGMP, leading to the expression of negative pathway actions such as vasodilation and inhibition of aggregation. In addition, cGMP can be generated by particulate guanylate cyclase, a membrane-bound glycoprotein. Identification of endogenous stimulants was made possible by the discovery of atrial natriuretic peptide (ANP).[32-35]

II. EFFECTS OF ANP ON CYCLIC NUCLEOTIDES IN EXTRACELLULAR FLUID, TISSUES, AND CULTURED CELLS

Increases of cGMP in urine, plasma, and kidney slices were initially observed in acidic extracts of atria, whereas ventricular extracts were without any effect. cAMP did not change during stimulation, although a late decrease could be discerned in the period following diuresis.[33,34] These initial findings[34] were confirmed with the synthetic peptide ANP(8-33) when it became available.[36] Increases of cGMP levels were prevented by the addition of anti-ANP antisera. It was also noted that the capacity of atrial extracts to augment cGMP rose throughout the process of ANP purification parallel to the biological activity of ANP, even when two widely different bioassay systems were used, i.e., to study diuresis in rats as an expression of the biological effects of ANP and cGMP increases in cultured cells for the determination of cGMP generation. These observations led to the proposal that cGMP may serve as a second messenger system for the expression of the actions of ANP. This initial finding was rapidly confirmed[35,37] and, in addition, it was demonstrated that ANP generates cGMP via its interaction with particulate guanylate cyclase, as described in detail in Chapter 7 of this book. Increases of plasma and urinary cGMP levels have since been reported in dogs,[38] monkeys,[39] and humans.[40] ANP-induced cGMP elevations are observed not only in tissues, but also in cultured cells such as vascular smooth muscle[41,42] and endothelial cells,[43] which became an invaluable tool in the exploration of the biological effects of ANP.

Although the inhibitory influence of ANP on adenylate cyclase activity has been well demonstrated in many tissues,[44-46] a significant modulation of cAMP levels is usually not evident or appears to occur beyond the time of expression of the ANP function.[34,47] At present, the specific implication of adenylate cyclase inhibition in the expression of the actions of ANP remains unresolved. It has also been suggested that ANP has an effect on potassium current,[48] on Na^+, K^+, and Cl^- co-transport,[49] and on phosphoinositol turnover,[50] as well as on calcium movement.[51,52] On the other hand, it has been shown that ANP makes no impact on basal cytosolic calcium levels in vascular smooth muscle cells,[53,54] using the fluorescent dye Quin-2, while opposite results on the effect of ANP on angiotensin II-induced increases of cytosolic calcium[53,54] have also been recorded. It has not been directly assessed whether these events are primary or secondary to modulation of cGMP levels.

With the description of the second messenger concepts outlined above, it is apparent that significant increases of cGMP could lead to the subsequent modification of ionic currents, calcium levels, and its movements, mainly by the known opposing effects of cGMP on the calcium-regulated positive pathways.[55-58]

III. DISTRIBUTION OF PARTICULATE GUANYLATE CYCLASE AND BIOLOGICAL EFFECTS OF ANP

The initial observation of co-distribution of particulate guanylate cyclase and increases of cGMP levels was made in isolated kidney fractions.[41] In enzymatically and mechanically separated fractions, including glomeruli, proximal and distal tubules, and collecting ducts, it is evident that the main target for ANP in the kidney is the glomeruli. ANP increases cGMP up to 50-fold in this organelle,[41] whereas only twofold elevations have been noted in the distal part of the tubule and in the medullary collecting ducts. No response to ANP has been demonstrated in the proximal tubule. These increases of cGMP correspond to the distribution of particulate guanylate cyclase, with the glomeruli being the richest.[41,59] Soluble guanylate cyclase is much less present in the glomeruli, leading accordingly to higher increases of cGMP when stimulated by ANP than by SNP, an agonist of soluble guanylate cyclase. The distribution of particulate guanylate cyclase corresponds to the distribution of ANP receptors.[60,61] The presence of particulate guanylate cyclase in the glomeruli was further explored by Ardaillou et al.,[62,63] who demonstrated that the enzyme is specifically located in endothelial cells, as opposed to the receptors for angiotensin-II, which are located predominantly on mesangial cells.

As with glomeruli, endothelial cells cultured from bovine aorta also mainly express particulate guanylate cyclase, leading to pronounced increases of cGMP by ANP, while the addition of SNP has no effect in this tissue with very little soluble guanylate cyclase.[39,43,64] Similarly, in zona glomerulosa of the adrenal cortex, particulate guanylate cyclase is also highly expressed[65,66] and could be involved in the ANP-induced inhibition of aldosterone secretion.[67-69] In vascular smooth muscle cells, soluble and particulate guanylate cyclases are just about equally expressed,[41] responding with increases of cGMP to both ANP, a particulate guanylate cyclase stimulant, and SNP, a soluble guanylate cyclase agonist. Both agents are known vasodilators.[70]

The opposite is observed in platelets. The role of cGMP in this cellular element is established in the expression of negative pathways, i.e., inhibition of aggregation by such agents as SNP.[71,72] cGMP, which serves as a negative feedback during positive pathway stimulation, has already been discussed. Platelets have large amounts of soluble guanylate cyclase,[73] but they are very poor in particulate enzyme content. ANP does not appear to significantly modulate any platelet function. It exerts no direct effect on platelet aggregation, nor is it able to potentiate or modulate the aggregation induced by thrombin or ADP or the inhibition evoked by prostaglandins.[39] This lack of ANP action is of interest since platelets apparently do possess receptors for ANP[74] and adenylate cyclase in this cellular element can also be inhibited by ANP.[149] The presence of this type of receptor can, therefore, be dissociated from the increases of cGMP and from any apparent function of platelets. In other tissues, such as the intestine, particulate guanylate cyclase is certainly present in the brush border.[75] It is not necessarily responsive to ANP,[150] but is sensitive to specific exogenous agents such as the heat stable toxin of *Escherichia coli*.[76] Although some modification of intestinal fluid transport has been observed,[77] it is not yet resolved whether these events are secondary to a direct action of ANP on the intestinal mucosa as a consequence of an indirect vascular effect.

In most of the tissues described, the effects of ANP are clearly hormonal, interacting with its receptors and followed by second messenger stimulation, i.e., cGMP generation. It is, however, conceivable that in some tissues, such as in the autonomic nervous system, particulate guanylate cyclase stimulation by ANP may be of a paracrine or autocrine, rather than an endocrine, character.[78] In the superior cervical ganglia, ANP appears to be localized and perhaps generated in particulate guanylate cyclase-rich tissue which is responsive to ANP.[78] The role of this potential paracrine and autocrine function of ANP is under intensive investigation.

IV. CYCLIC GMP AS A MARKER OF THE PHARMACOLOGICAL ACTION OF ANP

Pharmacological doses of ANP injected in rats and humans lead to increases of cGMP in plasma and urine[34,40] and to the expression of the biologic functions of ANP, namely, diuresis, natriuresis, and decreased blood pressure.[79] To fulfill the criteria of a second messenger, cGMP generation ought to appear prior to the onset of biological events related to hormonal action.[2] This criterion is certainly fulfilled in the case of stimulation of cGMP increases by ANP since low doses of ANP from 10 to 50 μg, injected in human subjects, produce cGMP increments in the absence of significant diuresis.[79]

Additional characteristics of cGMP increases have been observed with higher doses of ANP, which augment cGMP in plasma and urine, remaining elevated beyond the heightened plasma levels of ANP.[40,79] Thus, plasma and urinary cGMP rise for up to several hours beyond the time that ANP reaches the basal level. It is conceivable that this prolonged increase of cGMP has a biological consequence in the prolonged stimulation of diuresis and natriuresis, as observed in man. It has been suggested that the prolonged biological effects of ANP and cGMP generation are due to the prolonged stimulation of particulate guanylate cyclase.[80,81] Indeed, when cultured cells are exposed to ANP for only 2 min, followed by thorough washes to reduce ANP to undetectable levels, as measured by radioimmunoassay or the remaining radioactivity of spiked ANP-I[125], the production of cGMP continues for the same length of time and attains the same degree of elevation[39] as when ANP is continuously present. This prolonged stimulation of cGMP production corresponds to a persistent increase of particulate guanylate cyclase activity, which can be reproduced *in vitro* in particulate preparations exposed to ANP. The result is quite different from the observations with adenylate cyclase, where simple dilution or washing of the agonist returns the activity to its basal state. It appears that particulate guanylate cyclase can be specifically turned on by interaction with ANP.[80]

This prolonged production of cGMP after acute exposure to ANP contrasts with findings of chronic stimulation by low doses of ANP *in vivo*. Infusions of low doses of ANP in the rat[82] and monkey[83] lead to significant biological effects, including a decrease of blood pressure which, in normotensive monkeys, actually continues beyond the time of ANP infusion for another 48 h.[83] At the end of the ANP infusion, the plasma levels of cGMP are even significantly reduced. The kinetics of the cGMP turnover in these chronically stimulated situations is not understood at the present time. It should be remembered that the catabolism of cyclic nucleotides by phosphodiesterases is a regulated event,[84] which can adapt to new steady-state situations of chronically increased production of cyclic nucleotides.[84]

Various ANP analogs have been used to explore the relationship between structural requirements for the action of ANP and its capacity to generate cGMP.[85,86] Generally speaking, the analogs able to increase cGMP synthesis do so with an order of potency similar to that by which they can increase biological actions such as vasodilation, natriuresis, and diuresis. A series of analogs which bind to high-affinity ANP receptors are devoid of the capacity to stimulate cGMP synthesis. These analogs, studied by Maack et al.,[87] bind specifically to the high-affinity C-receptor not linked to particulate guanylate cyclase. However, when infused *in vivo*, they are able to induce biological actions, again in relationship to cGMP increases, perhaps due to the decreased clearance of endogenous ANP.

Met-O[110]-ANP, the oxidized analog of human ANP, was helpful in dissociating the diuretic and natriuretic actions of ANP. In doses which produce significant diuresis in the rat, this analog does not induce natriuresis or increase plasma or urinary cGMP.[88] *In vitro*, it is able to enhance cGMP synthesis in vascular smooth muscle cells, with much less effect on glomeruli and almost no impact in the distal part of the tubule. These studies suggest a heterogeneity of ANP receptors, as well as the involvement of at least two distinct sites in the kidney in the expression of the natriuretic and diuretic activities of ANP.[88] It is interesting to consider the reason why the diuretic activity of this analog is not accompanied by an elevation of urinary cGMP levels. Although this may be secondary to the fact that ANP may use another second messenger system for the expression of anti-ADH-like activity, it is also conceivable that, while some events related to ANP actions lead to increases of cGMP in urine, others may be related only to intracellular elevations. This type of situation is known for cAMP. Specifically, increases of cAMP induced by parathyroid hormone (PTH) in the proximal tubule augment urinary cAMP, which serves as a marker of the action of PTH on the tubule.[59] On the other hand, another agonist, ADH, which is able to stimulate adenylate cyclase in the distal part of the tubule,[89] does not lead to modifications of extracellular cAMP reflected in urine. It is possible that the egression of cyclic nucleotides in the distal tubule is different from that in glomeruli or proximal tubules.

With Mpr[105]-ANP,[86] another analog shortened at the N terminal and modified at position 105, it was possible to demonstrate increases of cGMP, as well as of diuresis superior to those elicited by the parent compound.[90] This analog apparently has a lower total binding affinity than its parent. Combination experiments with Met-O[110]-ANP, Mpr[105]-ANP, and the parent compound have demonstrated an antagonism, as well as potentiation, of the effects of these analogs on ANP-induced cGMP generation.[90] These studies are compatible with the presence of two types of ANP receptors with possible interactions between them. It is conceivable that the occupancy of high-affinity receptors unrelated to particulate guanylate cyclase leads to the modification of guanylate cyclase activity itself.[90]

To fully ascertain the utility of cGMP as a marker of the action of ANP, the cellular origin of plasma cGMP needs to be determined. As already mentioned, both endothelial and vascular smooth muscle cells respond to ANP by increases of cGMP levels. Endothelial responsiveness is actually higher than that of smooth muscle cells which, with their equal distribution of particulate and soluble guanylate cyclase, also respond to SNP. However, when the two agents are infused into human subjects at doses producing similar vasodilation, only ANP raises the plasma levels of cGMP, while no increase of this nucleotide is observed with SNP.[91] This observation underlines the importance of the site of origin of cGMP. Although both agonists can augment cGMP in smooth muscle cells, they are not responsible for cGMP increases in plasma. cGMP apparently cannot cross through another cellular layer without being destroyed by phosphodiesterases. Therefore, plasma cGMP increases seem to be a reflection of the interaction of ANP with endothelial cells, even though they may correlate with the biological activities of ANP elsewhere.

V. CYCLIC GMP AND PHYSIOLOGICAL EFFECTS OF ANP

If cGMP is a faithful marker of the biological effects of ANP, endogenous, physiologically-stimulated ANP should lead to cGMP increases parallel to its biological functions. Elevated levels of endogenous circulating ANP have been reported in the literature and some of them will be briefly considered here.

Endogenous ANP can be enhanced by injections of pharmacological doses of clonidine.[92] This leads to an increase of ANP, diuresis, and natriuresis, paralleled by cGMP elevations.[92] When ANP antibodies are preinjected prior to the clonidine injection, the cGMP increases are progressively decreased, as is the diuretic and natriuretic effect of ANP. These results suggest that endogenously-released ANP leads to cGMP increases, as well as to the diuretic and natriuretic response.[92]

Similar conclusions are reached when endogenous ANP is released by postural change. Assumption of the recumbent position causes increases of plasma ANP.[93-96] Recumbency is also accompanied by natriuresis and diuresis,[97,98] which could be explained, at least in part, by ANP. Upon detailed analysis of these physiological maneuvers by separating the posture from upright to sitting and from sitting to standing, the change from standing to sitting leads to natriuresis and diuresis, which is clearly ANP-independent since ANP or plasma or urinary cGMP levels do not change.[99] In this posture, the decrease of plasma renin activity and aldosterone is perhaps responsible for the diuretic and natriuretic response. However, the change from sitting to recumbency can be clearly linked to the ANP increases.[99]

Physical exercise is a similar physiologic maneuver. With this type of stimulant, ANP concentrations increase in the plasma of human subjects.[100,101] However, the biological effects of exercise are variable: an enhanced glomerular filtration rate is observed in some, but is absent in other, subjects. A similar variable is the antinatriuretic and antidiuretic effect of exercise. However, when human subjects are separated according to their ANP response to exercise, there is a significant increase of plasma and urinary cGMP and a rise in the glomerular filtration rate, as well as lesser antidiuresis and antinatriuresis in those with a higher ANP response. The most significant antinatriuresis and antidiuresis are observed in subjects lacking the ANP-cGMP response.[102]

All these stimulants which lead to increases of ANP appear to be reflected in heightened plasma and urinary cGMP levels, as well as in modified natriuretic and diuretic functions. Overall, these studies support the notion that ANP is physiologically involved in the regulation of water and salt homeostasis and that this function is related to the generation of cGMP.

VI. EGRESSION OF CYCLIC GMP

Throughout this chapter, we have discussed intracellular and extracellular cGMP levels. It has to be realized that cGMP is an intracellular messenger for ANP and that its extracellular appearance, although reflecting the degree of intracellular increase, is not directly related to any known function of the cyclic nucleotide. The effect of extracellular cyclic nucleotides has been demonstrated only in slime molds.[103] The mechanisms of egression of cyclic nucleotides have been studied and appear to be a regulated, energy-dependent process.[4] cGMP egression possesses several characteristics which are clearly distinct from those of cAMP. First, upon stimulation by ANP in cultured cells, cGMP continues to accumulate in the extracellular milieu for up to 24 h[39] after a brief increase of intracellular levels. As a result, the degree of accumulation of extracellular cGMP exceeds that of the intracellular elevation manyfold. This is quite distinct from cAMP increases in the same cells, where both intracellular and extracellular nucleotide levels peak at the same time, followed by a continuous decline.[104] cGMP levels in different tissues and cells are generally one to two orders of magnitude lower than those of cAMP. It is, therefore, somewhat surprising that the plasma levels of cGMP are of the same order of magnitude as cAMP. Continuous egression of this nucleotide is perhaps one of the relevant contributors of the relatively high plasma levels.

cGMP egression can be inhibited by lower temperatures and by organic acid transport inhibitors, such as probenecid, similar to that of cAMP.[4] It is impossible to saturate this egression process with cGMP, but huge increases of intracellular cAMP (which are several orders of magnitude higher than those of cGMP) obtained with the adenylate cyclase agonist, forskolin, can effectively prevent cGMP egression, resulting in a rise of cGMP intracellular levels.[104] This observation leads to the conclusion that cAMP and cGMP at least partially share the same egression system. It is not known at present whether the cyclic nucleotides have any function during their egression through the cellular membrane. The only known involvement of cGMP in membrane function is in the retinal transmission of the light signal. ANP causes greater cGMP egression than SNP.[104] This observation suggests the possibility that intracellular cGMP, when induced by SNP, may be more accessible to degradation by intracellular phosphodiesterases, while cGMP, when synthetized by particulate guanylate cyclase, may remain perimembranous and, thus, more easily egressed. Whether this mechanism contributes to some of the biological differences between the ANP and SNP effects is not known at the present time.

VII. CYCLIC GMP IN PATHOLOGICAL STATES IMPLICATING ANP

Abnormalities of ANP secretion, its plasma levels, or its metabolism have been reported in several disease states, including heart failure, renal failure, edema formation, cirrhosis, hypertension, and diabetes. Since most of the information accumulated is on heart failure, hypertension, and renal failure, these three pathological states and their relation to the cGMP system will be discussed in more detail.

A. RENAL FAILURE

Studies on ANP have received particular attention in relation to renal failure since this organ is well recognized as a target for ANP. Plasma ANP levels are significantly elevated in renal failure[105-111] and are decreased by dialysis.[93,112] These changes may be related to water and salt metabolism, but may also be secondary to a decreased capacity of the renal parenchyma to remove peptides, as in the case of increased levels of insulin, TSH, LH, FSH, and other peptides, which are well known to be augmented in renal failure.[113,114] Actually, akin to the increases of plasma ANP levels, there is an elevation of plasma cGMP in this condition, which again is significantly related to the decreased metabolic clearance of cGMP, as is the case in the reduced metabolic elimination of cAMP in renal insufficiency.[115]

Specific increases of plasma ANP also occur in hypertension involving the kidney, i.e., renovascular hypertension.[116] The pathophysiology of the elevated ANP levels in this situation is not fully understood but, again, the handling of cyclic nucleotides (at least of cAMP) has been demonstrated to be abnormal.[117]

B. HEART FAILURE

Increased ANP levels in the circulation have been noted in experimental and in human heart failure,[118-123] in induced[124] or spontaneous tachycardia,[125] and in other pathophysiological conditions of deficient heart function. A situation, therefore, exists in which there is an excess of a circulating diuretic and natriuretic hormone in a pathology involving water and sodium retention. The observation cannot be attributed to any down-regulation of receptors in a general sense since plasma cGMP levels are also increased.[118] It could, therefore, at least be hypothesized that there is a failure in the expression of the effector system, i.e., a post-cGMP defect.

C. HYPERTENSION

This area has received the greatest overall attention in ANP-related research. Although discrepancies persist about the degree of plasma ANP levels being either normal[116,126-129] or abnormal,[130-135] it appears that ANP is most effective in hypertension.[136,137] Several reports also point to a hyperresponsiveness of the cGMP effector system, with an increased accumulation of cGMP in plasma and urine in both spontaneously hypertensive rats[136] and human subjects.[138] An excessive responsiveness of cGMP generation has been observed, even *in vitro*, in passaged cells derived from spontaneously hypertensive rats.[139,140] It can, therefore, be suggested that there is a hyperreactivity of the vasodilatory, diuretic, and natriuretic systems in hypertension. This notion does not fit the prevailing hypothesis of hypertension being caused by an increase of peripheral vascular resistance. It is, nevertheless, conceivable that one of the pathogenetic events in hypertension is, indeed, an excess of the vasodilatory, natriuretic, and diuretic response occurring early in the development of hypertension and being only opposed by mechanisms retaining salt and water, leading secondarily to enhanced peripheral vascular resistance.

VIII. CELLULAR MECHANISMS OF ACTION OF CYCLIC GMP

In this chapter, we have reviewed the involvement of cGMP in the expression of the actions of ANP. cGMP fulfills several of the criteria required to be considered as a second messenger.[7] It can be generated prior to the expression of ANP function. ANP can stimulate its synthesis in broken cell preparations by a direct action on particulate guanylate cyclase, and cGMP increased by other means, at least in relevant cells such as vascular smooth muscle cells, leads to the expression of similar functions. Caution has to be taken when some of these criteria are applied — e.g., the lack of simulation of ANP function by SNP, which frequently has a different target cell responding to its action and leading, therefore, to effects quite distinct from those of ANP. cGMP analogs should also be used with care since they may affect all cells to which they are added, whereas ANP selectively influences only cells possessing particulate guanylate cyclase.

In addition, lessons learned from the specific cGMP-mediated effect in the retina[141] and from studies on the heart demonstrate that the analogs of cyclic nucleotides have to be carefully evaluated because of their ability to modulate phosphodiesterase, as well as to react to both cAMP- and cGMP-dependent protein kinases.[142] Thus, the lack of both specificity and metabolism of these analogs in their different effector systems needs to be considered before using them for evaluating the actions of ANP.

Generally speaking, the expression of cGMP is related, by analogy, to that of cAMP with the activation of specific cGMP-dependent protein kinases. However, it has yet to be demonstrated that the activation of this enzyme is required for all cGMP functions and is not only related to some specific events requiring phosphorylation of substrates. cGMP-dependent protein kinase has been detected in vascular and other tissues[142] and the influence of its increased activity upon the action of ANP has been described,[143] but the subsequent phosphorylation steps need more thorough study. It has also been suggested that, either directly or indirectly, ANP can modulate phosphodiesterase activity,[34] but whether this modulation can, over either the short or long term, change the expression of ANP function is not known at present.

Finally, as already mentioned, the best-described cGMP effector system is that of light transmission in the retina.[144,145] Photons modify rhodopsin via the intervention of transducin, a specific G-protein of the retina. As a consequence, cGMP hydrolysis by its specific phosphodiesterase is stimulated.[146] The modulation of cGMP levels in the retina is directly responsible for the rate of opening of sodium channels.[145,147] It has been clearly demonstrated by an electrophysiological approach with the patch-clamp technique that cGMP as a molecule, without any intervention of phosphorylation, provokes the opening of the sodium channels, and the hydrolysis of this nucleotide leads to its closure.[148] There is no reason to believe that such a specific effect of cGMP is confined to the retina. Yet, it is not clear at present that cGMP is involved in the regulation of ionic movement, without requiring phosphorylation, in other tissues. A better understanding of the expression of cGMP function is necessary for a more in depth knowledge of the activity of ANP if this nucleotide is, indeed, the principal messenger for this hormone.

ACKNOWLEDGMENTS

The studies described in this review have been supported in part by grants from the Medical Research Council of Canada to the Multidisciplinary Group on Hypertension Research (MA-9299), the Canadian Heart Foundation, and the Fonds de la Recherche en Santé du Québec. The authors thank Regis Tremblay, Bruno Lachance, Carole Long, Suzanne Cossette, and Monique Poirier-Dupuis for their technical help, Louise Chevrefils and Micheline Caron for their secretarial assistance, and Ovid Da Silva for editing this review.

REFERENCES

1. **Sutherland, E. W., Robison, G. A., and Butcher, R. W.,** Some aspects of the biological role of adenosine 3',5'-monophosphate (cyclic AMP), *Circulation,* 37, 279, 1968.
2. **Robison, G. A., Butcher, R. W., and Sutherland, E. W.,** Adenyl cyclase as an adrenergic receptor, *Ann. N.Y. Acad. Sci.,* 139, 703, 1967.
3. **Strada, S. J. and Thompson, W. J.,** in *Advances in Cyclic Nucleotide Protein Phosphorylation Research,* Vol. 16, Strada, S. J. and Thompson, W. J., Eds., Raven Press, New York, 1984.
4. **Brunton, L. L. and Mayer, S. E.,** Extrusion of cyclic AMP from pigeon erythrocytes, *J. Biol. Chem.,* 254, 9714, 1979.
5. **Walsh, D. A., Perkins, J. P., and Krebs, E. G.,** An adenosine 3',5'-monophosphate-dependent protein kinase from rabbit skeletal muscle, *J. Biol. Chem.,* 243, 3763, 1968.
6. **Birnbaumer, L., Pohl, S. L., Krans, M. J., and Rodbell, M.,** The actions of hormones on the adenyl cyclase system, in *Role of Cyclic AMP in Cell Function,* Vol. 3, Greengard, P. and Costa, E., Eds., Raven Press, New York, 1970, 185.
7. **Robison, G. A., Butcher, R. W., and Sutherland, E. W.,** in *Cyclic AMP,* Robison, G. A., Butcher, R. W., and Sutherland, E. W., Eds., Academic Press, New York, 1971.
8. **Rasmussen, H.,** Cellular calcium homeostasis and the calcium messenger system, *Semin. Liver Dis.,* 5, 110, 1985.
9. **Berridge, M. J.,** The interaction of cyclic nucleotides and calcium in the control of cellular activity, in *Advances in Cyclic Nucleotide Research,* Vol. 6, Greengard, P. and Robison, G. A., Eds., Raven Press, New York, 1975, 1.
10. **Nishizuka, Y.,** The role of protein kinase C in cell surface signal transduction and tumor promotion, *Nature (London),* 308, 693, 1984.
11. **Nishizuka, Y. and Takai, Y.,** Calcium and phospholipid turnover in a new receptor function for protein phosphorylation, in *Cold Spring Harbor Conferences on Cell Proliferation,* Vol. 8, Cold Spring Harbor Press, Cold Spring Harbor, New York, 1981, 237.
12. **Nishizuka, Y., Takai, Y., Kishimoto, A., Hashimoto, E., Inoue, M., Yamamoto, M., and Kuroda, Y.,** A role of calcium in the activation of a new protein kinase system, in *Advances in Cyclic Nucleotide Research,* Vol. 9, George, W. J. and Ignarro, L. J., Eds., Raven Press, New York, 1978, 209.
13. **Berridge, M. J. and Irvine, R. F.,** Inositol trisphosphate, a novel second messenger in cellular signal transduction, *Nature (London),* 312, 314, 1984.
14. **Michell, R. H.,** Inositol phospholipid breakdown cell activation and drug action, in *Control and Manipulation of Calcium Movement,* Parratt, J. R., Ed., Raven Press, New York, 1985, 51.
15. **Hokin, L. E. and Hokin, M. R.,** Metabolism of phospholipids in vitro, *Can. J. Biochem. Physiol.,* 34, 349, 1956.
16. **Kikkawa, U., Kaibuchi, K., Castagna, M., Yamanishi, J., Sano, K., Tanaka, Y., Miyake, R., Takai, Y., and Nishizuka, Y.,** Protein phosphorylation and mechanism of action of tumor-promoting phorbol esters, in *Advances in Cyclic Nucleotide Protein Phosphorylation Research,* Vol. 17, Greengard, P., Robison, G. A., Paoletti, R., and Nicosia, S., Eds., Raven Press, New York, 1984, 437.
17. **Price, T. D., Ashman, D. F., and Melicow, M. M.,** Organophosphates of urine, including adenosine 3',5'-monophosphate and guanosine 3',5'-monophosphate, *Biochim. Biophys. Acta,* 138, 452, 1967.
18. **Hardman, J. G., Schultz, G., and Sutherland, E. W.,** Cyclic GMP: vestige or another intracellular messenger?, in *cGMP Cell Growth and the Immune Response,* Braun, W., Lichtenstein, L. M., and Parker, C. W., Eds., Springer-Verlag, New York, 1974, 223.
19. **Goldberg, N. D. and Haddox, M. K.,** Cyclic GMP metabolism and involvement in biological regulation, *Annu. Rev. Biochem.,* 46, 823, 1977.
20. **Schultz, G., Hardman, J. G., Schultz, K., Baird, C. E., and Sutherland, E. W.,** The importance of calcium ions for the regulation of guanosine 3':5'-cyclic monophosphate levels, *Proc. Natl. Acad. Sci. U.S.A.,* 70, 3889, 1973.
21. **Schultz, K. D., Bohme, E., Kreye, V. A. W., and Schultz, G.,** Relaxation of hormonally stimulated smooth muscular tissues by the 8-bromo derivative of cyclic GMP, *Naunyn Schmiedeberg's Arch. Pharmacol.,* 306, 1, 1979.
22. **Schultz, K.-D., Schultz, K., and Schultz, G.,** Sodium nitroprusside and other smooth muscle-relaxants increase cyclic GMP levels in rat ductus deferens, *Nature (London),* 265, 750, 1977.
23. **Murad, F., Rapoport, R. M., and Fiscus, R.,** Role of cyclic-GMP in relaxations of vascular smooth muscle, *J. Cardiovasc. Pharmacol.,* 7 (Suppl. 3), S111, 1985.
24. **Murad, F.,** Cyclic guanosine monophosphate as a mediator of vasodilation, *J. Clin. Invest.,* 78, 1, 1986.
25. **Kukovetz, W. R., Holzmann, S., and Poch, G.,** Function of cGMP on acetylcholine-induced contraction of coronary smooth muscle, *Naunyn Schmiedeberg's Arch. Pharmacol.,* 319, 29, 1982.
26. **Axelsson, K. L. and Karlsson, J. O. G.,** Nitroglycerin tolerance in vitro: effect on cGMP turnover in vascular smooth muscle, *Acta Pharmacol. Toxicol.,* 55, 203, 1984.

27. **Gerzer, R., Hamet, P., Ross, A. H., Lawson, J. A., and Hardman, J. G.,** Calcium-induced release from platelet membranes of fatty acids that modulate soluble guanylate cyclase, *J. Pharmacol. Exp. Ther.,* 226, 180, 1983.

28. **Tremblay, J. and Hamet, P.,** Cyclic nucleotides and calcium in platelets, in *Platelets in Biology and Pathology,* Vol. 3, Gordon, J. L. and MacIntyre, D. E., Eds., Elsevier/North-Holland, Amsterdam, 1987, 433.

29. **Bohme, E., Graf, H., Hill, H. U., and Arsenow, W.,** Stimulation of guanylate cyclase by sodium nitroprusside, *Naunyn Schmiedeberg's Arch. Pharmacol.,* 297, R12, 1977.

30. **Ignarro, L. J. and Gruetter, C. A.,** Requirement of thiols for activation of coronary arterial guanylate cyclase by glyceryl trinitrate and sodium nitrite, *Biochim. Biophys. Acta,* 631, 221, 1980.

31. **Furchgott, R. F. and Zawadzki, J. V.,** The obligatory role of endothelial cells in the relaxation of arterial smooth muscle by acetylcholine, *Nature (London),* 288, 373, 1980.

32. **deBold, A. J.,** Atrial natriuretic factor: a hormone produced by the heart, *Science,* 230, 767, 1985.

33. **Hamet, P., Tremblay, J., Thibault, G., Garcia, R., Cantin, M., and Genest, J.,** Effect of atrial natriuretic factor on metabolism of cGMP, *Endocrinology,* 112, 289, 1983.

34. **Hamet, P., Tremblay, J., Pang, S. C., Garcia, R., Thibault, G., Gutkowska, J., Cantin, M., and Genest, J.,** Effect of native and synthetic atrial natriuretic factor on cyclic GMP, *Biochem. Biophys. Res. Commun.,* 123, 515, 1984.

35. **Waldman, S. A., Rapoport, R. M., and Murad, F.,** Atrial natriuretic factor selectively activates particulate guanylate cyclase and elevates cyclic GMP in rat tissues, *J. Biol. Chem.,* 259, 14332, 1984.

36. **Nutt, R. F., Brady, S. F., Lyle, T. A., Dylion-Colton, C., Paleveda, W. J., Ciccarone, T. M., Blaine, E. H., Winquist, R. J., Bennett, C. D., Hirschmann, R., and Veber, D. F.,** Synthesis of peptides with atrial natriuretic factor sequence, *Peptides,* 5, 513, 1984.

37. **Hirata, Y., Tomita, M., Yoshimi, H., and Ikeda, M.,** Specific receptors of atrial natriuretic factor (ANF) in cultured vascular smooth muscle cells of rat aorta, *Biochem. Biophys. Res. Commun.,* 125, 562, 1984.

38. **Seymour, A. A., Smith, S. G., Mazack, E. K., and Blaine, E. H.,** A comparison of synthetic rat and human atrial natriuretic factor in conscious dogs, *Hypertension,* 8, 211, 1986.

39. **Hamet, P., Tremblay, J., Pang, S. C., Skuherska, R., Schiffrin, E. L., Garcia, R., Cantin, M., Genest, J., Palmour, R., Ervin, F. R., Martin, S., and Goldwater, R.,** Cyclic GMP as mediator and biological marker of atrial natriuretic factor, *J. Hypertens.,* 4 (Suppl. 2), S49, 1986.

40. **Gerzer, R., Witzgall, H., Tremblay, J., Gutkowska, J., and Hamet, P.,** Rapid increase in plasma and urinary cGMP after bolus injection of atrial natriuretic factor in man, *J. Clin. Endocrinol. Metab.,* 61, 1217, 1985.

41. **Tremblay, J., Gerzer, R., Vinay, P., Pang, S. C., Beliveau, R., and Hamet, P.,** The increase of cGMP by atrial natriuretic factor correlates with the distribution of particulate guanylate cyclase, *FEBS Lett.,* 181, 17, 1985.

42. **Harris, D. W., Baker, C. A., Saneii, H. H., and Johnson, G. A.,** Stimulation of cyclic GMP formation in smooth muscle cells by atriopeptin II, *Life Sci.,* 37, 591, 1985.

43. **Schenk, D. B., Johnson, L. K., Schwartz, K., Sista, H., Scarborough, R. M., and Lewicki, J. A.,** Distinct atrial natriuretic factor receptor sites on cultured bovine aortic smooth muscle and endothelial cells, *Biochem. Biophys. Res. Commun.,* 127, 433, 1985.

44. **Anand-Srivastava, M. B., Franks, D. J., Cantin, M., and Genest, J.,** Atrial natriuretic factor inhibits adenylate cyclase activity, *Biochem. Biophys. Res. Commun.,* 121, 855, 1984.

45. **Anand-Srivastava, M. B., Cantin, M., and Genest, J.,** Inhibition of pituitary adenylate cyclase by atrial natriuretic factor, *Life Sci.,* 36, 1873, 1985.

46. **Anand-Srivastava, M. B., Genest, J., and Cantin, M.,** Inhibitory effect of ANF on adenylate cyclase activity in adrenal cortical membranes, *FEBS Lett.,* 181, 199, 1985.

47. **Leitman, D. C. and Murad, F.,** Atrial natriuretic factor receptor heterogeneity and stimulation of particulate guanylate cyclase and cyclic GMP accumulation, in *Endocrinology and Metabolism Clinics of North America,* Vol. 16, Rosenblatt, M. and Jacobs, J. W., Eds., W. B. Saunders, Philadelphia, 1987, 79.

48. **Garay, R., Rodrigue, F., Longchampt, M. O., DeFeray, J. C., Cantin, M., Genest, J., Meyer, P., and Braquet, P.,** Atrial natriuretic factor (ANF) inhibits Ca^{2+}-dependent, K^+-fluxes in cultured vascular smooth muscle cells, *J. Mol. Cell. Cardiol.,* 17 (Suppl. 3), 198, 1985.

49. **O'Donnell, M. E. and Owen, N. E.,** Role of cyclic GMP in atrial natriuretic factor stimulation of Na^+, K^+, Cl^- cotransport in vascular smooth muscle cells, *J. Biol. Chem.,* 261, 15461, 1986.

50. **Sasaguri, T., Hirata, M., and Kuriyama, H.,** Phosphatidylinositol 4,5-biphosphate phosphodiesterase and inositol 1,4,5-trisphosphate phosphatase of porcine coronary artery smooth muscle, *Jpn. J. Pharmacol.,* 39, 219P, 1985.

51. **Taylor, C. J. and Meisheri, K. D.,** The effects of synthetic atrial peptide (AP-II) on contractions and calcium fluxes in vascular smooth muscle, *Fed. Proc.,* 44, 1104, 1985.

52. **Chartier, L. and Schiffrin, E. L.,** Role of calcium in effects of atrial natriuretic peptide on aldosterone production in adrenal glomerulosa cells, *Am. J. Physiol.,* 252, E485, 1987.

53. **Knorr, M., Locher, R., Stimpel, M., Neyses, L., and Vetter, W.,** Cyclic GMP and cytosolic free calcium in the interaction between atrial natriuretic polypeptide and angiotensin II in smooth muscle cells, in *Natriuretic Hormones in Hypertension,* 11th Sci. Meet. Int. Soc. Hypertension, Heidelberg, September 7 to 9, 1986.

54. **Capponi, A. M., Lew, P. D., Wuthrich, R., and Vallotton, M. B.,** Effects of atrial natriuretic peptide on the stimulation by angiotensin II of various target cells, *J. Hypertens.,* 4 (Suppl. 2), S61, 1986.

55. **Popescu, L. M., Panoiu, C., Hinescu, M., and Nutu, O.,** The mechanism of cGMP-induced relaxation in vascular smooth muscle, *Eur. J. Pharmacol.,* 107, 393, 1985.

56. **Takai, Y., Kaibuchi, K., Sano, K., and Nishizuka, Y.,** Counteraction of calcium-activated, phospholipid-dependent protein kinase activation by cAMP and cGMP in platelets, *J. Biochem.,* 91, 403, 1982.

57. **Kawahara, Y., Yamanishi, J., and Fukuzaki, H.,** Inhibitory action of guanosine 3′,5′-monophosphate on thrombin-induced calcium mobilization in human platelets, *Thromb. Res.,* 33, 203, 1984.

58. **Nakashima, S., Tohmatsu, T., Hattori, H., Okano, Y., and Nozawa, Y.,** Inhibitory action of cyclic GMP on secretion, polyphosphoinositide hydrolysis and calcium mobilization in thrombin-stimulated human platelets, *Biochem. Biophys. Res. Commun.,* 135, 1099, 1986.

59. **Dousa, T. P., Shah, S. V., and Abboud, H. E.,** Potential role of cyclic nucleotides in glomerular pathophysiology, in *Advances in Cyclic Nucleotide Research,* Vol. 12, Hamet, P. and Sands, H., Eds., Raven Press, New York, 1980, 285.

60. **Bianchi, C., Gutkowska, J., Thibault, G., Garcia, R., Genest, J., and Cantin, M.,** Distinct localization of atrial natriuretic factor and angiotensin II binding sites in the glomerulus, *Am. J. Physiol.,* 251, F594, 1986.

61. **De Lean, A., Vinay, P., and Cantin, M.,** Distribution of atrial natriuretic factor receptors in dog kidney fractions, *FEBS Lett.,* 193, 239, 1985.

62. **Ardaillou, N., Nivez, M.-P., and Ardaillou, R.,** Stimulation of guanylate cyclase by atrial natriuretic factor in isolated human glomeruli, *FEBS Lett.,* 189, 8, 1985.

63. **Ardaillou, N., Nivez, M.-P., and Ardaillou, R.,** Stimulation of cyclic GMP synthesis in human cultured glomerular cells by atrial natriuretic peptide, *FEBS Lett.,* 204, 177, 1986.

64. **Leitman, D. C., Andresen, J. W., Kuno, T., Kamisaki, Y., Chang, J. K., and Murad, F.,** Identification of multiple binding sites for atrial natriuretic factor by affinity cross-linking in cultured endothelial cells, *J. Biol. Chem.,* 261, 11650, 1986.

65. **Tremblay, J., Gerzer, R., Pang, S. C., Cantin, M., Genest, J., and Hamet, P.,** ANF stimulation of detergent-dispersed particulate guanylate cyclase from bovine adrenal cortex, *FEBS Lett.,* 194, 210, 1986.

66. **Misono, K. S., Grammer, R. T., Rigby, J. W., and Inagami, T.,** Photoaffinity labeling of atrial natriuretic factor receptor in bovine and rat adrenal cortical membranes, *Biochem. Biophys. Res. Commun.,* 130, 994, 1985.

67. **Chartier, L., Schiffrin, E., and Thibault, G.,** Effect of atrial natriuretic factor (ANF)-related peptides on aldosterone secretion by adrenal glomerulosa cells: critical role of the intramolecular disulphide bond, *Biochem. Biophys. Res. Commun.,* 122, 171, 1984.

68. **Atarashi, K., Franco-Saenz, R., Mulrow, P. J., Snajdar, R., and Rapp, J. P.,** Inhibition of aldosterone production by atrial natriuretic factor, *J. Hypertens.,* 2, 293, 1984.

69. **De Lean, A., Racz, K., Gutkowska, J., Nguyen, T.-T., Cantin, M., and Genest, J.,** Specific receptor-mediated inhibition by synthetic atrial natriuretic factor of hormone-stimulated steroidogenesis in cultured bovine adrenal cells, *Endocrinology,* 115, 1636, 1984.

70. **Garcia, R., Thibault, G., Cantin, M., and Genest, J.,** Effect of a purified atrial natriuretic factor on rat and rabbit vascular strips and vascular beds, *Am. J. Physiol.,* 247, R34, 1984.

71. **Bohme, E., Graf, H., and Schultz, G.,** Effects of sodium nitroprusside and other smooth muscle relaxants on cyclic GMP formation in smooth muscle and platelets, in *Advances in Cyclic Nucleotide Research,* Vol. 9, George, W. J. and Ignarro, L. J., Eds., Raven Press, New York, 1978, 131.

72. **Bohme, E. and Jakobs, K. H.,** Guanosine-3:5-monophosphate in human platelets, *IRCS Med. Sci.,* 1, 8a, 1973.

73. **Bohme, E., Gerzer, R., Grossmann, G., Herz, J., Mulsch, A., Spies, C., and Schultz, G.,** Regulation of soluble guanylate cyclase activity, in *Hormones and Cell Regulation,* Vol. 7, Dumont, J. E., Nunez, J., and Denton, R. M., Eds., Elsevier, Amsterdam 1983, 147.

74. **Schiffrin, E. L., Deslongchamps, M., and Thibault, G.,** Platelet binding sites for atrial natriuretic factor in humans, *Hypertension,* 8 (Suppl. 2), 6, 1986.

75. **Ishikawa, E., Ishikawa, S., Davis, J. W., and Sutherland, E. W.,** Determination of guanosine 3′,5′-monophosphate in tissues and of guanyl cyclase in rat intestine, *J. Biol. Chem.,* 244, 6371, 1969.

76. **Field, M., Graf, L. H., Laird, W. J., and Smith, P. L.,** Heat-stable enterotoxin of Escherichia coli: *in vitro* effects on guanylate cyclase activity, cyclic GMP concentration, and ion transport in small intestine, *Proc. Natl. Acad. Sci. U.S.A.,* 75, 2800, 1978.

77. **O'Grady, S. M., Field, M., Nash, N. T., and Rao, M. C.,** Atrial natriuretic factor inhibits Na-K-Cl cotransport in teleost intestine, *Am. J. Physiol.,* 249, C531, 1985.

78. **Debinski, W., Gutkowska, J., Kuchel, O., Racz, K., Buu, N. T., Cantin, M., and Genest, J.,** ANF-like peptide(s) in the peripheral autonomic nervous system, *Biochem. Biophys. Res. Commun.,* 134, 279, 1986.

79. **Cusson, J. R., DuSouich, P., Hamet, P., Schiffrin, E. L., Kuchel, O., Tremblay, J., Cantin, M., Genest, J., and Larochelle, P.,** Effects and pharmacokinetics of bolus injections of atrial natriuretic factor in normal volunteers, *J. Cardiovasc. Pharmacol.,* 11, 635, 1988.

80. **Tremblay, J., Pang, S. C., Schiffrin, E. L., Gutkowska, J., Cusson, J., Larochelle, P., and Hamet, P.,** Particulate guanylate cyclase: target enzyme of ANF, in *Biologically Active Atrial Peptides,* Vol. 1, Brenner, B. M. and Laragh, J. H., Eds., Raven Press, New York, 1987, 255.

81. **Larochelle, P., Cusson, J., Hamet, P., DuSouich, P., Schiffrin, E. L., Genest, J., and Cantin, M.,** Pharmacodynamic effects of bolus administration of ANF in normal volunteers, in *Biologically Active Atrial Peptides,* Vol. 1, Brenner, B. M. and Laragh, J. H., Eds., Raven Press, New York, 1987, 451.

82. **Garcia, R., Thibault, G., Gutkowska, J., Horky, K., Hamet, P., Cantin, M., and Genest, J.,** Chronic infusion of low doses of atrial natriuretic factor (ANF Arg 101-Tyr 126) reduces blood pressure in conscious SHR without apparent changes in sodium excretion, *Proc. Soc. Exp. Biol. Med.,* 179, 396, 1985.

83. **Hamet, P., Testaert, E., Palmour, R., Larochelle, P., Cantin, M., Martin, S., Ervin, F., and Tremblay, J.,** Effect of prolonged infusion of ANF in normotensive and hypertensive monkeys, *Am. J. Hypertens.,* in press.

84. **Tremblay, J., Lachance, B., and Hamet, P.,** Activation of cyclic GMP-binding and cyclic AMP-specific phosphodiesterases of rat platelets by a mechanism involving cyclic AMP-dependent phosphorylation, *J. Cyclic Nucleotide Protein Phosphor. Res.,* 10, 397, 1985.

85. **Scarborough, R. M., Schenk, D. B., McEnroe, G. A., Arfsten, A., Kang, L. L., Schwartz, K., and Lewicki, J. A.,** Truncated atrial natriuretic peptide analogs, *J. Biol. Chem.,* 261, 12960, 1986.

86. **Schiller, P. W., Bellini, F., Dionne, G., Maziak, L. A., Garcia, R., De Lean, A., and Cantin, M.,** Synthesis and activity profiles of atrial natriuretic peptide (ANP) analogs with reduced ring size, *Biochem. Biophys. Res. Commun.,* 138, 880, 1986.

87. **Maack, T., Suzuki, M., Almeida, F. A., Nussenzveig, D., Scarborough, R. M., McEnroe, G. A., and Lewicki, J. A.,** Physiological role of silent receptors of atrial natriuretic factor, *Science,* 238, 675, 1987.

88. **Willenbrock, R. C., Tremblay, J., Garcia, R., and Hamet, P.,** Dissociation of natriuresis and diuresis and heterogeneity of the effector system of atrial natriuretic factor in rats, *J. Clin. Invest.,* 83, 482, 1989.

89. **Morel, F., Imbert-Teboul, M., and Chabardes, D.,** Cyclic nucleotides and tubule function, in *Advances in Cyclic Nucleotide Research,* Vol. 12, Hamet, P. and Sands, H., Eds., Raven Press, New York, 1980, 301.

90. **Tremblay, J. and Hamet, H.,** Role of action of particulate guanylate cyclase in the expression of biological actions of ANF, in *Biological and Molecular Aspects of Atrial Factors,* University of California, Los Angeles Symposia on Molecular Biology, Steamboat Springs, CO, 1988.

91. **Roy, L. F., Larochelle, P., Hamet, P., Ogilvie, R. I., and Leenen, F. H. H.,** Hemodynamic effects of atrial natriuretic factor (ANF) versus sodium nitroprusside (NIP) in healthy men, in 12th Int. Meet. Int. Soc. Hypertension, Kyoto, Japan, May 22 to 26, 1988.

92. **Baranowska, B., Gutkowska, J., and Tremblay, J.,** Clonidine stimulates atrial natriuretic factor (ANF) release in water-deprived rats, *Peptides,* 9 (Suppl. 1), 189, 1988.

93. **Anderson, J. V., Christofides, N. D., and Bloom, S. R.,** Plasma release of atrial natriuretic peptide in response to blood volume expansion, *J. Endocrinol.,* 109, 9, 1986.

94. **Hollister, A. S., Tanaka, I., Imada, T., Onrot, J., Biaggioni, I., Robertson, D., and Inagami, T.,** Sodium loading and posture modulate human atrial natriuretic factor plasma levels, *Hypertension,* 8 (Suppl. 2), 106, 1986.

95. **Walsh, M. F. J., Barakat, S. N., Zemel, M. B., Gualdoni, S. M., and Sowers, J. R.,** Postural changes in atrial natriuretic peptide in hypertensive and normal subjects: effect of varying sodium intake, in *Biologically Active Atrial Peptides,* Vol. 1, Brenner, B. M. and Laragh, J. H., Eds., Raven Press, New York, 1987, 574.

96. **Larose, P., Meloche, S., du Souich, P., De Lean, A., and Ong, H.,** Radioimmunoassay of atrial natriuretic factor: human plasma levels, *Biochem. Biophys. Res. Commun.,* 130, 553, 1985.

97. **Pearce, M. L., Newman, E. V., and Birmingham, M. R.,** Some postural adjustments of salt and water excretion, *J. Clin. Invest.,* 33, 1089, 1954.

98. **Epstein, F. H., Goodyer, A. V. N., Lawrison, F. D., and Relman, A. S.,** Studies of the antidiuresis of quiet standing: the importance of changes in plasma volume and glomerular filtration rate, *J. Clin. Invest.,* 30, 63, 1951.

99. **Cusson, J. R., Larochelle, P., Gutkowska, J., Tremblay, J., and Hamet, P.,** Role of ANF in physiological response to postural changes, *Am. J. Physiol.,* submitted.

100. **Somers, V. K., Anderson, J. V., Conway, J., Sleight, P., and Bloom, S. R.,** Atrial natriuretic peptide is released by dynamic exercise in man, *Horm. Metab. Res.,* 18, 871, 1986.

101. **Richards, A. M., Tonolo, G., Cleland, J. G. F., McIntyre, G. D., Leckie, B. J., Dargie, H. J., Ball, S. G., and Robertson, J. I. S.,** Plasma atrial natriuretic peptide concentrations during exercise in sodium replete and deplete normal man, *Clin. Sci.,* 72, 159, 1987.

102. **Blanchard, D., Verdy, M., Gutkowska, J., Tremblay, J., and Hamet, P.,** Role of ANF in the phys-iological response to exercise, paper presented at the Canadian Society for Clinical Investigation Annual Meeting, Ottawa, Ontario, 1988.

103. **Van Haastert, P. J. M.,** cAMP activates adenylate and guanylate cyclase of Dictyostelium discoideum cells by binding to different classes of cell-surface receptors. A study with extracellular Ca^{2+}, *Biochim. Biophys. Acta,* 846, 324, 1985.

104. **Hamet, P., Pang, S. C., and Tremblay, J.,** Atrial natriuretic factor induced-egression of cyclic guanosine 3':5' monophosphate in cultured vascular smooth muscle and endothelial cells, *J. Biol. Chem.,* 264, 1989 (in press.)

105. **Cole, B. R. and Needleman, P.,** Atriopeptins: volume regulatory hormones, *Clin. Res.,* 33, 389, 1985.

106. **Smith, S., Anderson, S., Ballermann, B. J., and Brenner, B. M.,** Role of atrial natriuretic peptide in adaptation of sodium excretion with reduced renal mass, *J. Clin. Invest.,* 77, 1395, 1986.

107. **Anderson, J. V., Raine, A. E. G., Proudler, A., and Bloom, S. R.,** Effect of haemodialysis on plasma concentrations of atrial natriuretic peptide in adult patients with chronic renal failure, *J. Endocrinol.,* 110, 193, 1986.

108. **Hasegawa, K., Matsushita, Y., Inoue, T., Morii, H., Ishibashi, M., and Yamaji, T.,** Plasma levels of atrial natriuretic peptide in patients with chronic renal failure, *J. Clin. Endocrinol. Metab.,* 63, 8ı9, 1986.

109. **Rascher, W., Tulassay, T., and Lang, R. E.,** Atrial natriuretic peptide in plasma of volume-overloaded children with chronic renal failure, *Lancet,* 2, 303, 1985.

110. **Tulassay, T., Rascher, W., Ganten, D., Scharer, K., and Lang, R. E.,** Atrial natriuretic peptide and volume changes in children, *Clin. Exp. Hypertens. A,* 8, 695, 1986.

111. **Wilkins, M. R.,** Endogenous digitalis: a review of the evidence, *Trends Pharmacol. Sci.,* 6, 206, 1985.

112. **Larochelle, P., Beroniade, V., Gutkowska, J., Cusson, J. R., Lécrivain, A., DuSouich, P., Cantin, M., and Genest, J.,** Influence of hemodialysis on the plasma levels of the atrial natriuretic factor in chronic renal failure, *Clin. Invest. Med.,* 10, 350, 1987.

113. **Martin, T. J., Melick, R. A., and De Luise, M.,** The effect of nephrectomy on the metabolism of labelled parathyroid hormone, *Clin. Sci.,* 37, 137, 1969.

114. **O'Brien, J. P. and Sharpe, A. R., Jr.,** The influence of renal disease on the insulin I^{131} disappearance curve in man, *Metab. Clin. Exp.,* 16, 76, 1967.

115. **Hamet, P., Stouder, D. A., Ginn, H. E., Hardman, J. G., and Liddle, G. W.,** Studies of the elevated extracellular concentration of cyclic AMP in uremic man, *J. Clin. Invest.,* 56, 339, 1975.

116. **Larochelle, P., Cusson, J. R., Gutkowska, J., Schiffrin, E. L., Hamet, P., Kuchel, O., Genest, J., and Cantin, M.,** Plasma atrial natriuretic factor concentrations in essential and renovascular hypertension, *Br. Med. J.,* 294, 1249, 1987.

117. **Kuchel, O., Messerli, F. H., Tolis, G., Hamet, P., Fraysse, J., Cartier, P., Roy, P., Boucher, R., and Genest, J.,** Renal vein plasma adenosine 3',5'-cyclic monophosphate in renovascular hypertension, *Can. Med. Assoc. J.,* 116, 992, 1977.

118. **Cantin, M., Thibault, G., Ding, J., Gutkowska, J., Garcia, R., Jasmin, G., Hamet, P., and Genest, J.,** ANF in experimental congestive heart failure, *Am. J. Pathol.,* under revision.

119. **Arendt, R. M., Gerbes, A. L., Ritter, D., Stangl, E., Bach, P., and Zahringer, J.,** Alpha-atrial natriuretic factor in cardiovascular disease, *J. Am. Coll. Cardiol.,* 7, 75A, 1986.

120. **Burnett, J. C., Jr. Kao, P. C., Hu, D. C., Heser, D. W., Heublein, D., Granger, J. P., Opgenorth, T. J., and Reeder, G. S.,** Atrial natriuretic peptide elevation in congestive heart failure in the human, *Science,* 231, 1145, 1986.

121. **Kouz, S., Bourassa, M. G., Laurier, J., Gutkowska, J., Genest, J., David, P. R., Dyrda, I., and Cantin, M.,** Plasma concentration of immunoreactive atrial natriuretic factor (IR-ANF) in patients with coronary artery disease, *J. Am. Coll. Cardiol.,* 7, 210A, 1986.

122. **Naruse, M., Naruse, K., Obana, K., Kurimoto, F., Sakurai, H., Honda, T., Higashida, T., Demura, H., Inagami, T., and Shizume, K.,** Immunoreactive alpha-human atrial natriuretic polypeptide in human plasma, *Peptides,* 7, 141, 1986.

123. **Pasternac, A., Kouz, S., Gutkowska, J., Petitclerc, R., Vellas, B., DeChamplain, J., Cantin, M., and Bourassa, M. G.,** Abnormal plasma levels of atrial natriuretic factor (ANF) in patients with symptomatic mitral valve prolapse, *J. Am. Coll. Cardiol.,* 7, 169A, 1986.

124. **Osborn, M. J., Hammill, S. C., and Burnett, J. C., Jr.,** Enhanced levels of circulating atrial natriuretic peptide during ventricular pacing in humans, *J. Am. Coll. Cardiol.,* 7, 192A, 1986.

125. **Schiffrin, E. L., Gutkowska, J., Kuchel, O., Cantin, M., and Genest, J.,** Plasma concentration of atrial natriuretic factor in a patient with paroxysmal atrial tachycardia, *N. Engl. J. Med.,* 312, 1196, 1985.

126. **Adelstein, R. S.,** Biochemical mechanism of contractility, in *Hypertension,* 2nd ed., Genest, J., Kuchel, O., Hamet, P., and Cantin, M., Eds., McGraw-Hill, New York, 1983, 524.

127. **Nakaoka, H., Kitahara, Y., Amano, M., Imataka, K., Fujii, J., Ishibashi, M., and Yamaji, T.,** Effect of β-adrenergic receptor blockade on atrial natriuretic peptide in essential hypertension, *Hypertension,* 10, 221, 1987.

128. **Muller, F. B., Bolli, P., Kiowski, W., Erne, P., Resink, T., Raine, A. E. G., and Buhler, F. R.,** Atrial natriuretic peptide is elevated in low-renin essential hypertension, *J. Hypertens.,* 4 (Suppl. 6), S489, 1986.

129. **Nillsson, P., Lindholm, L., Schersten, B., Horn, R., Melander, A., and Hesch, R. D.,** Atrial natriuretic peptide and blood pressure in a geographically defined population, *Lancet,* 2, 883, 1987.

130. **Sugawara, A., Nakao, K., Sakamoto, M., Morii, N., Yamada, T., Itoh, H., Shiono, S., and Imura, H.,** Plasma concentration of atrial natriuretic polypeptide in essential hypertension, *Lancet,* 2, 1426, 1985.

131. **Sugawara, A., Nakao, K., Kono, T., Morii, N., Yamada, T., Itoh, H., Shiono, S., Saito, Y., Mukoyama, M., Arai, H., and Imura, H.,** Implication of atrial natriuretic polypeptide in essential hypertension and primary aldosteronism, *Hypertension,* 9, 551, 1987.

132. **Sagnella, G. A., Markandu, N. D., Shore, A. C., and MacGregor, G. A.,** Raised circulating levels of atrial natriuretic peptides in essential hypertension, *Lancet,* 1, 179, 1986.

133. **MacGregor, G. A., Sagnella, G. A., Markandu, N. D., Shore, A. C., Buckley, M. G., Cappuccio, F. P., and Singer, D. R. J.,** Raised plasma levels of atrial natriuretic peptide in subjects with untreated essential hypertension, *J. Hypertens.,* 4 (Suppl. 6), S567, 1986.

134. **Montorsi, P., Tonolo, G., Polonia, J., Hepburn, D., and Richards, M. A.,** Correlates of plasma atrial natriuretic factor in health and hypertension, *Hypertension,* 10, 570, 1987.

135. **Kohno, M., Yasunari, K., Matsuura, T., Murakawa, K., and Takeda, T.,** Circulating atrial natriuretic polypeptide in essential hypertension, *Am. Heart J.,* 113, 1160, 1987.

136. **Pang, S. C., Hoang, M. C., Tremblay, J., Cantin, M., Garcia, R., Genest, J., and Hamet, P.,** Effect of natural and synthetic atrial natriuretic factor on arterial blood pressure, natriuresis and cyclic GMP excretion in spontaneously hypertensive rats, *Clin. Sci.,* 69, 721, 1985.

137. **Kondo, K., Kida, O., Kangawa, K., Matsuo, H., and Tanaka, K.,** Enhanced diuretic response to alpha-human atrial natriuretic polypeptide (alpha-hANP) in spontaneously hypertensive rats, *Nippon Jinzo Gakkai Shi,* 27, 1313, 1985.

138. **Cusson, J. R., Hamet, P., Gutkowska, J., Kuchel, O., Genest, J., Cantin, M., and Larochelle, P.,** Effects of atrial natriuretic factor on natriuresis and cGMP in patients with essential hypertension, *J. Hypertens.,* 5, 435, 1987.

139. **Takayanagi, R., Imada, T., Grammer, R. T., Misono, K. S., Naruse, M., and Inagami, T.,** Atrial natriuretic factor in spontaneously hypertensive rats: concentration changes with the progression of hypertension and elevated formation of cyclic GMP, *J. Hypertens.,* 4 (Suppl. 3), S303, 1986.

140. **Hamet, P. and Tremblay, J.,** Abnormalities of second messenger systems in hypertension, in *Blood Cells and Arteries in Hypertension and Atherosclerosis,* Heyer, P. and Marche, P., Eds., Raven Press, New York, 1988, 12, 171.

141. **Zimmerman, A. L., Yamanaka, G., Eckstein, F., Baylor, D. A., and Stryer, L.,** Interaction of hydrolysis-resistant analogs of cyclic GMP with the phosphodiesterase and light-sensitive channel of retinal rod outer segments, *Proc. Natl. Acad. Sci. U.S.A.,* 82, 8813, 1985.

142. **Lincoln, T. M. and Johnson, R. M.,** Possible role of cyclic-GMP-dependent protein kinase in vascular smooth muscle function, in *Advances in Cyclic Nucleotide Protein Phosphorylation Research,* Vol. 17, Greengard, P., Robison, G. A., Paoletti, R., and Nicosia, S., Eds., Raven Press, New York, 1984, 285.

143. **Fiscus, R. R., Rapoport, R. M., Waldman, S. A., and Murad, F.,** Atriopeptin II elevates cGMP, activates cGMP-dependent protein kinase and causes relaxation in rat thoracic aorta, *Biochim. Biophys. Acta,* 846, 179, 1985.

144. **Stryer, L.,** Cyclic GMP cascade of vision, *Annu. Rev. Neurosci.,* 9, 87, 1986.

145. **Fung, B. K. K., Hurley, J. B. and Stryer, L.,** Flow of information in the light-triggered cyclic nucleotide cascade of vision, *Proc. Natl. Acad. Sci. U.S.A.,* 78, 152, 1981.

146. **Yamazaki, A., Uchida, S., Stein, P. J., Wheeler, G. L., and Bitenski, M. W.,** Enzyme regulation and GTP binding protein: an algorithm of control that includes physical displacement of an inhibitory protein, in *Advances in Cyclic Nucleotide and Protein Phosphorylation Research,* Vol. 16, Strada, S. J. and Thompson, W. J., Eds., Raven Press, New York, 1984, 381.

147. **Pober, J. S. and Bitensky, M. W.,** Light-regulated enzymes of vertebrate retinal rods, in *Advances in Cyclic Nucleotide Research,* Vol. 11, Greengard, P. and Robison, G. A., Eds., Raven Press, New York, 1979, 265.

148. **Fesenko, E. E., Kolesnikov, S. S., and Lyubarsky, A. L.,** Induction by cyclic GMP of cationic conductance in plasma membrane of retinal rod outer segment, *Nature (London),* 313, 310, 1985.

149. **Anand-Srivastava, M. B.,** personal communication.

150. **Gerzer, R.,** personal communication.

Chapter 9

VASCULAR ACTIONS OF ANP

Nick C. Trippodo

TABLE OF CONTENTS

I. INTRODUCTION

When injected in bolus or continuously infused at pharmacologic doses for up to 1 or 2 h, ANP usually lowers arterial blood pressure. The hemodynamic pattern is complex and may involve decreased total peripheral resistance, decreased cardiac output, or both. Although reflex inhibition of the heart may contribute to the overall hemodynamic effect, the response to short-term administration of ANP is primarily initiated by direct or indirect actions of the peptide on peripheral blood vessels.

Nomenclature for the atrial peptides used in this chapter is based on published guidelines.[1]

II. ENDOGENOUS AGENTS OTHER THAN ANP

One of the characteristics of the vascular action of ANP is heterogeneity with respect to species, vascular bed, the contractant(s) maintaining vascular tone, the level of vascular tone, vessel segment, dose, and method of administration. Since heterogeneity of action is also a feature of other vasoactive agents, two autocoids that show strikingly mixed vascular effects are briefly reviewed for perspective.[2]

A. HISTAMINE

Histamine is predominantly a vasodilator of the microcirculation and a constrictor of large vessels. Both H_1 and H_2 receptors seem to be involved in the vasodilation, whereas the vasoconstriction may be mostly mediated by H_1 receptors. In isolated strips of human coronary arteries, histamine caused endothelium-dependent relaxation at low concentrations and endothelium-independent contraction at high concentrations.[3] The relaxation was mediated by H_2 receptors and presumably involved liberation of an endothelium-derived relaxing factor. The histamine-induced contraction in these human coronary arteries was mediated by H_1 receptors presumably on the smooth muscle cells. Even within the microcirculation there is evidence, albeit controversial, that arterioles and venules greater than 80 μm in diameter constrict in response to histamine.[2,4] Local intraarterial infusion of histamine produces marked increases in net fluid filtration, protein clearance, and the ratio of lymph-to-plasma protein concentration.[4] There is evidence that this increased permeability is mediated by an action of histamine on the postcapillary venules. The classic systemic hemodynamic response to intravenously administered histamine in moderate doses in man and some animals is one of decreased total peripheral resistance, decreased arterial blood pressure, and increased hematocrit. However, high systemic doses of histamine can cause increases in arterial blood pressure and total peripheral resistance in rabbits and rats. Dogs show a peculiar response to intravenous infusion of histamine and to agents that release endogenous histamine in that the veins draining blood from the liver constrict very intensely.[5] This creates a marked outflow resistance and blood pools within the liver, severely retarding venous return and ultimately decreasing cardiac output.

B. SEROTONIN

Serotonin (5-hydroxytryptamine) is also a large vessel constrictor and a small vessel dilator.[2,6] The net effect of serotonin in a given vascular bed is determined by the balance between its vasoconstrictor and vasodilator actions. Serotonin-induced vasodilation predominates in skeletal muscle, whereas its vasoconstrictor effect is more prominent in skin and kidney. Nonuniform vessel responsiveness to serotonin was dramatically demonstrated in the perfused canine forelimb, where intraarterial infusion of serotonin resulted in a unique pattern of changes in segmental cutaneous vascular resistances.[7] Although total vascular resistance increased, the resistance across the microcirculation actually decreased (Table 1). The marked vasoconstrictor response to serotonin was confined to the large vessels, with a

TABLE 1
Segmental Vascular Resistances across Cutaneous Bed
in Canine Forelimbs Perfused at Constant Flow

		TVR	R_a	R_v	R_{micro}
Saline	Arbitrary units	290	70	20	200
	% TVR	100%	24%	7%	69%
Serotonin	Arbitrary units	906	632	170	104
	% TVR	100%	70%	19%	11%

Note: Serotonin (25 µg base/min) was infused intraarterially for 3 to 5 min, causing perfusion pressure to increase from about 120 mmHg to approximately 200 mmHg. TVR, total vascular resistance. R_a, R_v, R_{micro}, resistances in large artery, large vein, and microcirculation (vessels smaller than about 500 µm in diameter, including arterioles, capillaries and venules), respectively. Infusion of serotonin displaced the location of the greatest vascular resistance from the microcirculation to the large vessels.

Data taken from Grega, G. J. and Adamski, S. W., *Fed. Proc.*, 46, 270, 1987. With permission.

significant proportion of the increase in total vascular resistance occurring in the large veins. Several types and subtypes of serotonin receptors have been hypothesized which may be located along the vascular tree in varying concentrations. Systemic administration of serotonin not surprisingly causes complex actions on the cardiovascular system which result from myriad opposing direct and reflex influences. In pithed animals, serotonin can cause a prompt rise in blood pressure despite inducing vasodilation in skeletal muscle. The hemodynamic response to serotonin in intact animals is variable and involves both pressor and depressor phases. Capillary permeability does not appear to be altered in most species, although it may increase in rats. Interestingly, serotonin initiates a coronary chemoreflex (Bezold-Jarisch reflex) characterized by inhibition of sympathetic outflow and increased activity of the efferent vagus to the heart, which produces a slowing of heart rate and hypotension.

III. ATRIAL NATRIURETIC PEPTIDE

It is evident that vasoactive agents can have diverse vascular actions, including constriction and relaxation, and to varying degrees, depending on a number of factors. The available evidence indicates that at pharmacologic doses ANP is an endothelium-independent vasodilator of large arteries, a dilator of certain agonist-contracted microcirculatory vessels, and a constrictor of postglomerular arterioles in the kidney. Most veins are relatively unresponsive to ANP. The vascular actions of ANP at physiological levels are unclear.

A. LARGE VESSELS *IN VITRO*
1. Characteristics
Winquist[8] summarized the major features of the vasorelaxant activity of ANP on blood vessels examined *in vitro*. Most of these studies have been carried out on relatively large vessels. ANP relaxes blood vessels contracted with a variety of receptor-mediated agonists, such as serotonin, histamine, methoxamine, and norepinephrine, with generally equal potency. That is, there are no consistent differences in the IC_{50}s of ANP (concentration of ANP producing 50% relaxation) for vessels contracted with different agonists. However, ANP was suggested as having a greater effect on angiotensin II-initiated contractions than

on those elicited by norepinephrine,[9] and this tendency appears to hold true in the exteriorized intestinal and skeletal muscle microcirculations.[10] Contractions elicited by high potassium concentration (20 to 80 mM) are inhibited by ANP less effectively than those stimulated by agonists. Various antagonists of vasoactive agents (adrenergic, cholinergic, histaminergic, and prostanoid) do not block the relaxant activity of ANP. ANP has a greater effect on the aorta and its main branches than on smaller, more distal arteries, which are generally refractory. Small renal preglomerular arteries (lumen diameter 250 μm) are an exception in that they relaxed to ANP with an IC$_{50}$ of about $8 \times 10^{-9} M$, whereas similarly sized arteries isolated from the mesenteric, femoral, cerebral, and coronary beds did not respond.[11,12] The selectivity of ANP in relaxing small renal preglomerular arteries (200 to 300 μm) was also demonstrated in vessels isolated from spontaneously hypertensive rats.[13]

Except for the facial vein of the rabbit[14] and the portal vein of the rat,[14,15] isolated veins from a variety of species and beds generally relax very little in the presence of ANP.[8] The responsiveness of the rabbit facial vein and the rat portal vein to ANP may have to do with the myogenic tone displayed by these vessels, with the former (tonic) being much more sensitive than the latter (phasic). The ineffectual action of ANP on veins *in vitro* contrasts with the effective venodilatory action of other relaxants such as beta adrenergic agonists and nitroglycerin;[15] however, this is consistent with the lack of evidence for ANP-induced venodilation *in vivo* (see below).

The pulmonary artery isolated from pig[16] and dog[17] is more sensitive to ANP than the renal artery, whereas in the rabbit, the renal artery is the more sensitive.[8] Variation among species can also occur in structure-activity relationships for different ANP peptides. Rat ANP(103—123) is much less potent than longer ANP peptides in relaxing the rabbit, dog, and monkey aorta, but equipotent on rat aorta.[18-20] Age, as well as the presence of hypertension, are other factors that might contribute to vessel responsiveness to ANP. ANP relaxation was greatest in arteries from younger rats, but similar in portal veins regardless of age.[19] Aortae isolated from spontaneously hypertensive rats and rats with renal hypertension showed decreased sensitivity to ANP,[21] but this is not a consistent finding.[13]

2. Biologic Importance

The biologic importance of the action of ANP on large blood vessels, as observed *in vitro*, is uncertain. For instance, the concentrations of ANP required to relax most vessels *in vitro* are well above physiological and pathophysiologic plasma levels of immunoreactive ANP (iANP) (Figure 1). Nevertheless, this does not exclude an effect of ANP on these vessels *in vivo*, where they may enjoy greater responsiveness. Indeed, the actual concentration of ANP in the baths used for studying vessels *in vitro* may be less than that calculated because of peptide loss due to adsorption and degradation. In any event, there is preliminary evidence that pharmacologic doses of ANP produced aortic relaxation in intact anesthetized rabbits.[25] Aortic dilation was suggested to cause a resetting of baroreceptors to lower pressure ranges by preventing the diameter of the aorta from decreasing during hypotensive doses of ANP and thus preventing the unloading of the aortic baroreceptors.[25] In general, it is evident that blood vessels larger than arterioles and venules contribute importantly to total vascular resistance, and in a given bed the contribution of each vascular section to total resistance can shift dramatically, depending on the balance of neural and circulatory influences.[7] As noted above, infusion of serotonin in the cutaneous bed changed the large artery contribution to total resistance from 24 to 70% and that of the large veins from 7 to 19% (Table 1). Similar studies with ANP have yet to be reported.

Convenient access to the larger arteries has allowed investigation of the molecular and biochemical mechanisms of ANP-induced relaxation in these vessels. Studies utilizing a number of *in vitro* systems have made substantial progress in characterizing specific ANP receptors and identifying intracellular second messengers and various regulatory molecules. This subject is covered in Chapters 7 and 8.

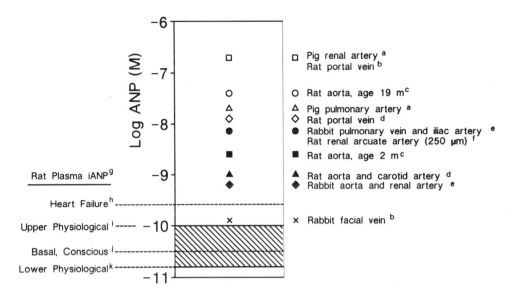

FIGURE 1. ANP IC_{50} values for relaxing blood vessels *in vitro* and rat plasma levels of immunoreactive ANP concentration. Key: [a]Jansen et al.;[16] [b]Winquist et al.;[14] [c]Emmick and Cohen;[19] [d]Cohen and Schenck;[15] [e]Winquist;[8] [f]Aalkjae et al.;[11] [g]immunoreactive ANP concentration; [h]Chien et al. 3 weeks after coronary artery ligation (750 pg/ml);[22] [i]Gotowska et al. 4-h immobilization stress (248 pg/ml);[23] [j]Gutkowska et al. 24 h after catheter implantation (94 pg/ml);[23] [k]Barbee and Trippodo, open-chest, Inactin-anesthetized (48 pg/ml).[24]

B. PERFUSED BEDS AND MICROCIRCULATION

1. Renal

Intraarterial infusion of ANP into several vascular beds in anesthetized dogs preferentially increased blood flow in the renal artery.[26] Others have reported immediate increases in renal blood flow that persisted,[27] waned,[28] or eventually decreased[29] during intrarenal arterial infusion of ANP in anesthetized dogs; renal vascular resistance decreased[27,28] or did not change.[29] Intraarterial administration of atrial extract in anesthetized rats elicited vasodilation in the autoperfused kidney, but caused no effect on vascular resistance in the hind limb,[30] again suggesting a selective vasodilatory effect of ANP in the renal bed. In contrast, intrarenal administration of ANP in conscious rats decreased renal blood flow in both the infused and contralateral, noninfused kidneys.[31] Although species difference may account for some of these disparate results, a number of other factors also come into play. The dose of ANP may be important not only because of dose-related direct renal actions, but also because of systemic hemodynamic effects due to spillover of ANP into the peripheral circulation. The peripheral actions of ANP could lead to a decrease in renal blood flow as a result of diminished cardiac output (see below) and/or reflex activation of renal sympathetic vasoconstrictor activity.[32] Nevertheless, local vasoconstrictor activity of ANP was also demonstrated in isolated perfused rat kidneys, whereas in the absence of constrictors in the perfusate, atrial extract or synthetic ANP produced a slow rise in renal vascular resistance.[33,34] The associated increase in glomerular filtration rate and filtration fraction suggested a direct or indirect preferential constriction of the postglomerular vessels.[33] However, with vasoconstrictors (norepinephrine, angiotensin II, or arginine vasopression) in the perfusate, atrial extract or ANP consistently lowered renal vascular resistance.[33,35] Thus, the level of preexisting vascular tone determines both the qualitative and quantitative effect of ANP on renal blood vessels.

The contention that ANP dilates afferent, but constricts efferent, renal arterioles is supported by observations on the *in vitro* perfused dog glomerulus, which allowed measurements in single, isolated glomerular units.[36] Following addition of ANP to the perfusate, glomerular filtration rate and glomerular capillary hydrostatic pressure increased without a rise in afferent or efferent arteriolar flow rate.[36] Similar results were obtained in micropuncture studies in Munich-Wistar rats[37] and can be interpreted as afferent dilation accompanied by efferent constriction.

More recently, intravital microscopy of split hydronephrotic kidneys in anesthetized rats showed that ANP relaxed various preglomerular vessels, including the arcuate artery (25 μm), interlobular artery (12 μm), and afferent arterioles (6 to 7 μm), whereas it constricted the efferent arterioles (12 to 17 μm).[38] These observations are consistent with data obtained in isolated perfused kidneys,[33,35] the isolated perfused glomerulus,[36] and the exteriorized kidney.[37] In contrast, ANP failed to relax superficial afferent (25 μm) and efferent (10 μm) arterioles isolated from rabbit kidneys, regardless of whether the vessels were contracted with norepinephrine (afferent) or angiotensin II (efferent).[39] Incubation of ANP alone with isolated rat glomeruli had no effect on glomerular cross-sectional area, but abolished the glomerular contraction induced by incubation with angiotensin II and platelet activating factor.[40] Similarly, ANP(103—126), but not ANP(103—123), inhibited angiotensin II-induced contraction of cultured glomerular mesangial cells.[41] Glomerular contraction by angiotensin, presumably mediated by interaction of this peptide with specific receptors located on the contractile mesangial cells, might attenuate the glomerular filtration rate by decreasing the ultrafiltration coefficient. Conceivably, ANP could counteract this action if its antagonistic action on glomerular contraction is operative *in vivo*. Taken together, most of the data so far on the renal micro-vasculature suggest that ANP relaxes agonist-induced contractions of preglomerular vessels and the glomerulus itself, but has constrictor activity on postglomerular vessels.

2. Other than Renal

ANP infused into the brachial artery of humans caused increased forearm blood flow, as determined by venous occlusion plethysmography[42,43] and increased forearm skin flux, as measured by laser doppler flowmetry.[43] The local concentration of ANP required to induce a meaningful arterial vasodilatory response was estimated as either physiologically relevant[42] or, contrarily, as well in excess of the normal range.[43] Dorsal hand veins contracted with norepinephrine showed no detectable dilation in response to intravenous infusion of ANP in humans.[43] Similarly, intravenous infusion of ANP into patients with congestive heart failure failed to dilate forearm veins.[44] Thus, unlike the nitrates, ANP shows arterial, but not venous, dilation in the human forearm. However, these data did not reveal whether the vasodilation was confined to the skin or included vessels in skeletal muscle as well. Intraarterial infusion of ANP in the vertebral, common carotid, coronary, and femoral arteries in anesthetized dogs caused very little change in blood flow through these beds.[26] ANP applied in massive doses to isolated perfused mammalian hearts caused immediate coronary vasoconstriction.[45] However, in physiologic or pharmacologic concentrations ($10^{-10.4}$ to $10^{-6.4}$ M), ANP failed to alter coronary flow or the chronotropic and inotropic functions of the isolated perfused rat heart.[46] Furthermore, when delivered directly into the left circumflex coronary artery in open-chest, anesthetized dogs, ANP (0.05 to 5 μg) increased coronary flow transiently and did not cause coronary vasoconstriction.[47] Similar transient dilation of the left circumflex coronary artery was observed following injection of ANP via a left atrial catheter in awake, chronically instrumented dogs.[48] Therefore, it is unlikely that myocardial depression resulting from direct coronary vasoconstriction participates importantly in the pharmacological or physiological action of ANP *in vivo* (see below).

Addition of ANP to the bathing medium did not alter the contractile responses of 228-μm mesenteric arteries isolated from stroke-prone, spontaneously hypertensive rats or Wistar-Kyoto rats to norepinephrine, serotonin, prostaglandin $F_2\alpha$, or electrical stimulation, regardless of whether ANP was added before or after the agonist.[12] Nor did ANP affect the myogenic tone, vasomotion, contractile response to serotonin and prostaglandin $F_2\alpha$, or relaxation in response to electrical stimulation of 212-μm cerebral arteries isolated from the same strains of rats.[12] Furthermore, there was no evidence that ANP relaxed mesenteric second-, third-, or fourth-order arterioles in the exteriorized mesentery of anesthetized Wistar rats, as observed through an intravital microscope.[49] Indeed, infusion of ANP into the superior mesenteric artery lowered arterial blood pressure, decreased arteriolar red blood cell velocity, and caused a decrease in diameter of second-order arterioles.[49] ANP did, however, selectively reduce, but did not abolish, the constriction of isolated rat intestinal (60 μm) and skeletal muscle (25 μm) arterioles caused by angiotensin II.[10] The microcirculatory dilator action of ANP was selective in that no relaxation occurred in these vessels in the absence of agonist or in the presence of contractile doses of norepinephrine or arginine vasopressin.[10] This suggests that various agonists may induce contraction of vascular smooth muscle through separate mechanisms, some of which are antagonized by the action of ANP, whereas others are not. The selectivity of ANP to cause relaxation only in the angiotensin II-contracted microcirculation is in marked contrast to the effectiveness of ANP to antagonize the vaso-constriction induced by a variety of agonists in large, isolated vessels and isolated kidneys (see above). In any event, other than antagonizing the arteriolar constriction induced by angiotensin II, there is currently little direct evidence that ANP relaxes vessels in the microcirculation outside of the kidney.

3. Permeability

There is also a paucity of information with regard to possible direct effects of ANP on permeability in the microcirculation. Conflicting data have been reported with regard to the kidney. ANP increased the glomerular capillary ultrafiltration coefficient in the isolated perfused dog glomerulus,[36] but had no effect on this variable in surface glomeruli of Munich-Wistar rats.[37] ANP was found to increase single capillary hydraulic conductivity of isolated frog mesenteric vessels.[50] However, the concentration of ANP used in the frog study (10^{-5} M) was 100,000 times that of the upper physiological plasma level in rats (Table 1). Furthermore, studies utilizing intravital microscopy indicate that permeability changes me-diated by various vasoactive substances in the microvessels of mammals did not occur in the microvessels of frogs, suggesting different microcirculatory characteristics between warm-blooded and cold-blooded animals.[51] Intravital fluorescence microscopy of rat mesenteric microvessels demonstrated that ANP lacked histamine-like action.[49] That is, intravenous infusion of ANP lowered arterial blood pressure, but caused no extravasation of fluorescein-labeled albumin, whereas histamine caused immediate, massive vascular leakage.[49]

C. HEMODYNAMICS *IN VIVO*
1. Long-Term Effects

Continuous intravenous infusion of ANP into experimental animals for 5 to 7 d can produce a sustained hypotensive effect that is not initiated by urinary fluid and salt loss.[13,52-60] Knowledge about long-term cardiovascular effects of ANP is crucial to under-standing the importance of this hormone in regulating body fluid volume and arterial blood pressure and to the assessment of its potential as an analog for developing therapeutic agents. However, a number of questions still remain unanswered. For instance, the time course over several days of the hemodynamic actions (cardiac output vs. peripheral vascular resistance) of ANP has not been established. There are conflicting data with respect to the effectiveness of ANP to lower blood pressure during prolonged administration in normotensive subjects. Some studies indicate that ANP lowered blood pressure in hypertensive rats, but not in the normotensive controls,[13,53,54] whereas others report a hypotensive response in both.[55,56] ANP also decreased mean arterial pressure in normotensive dogs during a 5-d infusion.[52] Increased diuresis during prolonged infusion of ANP has been observed in some studies,[13,55,56] but not in others,[57-60] although most investigators believe that urinary fluid loss is not required for the hypotensive effect. There is no clear relationship between dose and plasma concentration of iANP during prolonged infusion and, thus, a meaningful relationship between iANP plasma concentration and response is unavailable. Perhaps part of the reason for the discordant data stems from methodological problems. Indirect blood pressure measurements in heated, restrained rats, the use of anesthesia for collecting blood samples, and intermittently removing animals from metabolic cages, thus interrupting urine collection, could introduce errors in the measurements. Uniform delivery of chemically intact peptide from implanted osmotic pumps also needs verification.

A 3-d infusion of ANP at 40 pmol·min⁻¹·kg⁻¹ attenuated the hypertension caused by infusion of norepinephrine,[57] angiotensin II,[58] or vasopressin.[59] This is similar to the indiscriminate relaxation by ANP of agonist-contracted large vessels *in vitro*[8] and of agonist-constricted vasculature in isolated kidneys.[33] Yet ANP relaxed intestinal and skeletal muscle arterioles (20 to 70 μm) *in vitro* only when contracted by angiotensin II and not by norepinephrine or vasopressin.[10] This suggests that the 3-d antihypertensive action of ANP was not mediated by blocking the action of these vasoconstrictors on arterioles in the intestine or skeletal muscle.

2. Short-Term Effects

Acute administration of ANP to man and lower forms of animals as intravenous bolus or continuous infusion in pharmacological doses usually, but not always, lowers arterial blood pressure. The hypotensive response to ANP is most often associated with decreased cardiac output and varied changes in total peripheral resistance; increased or unchanged cardiac output has also been observed.[61-65] The heart rate response to ANP is variable, with lowered heart rate frequently being observed.[66-68] Although infusion of ANP into humans usually causes hypotension and apparent reflex tachycardia,[69-71] occasionally some subjects develop a marked decrease in blood pressure with unchanged or slowed heart rate.[70] One of the most consistent effects of ANP, regardless of the directional change in cardiac output, is decreased cardiac filling pressure (central venous, right atrial, and left atrial pressures), which occurs in man and lower forms of animals under a variety of conditions, including consciousness, anesthesia, hypertension, and heart failure.[61-63,65,68] Decreased cardiac filling pressure can be observed without concurrent changes in other hemodynamic variables.[62,68] Except for the renal vascular bed, changes in regional hemodynamics after intravenous administration of ANP generally correspond to the systemic hemodynamic effects. For instance, under conditions whereby ANP causes diminished cardiac output, blood flows to most organs are similarly decreased and regional resistances increased.[61,72-74] However, the renal vascular response to the systemic infusion of ANP is quite variable and can be one of initial vasodilation, which either persists[27,75] or eventually converts to vasoconstriction associated with reduced renal blood flow.[31,70,71,74] The transient increase in renal blood flow, when it occurs, might be associated with a transient increase in cardiac output.[76,77] Infusion of ANP usually increases hematocrit and plasma protein concentration[62,68,70,71] and decreases plasma volume.[78,79] These changes can also be observed in acutely nephrectomized animals, suggesting enhanced net filtration of plasma fluid into the tissues.[78-81]

a. Factors Influencing Acute Hemodynamic Responses

There are few definite differences among mammalian species with respect to systemic hemodynamic responses to ANP. However, tachycardia seems to occur more often in conscious humans after ANP administration than in other awake species, which often display no change in or a slowed heart rate. On the other hand, dose, duration, and mode of administration of ANP are all important in determining the cardiovascular responses to this peptide. Bolus injection of ANP into conscious, spontaneously hypertensive rats resulted in

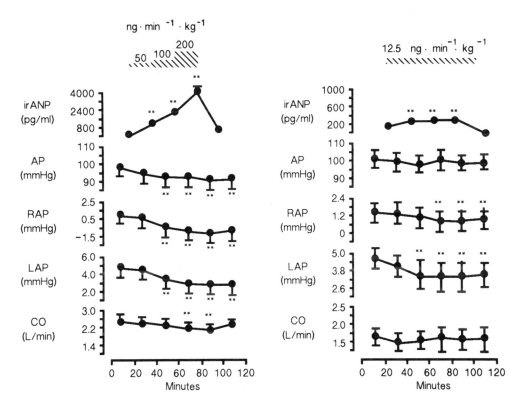

FIGURE 2. Effects of intravenous step-up (left side) and constant (right side) infusions of human ANP(99—126) in awake dogs. Dosage rates and periods of infusions of ANP are indicated at the top. Abbreviations: irANP, immunoreactive ANP plasma concentration; AP, aortic pressure; RAP, right atrial pressure; LAP, left atrial pressure; CO, cardiac output. (Data taken from Bie, P., Wang, B. C., Leadley, R. J., Jr., and Goetz, K. L., *Am. J. Physiol.*, 254, R161, 1988. With permission.)

marked, but transient (10 to 40 s), decreased renal vascular resistance and, at high doses, transient decreases in hindquarter and mesenteric vascular resistances.[82] A similar transient decrease in total peripheral resistance was observed in normotensive rats after bolus injection of ANP.[76] In contrast, continuous intravenous infusion of ANP often produces increases in regional[31,72,82] and systemic[68,72,83] vascular resistances. The duration of infusion is also critical when interpreting the dose-response effects of ANP. For example, when Bie et al.[68] infused ANP into conscious dogs in a "step-up" fashion at successive rates of 50, 100, and 200 ng·min^{-1}·kg^{-1} for 20 min at each dose, there were no significant hemodynamic changes during the 20-min period of the lowest dose (Figure 2, left side). However, when ANP was infused continuously at a given dose for 1 h, delayed, but significant, decreases in left and right atrial pressures occurred even at 12.5 ng·min^{-1}·kg^{-1} (Figure 2, right side). A similar time lag in the natriuretic and depressor actions of ANP have been observed in experimental animals[24,68] and in humans,[84,85] despite rapid attainment of plasma ANP plateau levels. These findings have certain implications with regard to mechanisms of action (see below), but also illustrate that when analyzing dose-related actions, it is important to carry out infusions of ANP long enough to allow various responses to develop.

The level of baseline blood pressure may determine to some extent the magnitude of the hypotensive response to ANP since blood pressure decreased more in spontaneously hypertensive rats than in normotensive Wistar-Kyoto rats.[86-88] However, this does not always hold true; patients with essential hypertension do not show a more sensitive hypotensive response to ANP than do normotensive subjects.[89,90] The mechanisms underlying the hypertension are probably more important in determining the hemodynamic response to ANP. For instance, rats with renin-dependent renal hypertension were more sensitive to the hypotensive action of ANP than the normotensive controls or rats with deoxycorticosterone (DOC)-salt hypertension.[91] This is consistent with the predilection of ANP for antagonizing vasoconstriction induced by angiotensin II *in vitro*, compared with other agonists.[9,10] Furthermore, whereas the DOC-salt hypertensive rats responded with marked decreases in cardiac output to the intermediate and high doses of ANP, the renal hypertensive animals showed a mixed hemodynamic response, with decreased total peripheral resistance during infusion of the intermediate dose and decreased cardiac output during infusion of the high dose of ANP.[91] Thus, at low doses, ANP preferentially caused peripheral vasodilation in the renin-dependent animals, but at high doses it caused a decrease in cardiac output. The level of circulating angiotensin II seems particularly important with respect to the renal hemodynamic response to ANP. ANP infusion into conscious rats usually increases renal vascular resistance,[72,82] but when administered to conscious rats receiving prolonged infusion of angiotensin II, ANP resulted in decreased renal vascular resistance.[92] In anesthetized dogs, the decrease in renal blood flow resulting from acutely infused angiotensin II was increased toward baseline level by superimposed infusion of ANP.[93] On the other hand, a high circulating level of angiotensin II does not appear to greatly alter the systemic vascular response to ANP outside of the kidney since pharmacologic doses of ANP still caused increased mesenteric vascular resistance in the angiotensin II-infused rats[92] and decreased cardiac output in the angiotensin-II-infused dogs.[93]

There is a striking difference in the hemodynamic response to ANP administration between patients with congestive heart failure and healthy subjects. Unlike the decreased cardiac output often observed in healthy experimental animals,[61] a consistent increase in cardiac output has been observed in patients with congestive heart failure after ANP administration.[62-65] ANP appears to have a prominent effect on cardiac afterload in these patients and thus improves cardiac performance by reducing peripheral vascular resistance. Since cardiac output increases in patients with congestive heart failure following ANP administration, venous return must also be increased and the lowering of cardiac filling pressure probably results in part from improved cardiac emptying against a reduced afterload.

b. Acute Circulatory Mechanisms

The overall hemodynamic response to pharmacologic doses of ANP is initiated by direct and indirect dilatory and constrictor actions on blood vessels, with the magnitude and type of response depending on dose and preexisting conditions.[61] Changes in cardiac function occur mostly indirectly via peripheral vascular actions and through an ANP-induced blunting of autonomic reflexes to the heart.[61,94] Although some of the factors influencing the cardiovascular response to ANP were discussed above, it is far from clear why in some situations ANP enhances cardiac output and decreases peripheral vascular resistance, while in others it suppresses cardiac output. A high level of circulating angiotensin II, as occurs in congestive heart failure and renin-dependent hypertension, might predispose the vasculature to the arteriolar dilatory action of ANP. However, as discussed above, in studies that examined the hemodynamic effects of ANP in rats[92] and dogs[93] receiving exogenous angiotensin II, vasodilation occurred only in the kidneys and cardiac output actually decreased.[93] Perhaps careful determination of dose-response relationships using continuous infusion of ANP for long enough durations for responses to fully develop will help determine the hemodynamic interactions of ANP with angiotensin II and other vasoactive hormones.

In any event, when ANP increases cardiac output, such as in congestive heart failure, it is apparent that the resistance-vessel dilatory action of the peptide predominates. The hemodynamic events that account for an ANP-induced decrease in cardiac output are less clear. Decreased cardiac filling pressure is one of the most consistent effects of ANP and it is evident that diminished venous return, rather than cardiac depression, is largely responsible for reducing the cardiac output.[61,94] ANP can decrease cardiac filling pressure at doses that have no measurable effects on arterial pressure, cardiac output (Figure 2, right side), or hematocrit.[68] suggesting that the decrease in cardiac filling pressure is a primary event and is not initiated by decreased blood volume resulting from diuresis or transfer of plasma fluid to the tissues.

Two hypotheses explaining the sequence of hemodynamic changes leading to diminished venous return and cardiac output following ANP administration are illustrated in Figure 3. According to the venodilator hypothesis (Figure 3B), the initial event is venodilation causing increased compliance of the capacitance vessels; this results in peripheral pooling and an immediate decrease in right atrial pressure. Increased urine output and extravasation of plasma fluid due to increased capillary permeability cause blood volume to contract and right atrial pressure to decline further. Cardiac output then diminishes, lowering arterial volume and arterial pressure. Finally, unloading of the cardiopulmonary and arterial baroreceptors leads to a reflex increase in total peripheral resistance. The major criticism of the venodilator hypothesis is the lack of evidence that ANP increases circulatory compliance *in vivo*. Indeed, studies in man,[43,44] dogs,[96] and rats[76,78,79] indicate that ANP does not dilate capacitance vessels (Figure 4). Furthermore, if the venodilation was also manifested as decreased postcapillary resistance, capillary hydrostatic pressure would be lowered, favoring net absorption and resulting in decreased hematocrit and plasma protein concentration. But, in fact, ANP usually decreases plasma volume, increases plasma protein concentration, and increases hematocrit.[62,68,70,71,78-81] These observations are incompatible with the proposed venodilation and increased capillary permeability.

According to the venoconstrictor hypothesis (Figure 3C), the initial event following ANP administration is increased postcapillary resistance resulting from either a direct action of the peptide on venous smooth muscle or from activation of an endogenous venoconstrictor.[61,78,83,94] The increased resistance to venous return causes an immediate slowing of blood flow into the right atrium and lowers cardiac filling pressure. Increased postcapillary resistance also raises capillary hydrostatic pressure, which enhances net capillary filtration or retards net absorption (depending on the amount of fluid loss through diuresis).[79] A decrease in blood volume causes a further lowering of cardiac filling pressure and diminishes cardiac output, arterial volume, and arterial pressure. A reflex increase in arteriolar resistance ensues, causing a further increase in total peripheral resistance. The venoconstrictor hypothesis is compatible with the ANP-induced increase in plasma protein concentration and hematocrit, but its major drawback is the lack of direct evidence for increased postcapillary resistance and increased capillary hydrostatic pressure, other than in the kidney. However, few studies on the effects of ANP in the microcirculation have been aimed at such information. Finally, it is possible that a more sophisticated concept of the circulation, such as the two-compartment, parallel circuit model,[95] will be required to explain the hemodynamic actions of ANP. However, change in cardiac output distribution among organs with different resistance-capacitance characteristics does not appear to be a prominent effect of ANP.[83,94]

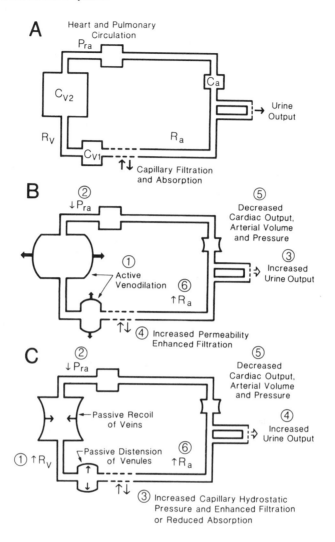

FIGURE 3.   (A) Model of the circulation showing resistances and compliances in series. Pra, right atrial pressure; Ca, precapillary compliance (arterial); Ra, precapillary resistance (arterial); Cv1, postcapillary compliance (venous); Rv, postcapillary resistance (venous); Cv2, postcapillary compliance (venous). The precise anatomic structures corresponding to Cv1 and Cv2 are unclear. (Modified from Gow, B. S., *Handbook of Physiology,* Vol. 2, American Physiological Society, Bethesda, 1977, 353.) (B) Venodilator hypothesis of ANP-induced decreased cardiac output. (1) Venodilation and increased compliance of capacitance vessels initiates diminished venous return, causing (2) decreased Pra. (3) Increased urinary fluid loss and (4) extravasation of plasma fluid due to increased capillary permeability cause a further decline in venous return and eventually (5) diminish cardiac output, arterial volume, and arterial pressure. Unloading of the baroreceptors leads to reflex (6) increased peripheral vascular resistance. (C) Venoconstrictor hypothesis of ANP-induced decreased cardiac output. (1) Increased postcapillary resistance traps a small volume of blood in the microcirculation, causing (2) decreased Pra and (3) increased capillary hydrostatic pressure. Decreased blood volume resulting from (4) increased urinary fluid loss and enhanced capillary filtration cause a further decline in venous return. (5) Cardiac output, arterial volume, and arterial pressure decrease, unloading the baroreceptors. A reflex (6) increase in arteriolar resistance leads to a further increase in peripheral vascular resistance.

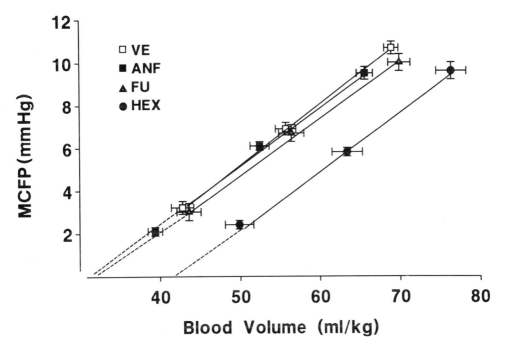

FIGURE 4. Mean circulating filling pressure (MCFP) — blood volume relationship in anesthetized rats infused with vehicle: VE (0.9% sodium chloride, 0.02 ml/min); rat ANP(99—126), ANF (0.5 $\mu g\cdot min^{-1}\cdot kg^{-1}$); furosemide, FU (10 $\mu g/min^{-1}\cdot kg^{-1}$); or hexamethonium, HEX (0.5 $mg\cdot min^{-1}\cdot kg^{-1}$). MCFP was measured from arterial and central venous pressures during brief circulatory arrest effected by inflating a balloon in the right atrium. MCFP and blood volume were determined at baseline and immediately after infusing or withdrawing 5 ml of blood. Compared with VE, the ganglionic blocking agent, HEX, displaced the MCFP-blood volume relationship toward the volume axis ($p < 0.01$); this indicated venodilation. No displacement of this relationship and, hence, no indication of venodilation was observed during ANF or FU infusion. (From Trippodo, N. C. and Barbee, R. W., *Am. J. Physiol.*, 252, R915, 1987. With permission.)

REFERENCES

1. Report of the Joint Nomenclature and Standardization Committee of the International Society of Hypertension, the American Heart Association, and the World Health Organization, *Hypertension*, 10, 461, 1987.
2. **Douglas, W. W.**, Histamine and 5-hydroxytryptamine (serotonin) and their antagonists, in *The Pharmacological Basis of Therapeutics*, Gilman, A. G., Goodman, L. S., Rall, T. W. and Murad, F., Eds., Macmillan, New York, 1985, 605.
3. **Toda, N.**, Mechanism of histamine actions in human coronary arteries, *Circ. Res.*, 61, 280, 1987.
4. **Grega, G. J., Adamski, S. W., and Dobbins, D. E.**, Physiological and pharmacological evidence for the regulation of permeability, *Fed. Proc.*, 45, 96, 1986.
5. **Emerson, T. E., Jr.**, Effects of acetylcholine, histamine, and serotonin infusion on venous return in dogs, *Am. J. Physiol.*, 215, 41, 1968.
6. **Van Nueten, J. M.**, 5-Hydroxytryptamine and precapillary vessels, *Fed. Proc.*, 42, 223, 1983.
7. **Grega, G. J. and Adamski, S. W.**, Patterns of constriction produced by vasoactive agents, *Fed. Proc.*, 46, 270, 1987.
8. **Winquist, R. J.**, Pharmacologic effects of atrial natriuretic peptide, *Endocrinol. Metab. Clin. N. Am.*, 16, 163, 1987.
9. **Kleinert, H. D., Maack, T., Atlas, S. A., Januszewicz, A., Sealey, J. E., and Laragh, J. H.**, Atrial natriuretic factor inhibits angiotensin-, norepinephrine-, and potassium-induced vascular contractility, *Hypertension*, 6 (Suppl. 1), 143, 1984.
10. **Proctor, K. G. and Bealer, S. L.**, Selective antagonism of hormone-induced vasoconstriction by synthetic atrial natriuretic factor in the rat microcirculation, *Circ. Res.*, 61, 42, 1987.

11. **Aalkjaer, C., Mulvany, M. J., and Nyborg, N. C. B.,** Atrial natriuretic factor causes specific relaxation of rat renal arcuate arteries, *Br. J. Pharmacol.,* 86, 447, 1985.

12. **Osol, G., Halpern, W., Tesfamariam, B., Nakayama, K., and Weinberg, D.,** Synthetic atrial natriuretic factor does not dilate resistance-sized arteries, *Hypertension,* 8, 606, 1986.

13. **De Mey, J. G., Defreyn, G., Lenaers, A., Calderon, P., and Roba, J.,** Arterial reactivity, blood pressure, and plasma levels of atrial natriuretic peptides in normotensive and hypertensive rats: effects of acute and chronic administration of atriopeptin III, *J. Cardiovasc. Pharmacol.,* 9, 525, 1987.

14. **Winquist, R. J., Faison, E. P., and Nutt, R. F.,** Vasodilator profile of synthetic atrial natriuretic factor, *Eur. J. Pharmacol.,* 102, 169, 1984.

15. **Cohen, M. L. and Schenck, K. W.,** Atriopeptin II: differential sensitivity of arteries and veins from the rat, *Eur. J. Pharmacol.,* 108, 103, 1985.

16. **Jansen, T. L. Th. A., Morice, A. H., and Brown, M. J.,** A comparison of the vasodilator response to atrial peptides in the pulmonary and renal arteries of the pig *in vitro, Br. J. Pharmacol.,* 91, 687, 1987.

17. **Ishikawa, N., Hayakawa, A., Uematsu, T., and Nakashima, M.,** Heterogeneity in vasorelaxant effects of α-human atrial natriuretic polypeptide in the dog, *Jpn. J. Pharmacol.,* 44, 515, 1987.

18. **Winquist, R. J.,** The relaxant effects of atrial natriuretic factor on vascular smooth muscle, *Life Sci.,* 37, 1081, 1985.

19. **Emmick, J. T. and Cohen, M. L.,** Aging and vasodilation to atrial peptides, *Clin. Exp. Theory Pract.,* A8(1), 75, 1986.

20. **Nutt, R. F. and Veber, D. F.,** Chemical synthesis and structure-activity relations for ANF analogues, *Endocrinol. Metab. Clin. N. Am.,* 16, 19, 1987.

21. **de Leon, H., Castaneda-Hernandez, G., and Hong, E.,** Decreased ANF atrial content and vascular reactivity to ANF in spontaneous and renal hypertensive rats, *Life Sci.,* 41, 341, 1987.

22. **Chien, Y. W., Barbee, R. W., MacPhee, A. A., Frohlich, E. D., and Trippodo, N. C.,** Increased ANF secretion after volume expansion is preserved in rats with heart failure, *Am. J. Physiol.,* 254, R185, 1988.

23. **Gutkowska, J., Genest, J., Thibault, G., Garcia, R., Larochelle, P., Cusson, J. R., Kuchel, O., Hamet, P., De Lean, A., and Cantin, M.,** Circulating forms and radioimmunoassay of atrial natriuretic factor, *Endocrinol. Metab. Clin. N. Am.,* 16, 183, 1987.

24. **Barbee, R. W. and Trippodo, N. C.,** The contribution of atrial natriuretic factor to acute volume natriuresis in rats, *Am. J. Physiol.,* 253, F1129, 1987.

25. **Hirooka, Y., Takeshita, A., Imaizumi, T., Nakamura, N., Tomoike, H., and Nakamura, M.,** Effects of α-human atrial natriuretic peptide on the interrelationship of arterial pressure, aortic nerve activity, and aortic diameter, *Circ. Res.,* 63, 987, 1988.

26. **Ishihara, I., Aisaka, K., Hattori, K., Hamasaki, S., Morita, M., Noguchi, T., Kangawa, K., and Matsuo, H.,** Vasodilatory and diuretic actions of α-human atrial natriuretic polypeptide (α-hANP), *Life Sci.,* 36, 1205, 1985.

27. **Wakitani, K., Cole, B. R., Geller, D. M., Currie, M. G., Adams, S. P., Fok, K. F., and Needleman, P.,** Atriopeptins: correlation between renal vasodilation and natriuresis, *Am. J. Physiol.,* 249, F49, 1985.

28. **Yukimura, T., Ito, K., Takenaga, T., Yamamoto, K., Kangawa, K., and Matsuo, H.,** Possible tubular site of action in anesthetized dogs of a synthetic α-human atrial natriuretic polypeptide, *J. Pharmacol. Exp. Ther.,* 238, 707, 1986.

29. **Burnett, J. C., Jr., Granger, J. P., and Opgenorth, T. J.,** Effects of synthetic atrial natriuretic factor on renal function and renin release, *Am. J. Physiol.,* 247, F863, 1984.

30. **Oshima, T., Currie, M. C., Geller, D. M., and Needleman, P.,** An atrial peptide is a potent renal vasodilator substance, *Circ. Res.,* 54, 612, 1984.

31. **Smits, J. F. M., van Essen, H., Struyker-Boudier, H. A. J., and Lappe, R. W.,** Lack of renal vasodilation during intrarenal infusion of synthetic atriopeptin II in conscious intact SHR, *Life Sci.,* 38, 81, 1986.

32. **Lappe, R. W., Todt, J. A., and Wendt, R. L.,** Mechanism of action of vasoconstrictor responses to atriopeptin II in conscious SHR, *Am. J. Physiol.,* 249, R781, 1985.

33. **Camargo, M. J. F., Kleinert, H. D., Atlas, S. A., Sealey, J. E., Laragh, J. H., and Maack, T.,** Ca-dependent hemodynamic and natriuretic effects of atrial extract in isolated rat kidney, *Am. J. Physiol.,* 246, F447, 1984.

34. **Murray, R. D., Itoh, S., Inagami, T., Misono, K., Seto, S., Scicli, A. G., and Carretero, O. A.,** Effects of synthetic atrial natriuretic factor in the isolated perfused rat kidney, *Am. J. Physiol.,* 249, F603, 1985.

35. **Wakitani, K., Currie, M. G., Geller, D. M., and Needleman, P.,** Vasodilator properties of a family of bioactive atrial peptides in isolated perfused rat kidneys, *J. Lab. Clin. Med.,* 105, 349, 1985.

36. **Fried, T. A., McCoy, R. N., Osgood, R. W., and Stein, J. H.,** Effect of atriopeptin II on determinants of glomerular filtration rate in the in vitro perfused dog glomerulus, *Am. J. Physiol.,* 250, F1119, 1986.

37. **Dunn, B. R., Ichikawa, I., Pfeffer, J. M., Troy, J. L., and Brenner, B. M.,** Renal and systemic hemodynamic effects of synthetic atrial natriuretic peptide in the anesthetized rat, *Circ. Res.,* 59, 237, 1986.

38. **Marin-Grez, M., Fleming, J. T., and Steinhausen, M.,** Atrial natriuretic peptide causes pre-glomerular vasodilatation and post-glomerular vasoconstriction in rat kidney, *Nature (London),* 324, 473, 1986.

39. **Edwards, R. M. and Weidley, E. F.,** Lack of effect of atriopeptin II on rabbit glomerular arterioles in vitro, *Am. J. Physiol.,* 252, F317, 1987.

40. **Barrio, V., De Arriba, G., Lopez-Novoa, J. M., and Rodriguez-Puyol, D.,** Atrial natriuretic peptide inhibits glomerular contraction induced by angiotensin II and platelet activating factor, *Eur. J. Pharmacol.,* 135, 93, 1987.

41. **Appel, R. G., Wang, J., Simonson, M. S., and Dunn, M. J.,** A mechanism by which atrial natriuretic factor mediates its glomerular actions, *Am. J. Physiol.,* 251, F1036, 1986.

42. **Bolli, P., Muller, F. B., Linder, L., Raine, A. E. G., Resink, T. J., Erne, P., Kiowski, W., Ritz, R., and Buhler, F. R.,** The vasodilator potency of atrial natriuretic peptide in man, *Circulation,* 75, 221, 1987.

43. **Webb, D., Benjamin, N., Allen, M., Brown, J., and Cockcroft, J.,** Atrial natriuretic peptide is a weak arteriolar dilator in the human forearm with no effect on dorsal hand veins, *Clin. Sci.,* 73 (Suppl. 17), 38p, 1987.

44. **Ikenouchi, H., Sato, H., Serizawa, T., Iizuka, M., and Sugimoto, T.,** Alpha human atrial natriuretic polypeptide has no venodilating effect in congestive heart failure patients, *Circulation,* 76 (Suppl. 4), 72, 1987.

45. **Wangler, R. D., Breuhaus, B. A., Otero, H. O., Hastings, D. A., Holzman, M. D., Saneii, H. H., Sparks, H. V., Jr., and Chimoskey, J. E.,** Coronary vasoconstrictor effects of atriopeptin II, *Science,* 230, 558, 1985.

46. **Burnett, J. C., Jr., Rubanyi, G. M., Edwards, B. S., Schwab, T. R., Zimmerman, R. S., and Vanhoutte, P. M.,** Atrial natriuretic peptide decreases cardiac output independent of coronary vasoconstriction, *Proc. Soc. Exp. Biol. Med.,* 186, 313, 1987.

47. **Bauman, R. P., Rembert, J. C., Himmelstein, S. I., Klotman, P. E., and Greenfield, J. C., Jr.,** Effect of atrial natriuretic factor on transmural myocardial blood flow distribution in the dog, *Circulation,* 76, 705, 1987.

48. **Chu, A. and Cobb, F. R.,** Effects of atrial natriuretic peptide on proximal epicardial coronary arteries and coronary blood flow in conscious dogs, *Circ. Res.,* 61, 485, 1987.

49. **Smits, J., le Noble, J., van Essen, H., and Slaaf, D.,** Microcirculatory effects of synthetic atrial natriuretic factor (hANF; WY 47,663) in rat mesentery, *Fed. Proc.,* 46, 1142, 1987.

50. **Huxley, V. H., Tucker, V. L., Verburg, K. M., and Freeman, R. H.,** Increased capillary hydraulic conductivity induced by atrial natriuretic peptide, *Circ. Res.,* 60, 304, 1987.

51. **Taylor, A. E. and Granger, D. N.,** Exchange of macromolecules across the microcirculation, in *Handbook of Physiology — The Cardiovascular System,* Vol. 4, American Physiological Society, Bethesda, MD, 1977, 467.

52. **Granger, J. P., Opgenorth, T. J., Salazar, J., Romero, J. C., and Burnett, J. C., Jr.,** Long-term hypotensive and renal effects of atrial natriuretic peptide, *Hypertension,* 8 (Suppl. 2), 112, 1986.

53. **Garcia, R., Cantin, M., Genest, J., Gutkowska, J., and Thibault, G.,** Body fluids and plasma atrial peptide after its chronic infusion in hypertensive rats, *Proc. Soc. Exp. Biol. Med.,* 185, 352, 1987.

54. **Forslund, T., Tikkanen, T., Tikkanen, I., and Fyhrquist, F.,** Effect of separate and simultaneous infusions of atrial natriuretic peptide (ANP) and angiotensin II (A II) on blood pressure in rats, in Program 2nd World Congr. Biologically Active Atrial Peptides, New York, May 16 to 21, 1987, 215.

55. **Kondo, K., Kida, O., Sasaki, A., Kato, J., and Tanaka, K.,** Natriuretic effect of chronically administered α-human atrial natriuretic polypeptide in sodium depleted or repleted conscious spontaneously hypertensive rats, *Clin. Exp. Pharmacol. Physiol.,* 13, 417, 1986.

56. **Kida, O., Kondo, K., and Tanaka, K.,** Natriuretic and hypotensive effects of chronically administered α-human atrial natriuretic polypeptide in sodium-deplete or replete conscious spontaneously hypertensive rats, *J. Hypertens.,* 4 (Suppl. 6), S529, 1986.

57. **Yasujima, M., Abe, K., Kohzuki, M., Tanno, M., Kasai, Y., Sato, M., Omata, K., Kudo, K., Tsunoda, K., Takeuchi, K., Yoshinaga, K., and Inagami, T.,** Atrial natriuretic factor inhibits the hypertension induced by chronic infusion of norepinephrine in conscious rats, *Circ. Res.,* 57, 470, 1985.

58. **Yasujima, M., Abe, K., Kohzuki, M., Tanno, M., Kasai, Y., Sato, M., Omata, K., Kudo, K., Takeuchi, K., Hiwatari, M., Kimura, T., Yoshinaga, K., and Inagami, T.,** Effect of atrial natriuretic factor on angiotensin II-induced hypertension in rats, *Hypertension,* 8, 748, 1986.

59. **Yasujima, M., Abe, K., Kohzuki, M., Tanno, M., Kasai, Y., Sato, M., Omata, K., Kudo, K., Takeuchi, K., and Yoshinaga, K.,** Antihypertensive effect of synthetic atrial natriuretic factor in vasopressin-infused rats, *Jpn. Circ. J.,* 50, 1185, 1986.

60. **Kohzuki, M., Abe, K., Yasujima, M., Tanno, M., Kasai, Y., Sato, M., Omata, K., Kudo, K., Takeuchi, K., and Yoshinaga, K.,** Chronic effect of a synthetic atrial natriuretic factor on the development of hypertension in young spontaneously hypertensive rats, *J. Hypertens.,* 4 (Suppl. 3), S487, 1986.

61. **Trippodo, N. C., Cole, F. E., MacPhee, A. A., and Pegram, B. L.,** Biologic mechanisms of atrial natriuretic factor, *J. Lab. Clin. Med.,* 109, 112, 1987.

62. **Cody, R. J., Atlas, S. A., Laragh, J. H., Kubo, S. H., Covit, A. B., Ryman, K. S., Shaknovich, A., Pondolfino, K., Clark, M., Camargo, M. J. F., Scarborough, R. M., and Lewicki, J. A.,** Atrial natriuretic factor in normal subjects and heart failure patients. Plasma levels and renal, hormonal, and hemodynamic responses to peptide infusion, *J. Clin. Invest.,* 78, 1362, 1986.

63. **Crozier, I. G., Ikram, H., Gomez, H. J., Nicholls, M. G., Espiner, E. A., and Warner, N. J.,** Haemodynamic effects of atrial peptide infusion in heart failure, *Lancet,* 2, 1242, 1986.

64. **Riegger, G. A. J., Kromer, E. P., and Kochsiek, K.,** Human atrial natriuretic peptide: plasma levels, hemodynamic, hormonal, and renal effects in patients with severe congestive heart failure, *J. Cardiovasc. Pharmacol.,* 8, 1107, 1986.

65. **Saito, Y., Nakao, K., Nishimura, K., Sugawara, A., Okumura, K., Obata, K., Sonoda, R., Ban, T., Yasue, H., and Imura, H.,** Clinical application of atrial natriuretic polypeptide in patients with congestive heart failure: beneficial effects on left ventricular function, *Circulation,* 76, 115, 1987.

66. **Allen, D. E. and Gellai, M.,** Cardioinhibitory effect of atrial peptide in conscious rats, *Am. J. Physiol.,* 252, R610, 1987.

67. **Baum, T., Sybertz, E. J., Watkins, R. W., Nelson, S., Coleman, W., Pula, K. K., Prioli, N., Rivelli, M., and Grossman, A.,** Hemodynamic actions of a synthetic atrial natriuretic factor, *J. Cardiovasc. Pharmacol.,* 8, 898, 1986.

68. **Bie, P., Wang, B. C., Leadley, R. J., Jr., and Goetz, K. L.,** Hemodynamic and renal effects of low-dose infusions of atrial peptide in awake dogs, *Am. J. Physiol.,* 254, R161, 1988.

69. **Richards, A. M., Ikram, H., Yandle, T. G., Nicholls, M. G., Webster, M. W. I., and Espiner, E. A.,** Renal, haemodynamic, and hormonal effects of human alpha atrial natriuretic peptide in healthy volunteers, *Lancet,* 1, 545, 1985.

70. **Weidmann, P., Hasler, L., Gnadinger, M. P., Lang, R. E., Uehlinger, D. E., Shaw, S., Rascher, W., and Reubi, F. C.,** Blood levels and renal effects of atrial natriuretic peptide in normal man, *J. Clin. Invest.,* 77, 734, 1986.

71. **Ishii, M., Sugimoto, T., Matsuoka, H., Ishimitsu, T., Atarashi, K., Hirata, Y., Sugimoto, T., Kangawa, K., and Matsuo, H.,** Blood pressure, renal and endocrine responses to α-human atrial natriuretic polypeptide in healthy volunteers, *Jpn. Heart J.,* 27, 777, 1986.

72. **Lappe, R. W., Smits, J. F. M., Todt, J. A., Debets, J. J. M., and Wendt, R. L.,** Failure of atriopeptin II to cause arterial vasodilation in the conscious rat, *Circ. Res.,* 56, 606, 1985.

73. **Pegram, B. L., Kardon, M. B., Trippodo, N. C., Cole, F. E., and MacPhee, A. A.,** Atrial extract: hemodynamics in Wistar-Kyoto and spontaneously hypertensive rats, *Am. J. Physiol.,* 249, H265, 1985.

74. **Biollaz, J., Waeber, B., Nussberger, J., Porchet, M., Brunner-Ferber, F., Otterbein, E. S., Gomez, H. J., and Brunner, H. R.,** Atrial natriuretic peptides: reproducibility of renal effects and response of liver blood flow, *Eur. J. Clin. Pharmacol.,* 31, 1, 1986.

75. **Kimura, T., Abe, K., Shoji, M., Tsunoda, K., Matsui, K., Ota, K., Inoue, M., Yasujima, M., and Yoshinaga, K.,** Effects of human atrial natriuretic peptide on renal function and vasopressin release, *Am. J. Physiol.,* 250, R789, 1986.

76. **Trippodo, N. C., Kardon, M. B., Pegram, B. L., Cole, F. E., and MacPhee, A. A.,** Acute haemodynamic effects of the atrial natriuretic hormone in rats, *J. Hypertens.,* 4 (Suppl. 2), S35, 1986.

77. **Shapiro, J. T., DeLeonardis, V. M., Needleman, P., and Hintze, T. H.,** Integrated cardiac and peripheral vascular response to atriopeptin 24 in conscious dogs, *Am. J. Physiol.,* 251, H1292, 1986.

78. **Trippodo, N. C., Cole, F. E., Frohlich, E. D., and MacPhee, A. A.,** Atrial natriuretic peptide decreases circulatory capacitance in areflexic rats, *Circ. Res.,* 59, 291, 1986.

79. **Trippodo, N. C. and Barbee, R. W.,** Atrial natriuretic factor decreases whole-body capillary absorption in rats, *Am. J. Physiol.,* 252, R915, 1987.

80. **Fluckiger, J. P., Waeber, B., Matsueda, G., Delaloye, B., Nussberger, J., and Brunner, H. R.,** Effect of atriopeptin III on hematocrit and volemia of nephrectomized rats, *Am. J. Physiol.,* 251, H880, 1986.

81. **Almeida, F. A., Suzuki, M., and Maack, T.,** Atrial natriuretic factor increases hematocrit and decreases plasma volume in nephrectomized rats, *Life Sci.,* 39, 1193, 1986.

82. **Lappe, R. W., Todt, J. A., and Wendt, R. L.,** Hemodynamic effects of infusion versus bolus administration of atrial natriuretic factor, *Hypertension,* 8, 866, 1986.

83. **Chien, Y. W., Frohlich, E. D., and Trippodo, N. C.,** Atrial natriuretic peptide increases resistance to venous return in rats, *Am. J. Physiol.,* 252, H894, 1987.

84. **Biollaz, J., Callahan, L. T., Nussberger, J., Waeber, B., Gomez, H. J., Blaine, E. H., and Brunner, H. R.,** Pharmacokinetics of synthetic atrial natriuretic peptides in normal men, *Clin. Pharmacol. Ther.,* 41, 671, 1987.

85. **Anderson, J. V., Donckier, J., Payne, N. N., Beacham, J., Slater, J. D. H., and Bloom, S. R.,** Atrial natriuretic peptide: evidence of action as a natriuretic hormone at physiological plasma concentrations in man, *Clin. Sci.,* 72, 305, 1987.

86. **Gellai, M., DeWolf, R. E., Kinter, L. B., and Beeuwkes, R., III,** The effect of atrial natriuretic factor on blood pressure, heart rate, and renal functions in conscious, spontaneously hypertensive rats, *Circ. Res.,* 59, 56, 1986.

87. **Pang, S. C., Hoang, M.-C., Tremblay, J., Cantin, M., Garcia, R., Genest, J., and Hamet, P.,** Effect of natural and synthetic atrial natriuretic factor on arterial blood pressure, natriuresis and cyclic GMP excretion in spontaneously hypertensive rats, *Clin. Sci.,* 69, 721, 1985.

88. **Marks, E. S., Zukowska-Groject, Z., Ropchak, T., and Keiser, H. R.,** Alterations in systemic haemodynamics induced by atriopeptin III, *J. Hypertens.,* 5, 39, 1987.

89. **Richards, A. M., Nicholls, M. G., Espiner, E. A., Ikram, H., Yandle, T. G., Joyce, S. L., Cullens, M. M.,** Effects of α-human atrial natriuretic peptide in essential hypertension, *Hypertension,* 7, 812, 1985.

90. **Ishii, M., Sugimoto, T., Matsuoka, H., Hirata, Y., Ishimitsu, T., Fukui, K., Sugimoto, T., Kanagawa, K., and Matsuo, H.,** A comparative study on the hemodynamic, renal and endocrine effects of α-human atrial natriuretic polypeptide in normotensive persons and patients with essential hypertension, *Jpn. Circ. J.,* 50, 1181, 1986.

91. **Volpe, M., Sosa, R. E., Muller, F. B., Camargo, M. J. F., Glorioso, N., Laragh, J. H., Maack, T., and Atlas, S. A.,** Differing hemodynamic responses to atrial natriuretic factor in two models of hypertension, *Am. J. Physiol.,* 250, H871, 1986.

92. **Lappe, R. W., Todt, J. A., and Wendt, R. L.,** Effects of atrial natriuretic factor on the vasoconstrictor actions of the renin-angiotensin system in conscious rats, *Circ. Res.,* 61, 134, 1987.

93. **Edwards, B. S., Schwab, T. R., Zimmerman, R. S., Heublein, D. M., Jiang, N.-S., and Burnett, J. C., Jr.,** Cardiovascular, renal, and endocrine response to atrial natriuretic peptide in angiotensin II mediated hypertension, *Circ. Res.,* 59, 663, 1986.

94. **Trippodo, N. C.,** Increased resistance to venous return: postulate for atrial natriuretic factor-induced decrease in cardiac preload, in *Biologically Active Atrial Peptides,* Vol. 1, Brenner, B. M. and Laragh, J. H., Eds., Raven Press, New York, 1987, 81.

95. **Gow, B. S.,** Circulatory correlates: vascular impedance, resistance, and capacity, in *Handbook of Physiology, Vol. 2,* American Physiological Society, Bethesda, 1977, 353.

96. **Holtz, J., Stewart, D. J., Elsner, D., and Bassenge, E.,** In vivo atrial peptide-venodilation: minimal potency relative to nitroglycerin in dogs, *Life Sci.,* 39, 2177, 1986.

Chapter 10

ATRIAL NATRIURETIC PEPTIDE AND THE RENIN-ANGIOTENSIN SYSTEM

Tadashi Inagami, Mitsuhide Naruse, and Kazuo Shizume

TABLE OF CONTENTS

I. INTRODUCTION

The recent discovery of atrial natriuretic peptide (ANP) or atrial natriuretic factor (ANF) from mammalian atrial tissue has attracted many investigators in various fields and has provoked an enormous quantity of research which attempts to assess its physiological significance. It has been well established that this novel peptide is a circulating hormone which causes potent diuresis, natriuresis, vasorelaxation, and changes in renal hemodynamics. Another intriguing aspect of this peptide is its interactions with other endocrine systems involved in the maintenance of homeostasis, especially that of the renin-angiotensin-aldosterone system which exerts major control over blood pressure and electrolyte homeostasis. Laragh[1] overviewed this issue and proposed that ANP has a major complementary role in the long-term regulation of blood pressure and electrolyte homeostasis through its counteraction against the renin-angiotensin system. This hypothesis is of great interest and of potential importance in view of the integrity of the regulatory system for maintaining body fluid volume and blood pressure homeostasis. Great controversies, however, still exist in this context.

The effects of ANP on the renin-angiotensin system have two major aspects: (1) antagonism of angiotensin II actions and (2) inhibition of renin secretion. ANP has been reported to antagonize both angiotensin II-induced vascular contraction and aldosterone secretion. ANP was also demonstrated to block the central action of angiotensin II, dipsogenic action, pressure response, and vasopressin secretion. Such interactions of ANP with angiotensin II actions have been discussed elsewhere. On the other hand, no recognizable interaction with other components of the renin-angiotensin system (i.e., angiotensinogen, angiotensin-converting enzyme, and angiotensinases) have been reported. Thus, the main focus of this review is the effect of ANP on renin secretion.

II. EFFECTS OF ANP ON RENIN SECRETION *IN VIVO*

Results of *in vivo* studies in animals and in humans are summarized in Tables 1 and 2, respectively. The earlier *in vivo* work of Atlas et al.,[2] Burnett et al.,[3] and Maack et al.[4] demonstrated that synthetic rat ANP suppresses plasma renin activity and/or the renin secretion rate in anesthetized, normal dogs. Similar ANP action was reported by subsequent studies in anesthetized control dogs, those with acute low output failure,[5] and conscious control dogs,[6] dogs with chronic heart failure by inferior vena cava constriction,[7] and those with coarctation of the aorta.[8] This ANP action was shown to be dose-dependent[6,7] and reversible.[2-4,6,7] However, contradicting observations were also reported in which ANP acutely decreased renin secretion, either in anesthetized[9] or conscious[7,10] control dogs, although there was a slight tendency of renin secretion to fall.[7,9] Sosa et al.[11] also found that ANP does not affect renin secretion in dogs with acute unilateral renal artery constriction.

In addition, a significant decrease in plasma renin activity was observed by the long-term infusion of ANP into conscious rats with saralasin-sensitive (therefore, renin-angiotensin dependent) hypertension: two-kidney, one-clip (2K, 1C) hypertensive rats,[12-14] and sodium-depleted, one-kidney, one-clip (1K, 1C) hypertensive rats.[15] Plasma renin activity was unaffected by the identical infusion of ANP by identical protocols into control rats[12,13,15-20] (saralasin-resistant 2K, 1C hypertensive rats[14,15,17,18] or sodium-repleted 1K, 1C hypertensive rats[15,17,18]). These results seem to imply that ANP-induced inhibition of renin release is more pronounced in the high renin state. Inhibition of plasma renin activity observed in the aforementioned dog experiments[2-5] and in control rats[21] may be related to the preactivated renin state under anesthesia.

In contrast to the results of the long-term experiment by Garcia et al.,[12-14] Volpe et al.[15,17,18] showed that acute administration of ANP produced a further increase in the already

TABLE 1

Effect of ANP on Plasma Renin Activity (PRA) and/or Renin Secretion Rate (RSR) in Experimental Animals

Species	Anesthesia (+, −)/ type of treatment[a]	Administration of ANP				Changes in renin(%)[c]		Ref.
		Peptide	Dose	Duration	Route[b]	PRA	RSR	
Dog	+, Normal	rANP(102—125)	0.1 μg/kd·min	40 min	i.v.	↓(41)	↓(71)	2
	+, Normal	rANP(101—126)	0.3 μg/kg·min	45 min	i.r.a.		↓(94)	3
	+, Normal	rANP(102—125)	1 μg/kg + 0.1 μg/kg·min	60 min	i.v.	↓(69)	↓(72)	4
	−, Normal Chronic caval constriction	rANP(99—126)	0.175, 0.35 μg/kg·min	30 min	i.v.	NC ↓(42)		7
	+, Nonfiltering kidney	rANP(101—126)	0.3 μg/kg·min		i.r.a.		NC	44
	+, Normal Acute low output, heart failure	rANP(101—126)	0.3 μg/kg·min	45 min	i.r.a.		↓(86) ↓(82)	5
	+, Normal	rANP(101—126)	1.2 to 156 pmol/kg·min	10 min	i.r.a.	NC	NC	9
	+, Acute renal artery constriction	rANP(102—125)	2 μg/kg + 0.3 μg/kg·min	30 min	i.v.	NC	NC	11
	−, Normal	rANP(103—126)	3 μg/kg·min	30 min	i.v.	NC		10
	+, Filtering kidney Nonfiltering kidney	rANP(101—126)	0.3 μg/kg·min	45 min	i.r.a.	↓(84)		45
	−, Normal	rANP(101—126) hANP(99—126)	50 to 200 pmol/kg·min 100 pmol/kg·min	20 min	i.v.	NC		6
	+, Filtering kidney Nonfiltering kidney	rANP(99—126)	2 μg/kg + 0.2, 0.4 μg/kg·min	20 min	i.v., i.r.a.	↓(57) ↓(75) ↓(81) ↓(77)		47
	+, Nonfiltering kidney	rANP(101—126)	0.3 μg/kg·min	18 min	i.r.a.	NE, NC prosta.		46
	−, Coarctation of the aorta	rANP(99—126)	5 ng/kg·min	120 min	i.v.	↓(?)		8
Rat	−, Normal	rANP(101—126)	50 ng/min	30 min	i.v.	NC		16
	−, 1K or 2K sham 1K,1C 2K,1C saral. resist. saral. resp.	rANP(102—125)	2 μg/kg + 0.3 μg/kg·min	60 min	i.v.	NC NC NC ↑(65, 39)		15, 17, 18
	−, 2K,1C sham 2K,1C	rANP(101—126)	1 μg/h	7 d	i.v.	NC ↓(79)		12
	−, Normal	hANP(99—126)	0.17, 0.67 μg/kg·min	30 min	i.v.	NC		19

TABLE 1 (continued)
Effect of ANP on Plasma Renin Activity (PRA) and/or Renin Secretion Rate (RSR) in Experimental Animals

Species	Anesthesia (+,−)/ type of treatment[a]	Administration of ANP				Changes in renin(%)[c]		Ref.
		Peptide	Dose	Duration	Route[b]	PRA	RSR	
	+, Normal	rANP(99—126)	8 µg/kg		i.v.	↓(49)		21
	−, 1K,1C, sodium depleted	rANP(101—125)	2 µg/kg + 0.3 µg/kg·min	60 min	i.v.	↓(36)		15
	−, 2K,1C sham	rANP(101—126)	35 pmol/h	13 d	i.v.	NC		13
	2k,1C					↓(57)		
	−, Normal	rANP(103—126)	1 µg/min	30 min	i.v.	NC		20
	−, 2K,1C saral. resist. saral. resp.	rANP(101—126)	0.1 µg/h	6 d	i.v.	NC ↓(66)		14

a Sham, sham operation; 1K,1C, one-kidney, one-clip Goldblatt hypertension; 2K,1C, two-kidney, one-clip Goldblatt hypertension; saral. resist., saralasin resistant; saral. resp., saralasin responsive.

b i.v., intravenous; i.r.a., intra renal artery.

c NC, not changed; NE, norepinephrine; prosta., prostacyclin.

TABLE 2
Effect of ANP on Plasma Renin Activity (PRA) in Humans

Subjects[a]	Salt intake and posture[b]	Administration of ANP Peptide	Dose	Duration	Changes in PRA[c] (%)	Ref.
Normal	10, 200 mmol/d	hANP(99—126)	3 µg/min	60 min	NC	28
Normal	r	hANP(99—126)	0.025 to 0.1 µg/kg·min	20 min	↑(121)	38
EH	120 mmol/d, s	hANP(99—126)	100 µg		NC	35
Normal	120 mmol/d, s	hANP(99—126)	100 µg		NC	29
Normal	Usual diet, r	hANP(99—126)	125 ng/kg + 0.05 µg/kg·min	30 min	NC	30
Normal	Usual diet, r + 5 g/d	rANP(101—126)	0.5, 5 µg/min	4 h	NC	31
Normal	Usual diet, s	rANP(102—126)	0.1 µg/kg·min	60 min	↓(34)	25
CHF	10, 100 mmol/d				↓(26)	
CHF	80 mmol/d, r	rANP(101—126)	5 µg/min	4 h	NC	36
Normal	200 mmol/d, s	hANP(99—126)	200 µg/h	60 min	↓(?)	26
	10 mmol/d				↓(30)	
Normal	8 to 10 g/d, r	hANP(99—126)	0.025 to 0.1 µg/kg·min	20 min	↑(133)	39
Normal	12 g/d, r	hANP(99—126)	0.1 µg/kg·min	20 min	NC	32
Normal	Usual diet, s	hANP(99—126)	1.5, 15 pmol/kg·min	30 min	↓(12)	27
Normal	Usual diet, r + 3 g/d	hANP(99—126)	175 to 775 µg	6 h	NC*	33
Normal	17 mmol/d, r	hANP(99—126)	50 µg + 0.1 µg/kg·min	45 min	↑(53—96)	40
	140 mmol/d					
	310 mmol/d					
EH	Usual diet, r	hANP(99—126)	50 µg + 0.1 µg/kg·min	45 min	↑(90)	41
Normal	Usual diet, r	hANP(99—126)	50 µg + 6.25 µg/min	45 min	NC	34
CHF	r	hANP(99—126)	0.1 µg/kg·min	30 min	NC	37

[a] EH, essential hypertension; CHF, congestive heart failure.

[b] s, sitting; r, recumbent.

[c] NC, not changed; *, plasma renin concentration.

elevated plasma renin activity of saralasin-responsive 2K, 1C hypertensive rats. Acute reduction of renal perfusion pressure secondary to the decrease in systemic blood pressure (as well as a failure of ANP to increase sodium load in the ischemic kidney) could increase renin secretion. Concurrently, direct stimulation of renin secretion by ANP cannot be ruled out.[22] Although the antagonism by ANP of AII feedback inhibition of renin secretion should be taken into account, *in vitro* studies using rat kidney slices do not support this possibility.[23,24]

Human studies provide a further inconsistency in results. ANP has been reported to suppress plasma renin activity in normal subjects[25-27] and, to a lesser extent, in patients with congestive heart failure.[25] It was reported not to affect plasma renin activity in normal subjects,[28-34] in patients with essential hypertension,[35] and in patients with congestive heart failure.[36,37] This failure to show suppression of renin secretion in normal subjects could be ascribed to the supine position[30-34] and/or salt loading.[31,33] Under these conditions, plasma renin is already relatively suppressed and is probably too low for ANP to show a further depressor effect. Attenuated suppression of renin in patients with congestive heart failure[23,35] might be attributed to the attenuated renal response to ANP since inhibition of renin secretion by ANP has been postulated to depend on the renal responsiveness to ANP.[11,15,18] In addition, it was even reported to stimulate plasma renin activity in normal subjects[38-40] and in patients with essential hypertension.[41]

These varied results may not contradict each other. Administration of a high dose of ANP elicits a marked fall in systemic arterial pressure, baroreceptor-mediated reflex augmentation of sympathetic activity, and volume contraction associated with diuresis and natriuresis. All of these effects trigger the release of renin.[42,43] Therefore, the renin secretion rate and plasma renin levels are possibly determined by the cumulative effect of various opposing ANP actions. Unchanged plasma renin activity may result from the counterbalancing of both inhibitory and stimulatory effects, whereas increased plasma renin activity may indicate that the stimulatory effect (secondary to the hemodynamic effects of ANP) is exceeding its inhibitory effect on renin secretion. Implicitly, ANP might have precluded a greater rise in plasma renin activity through its inhibitory action on renin secretion. Supporting this view, infusion of a lower dose of ANP (which elicits a change of plasma ANP levels within a physiological range, but does not have any marked effect on systemic hemodynamics) was demonstrated to suppress plasma renin activity.[8,27] In addition, an increase in plasma renin activity was observed during the recovery phase after ANP infusion, which strongly suggests that ANP nevertheless had an inhibitory effect on its secretion.[7,9,31]

These explanations still do not completely account for the different results seen among these studies (particularly, human studies). One possible explanation is the different experimental conditions employed. As shown in Tables 1 and 2, at least six different kinds of synthetic ANP-related peptides have been used with varying routes of administration and dosage. Additionally, the sodium status and the activity of the renin-angiotensin system (under which each study was performed) varied from study to study. Yet a discrepancy appears to exist among the results in which similar experimental protocols have been used. The exact explanation for this difference is not available presently.

III. MECHANISM OF ANP-INDUCED INHIBITION OF RENIN SECRETION

The mechanism by which ANP suppresses renin secretion and plasma renin activity remains unclear. ANP supposedly enhances the delivery of sodium chloride to the *macula densa* by increasing the filtered load of sodium and/or decreasing proximal tubular reabsorption, as estimated from the increased fractional lithium excretion.[5] It is well known that increased tubular delivery of sodium chloride to the *macula densa* decreases renin release.[42,43]

Thus, early observations in dogs[2-4] have led to the hypothesis that ANP inhibits renin secretion through the *macula densa*-mediated mechanism. Subsequently, Opgenorth et al.[44,45] found that continuous intrarenal infusion of ANP inhibits renin secretion in the intact filtering kidney (in which urinary sodium excretion was significantly increased), but not in the nonfiltering kidney (in which no such functional *macula densa* exists). It was also found that intrarenal infusion of ANP failed to alter either basal, norepinephrine- or prostacyclin-induced renin release in the nonfiltering dog kidneys.[46] Adenosine (known to directly inhibit renin secretion) retained its action in the nonfiltering model.[45,46] All these results support the *macula densa* as an important contributor to ANP inhibition in renin secretion.

In contrast, Villarreal et al.[47] reported that both intravenous and intrarenal arterial infusion of similar doses of ANP resulted in a marked inhibition of renin secretion in dogs with a single denervated, nonfiltering kidney, as well as in dogs with filtering kidneys; this suggests that an increase in the sodium load to the *macula densa* is not an indispensable mechanism for the ANP-induced suppression of renin secretion. Suppressed plasma renin activity (in the absence of increased urinary sodium excretion[7,14,27]) is in agreement with this concept. Infusions of ANP produced a sustained increase in renal blood flow.[2-4,9,44,47] Since the dilatation of renal afferent arterioles would be expected to elicit an inhibitory signal from the renal vascular receptor to inhibit renin release,[42] the interaction of ANP with the renal vascular receptor might possibly mediate the ANP action. This is further supported by the finding that ANP failed to decrease renin secretion from the kidney with renal artery constriction.[11] An alternative explanation for the suppression of renin release is a direct action by ANP on the juxtaglomerular cells. In support of this, the inhibitory effect of ANP on renin release was demonstrated in the isolated perfused rat kidney[48] by Narumi et al.

IV. EFFECTS OF ANP ON RENIN RELEASE *IN VITRO*

Studies reporting the effect of ANP on renin release *in vitro* are summarized in Table 3. We investigated the effect of ANP on renin release from rat kidney slices *in vitro*. ANP inhibited both basal and isoproterenol-induced renin release in a dose-dependent fashion, which suggested a direct action by ANP on the juxtaglomerular cells.[21] Moreover, ANP does not have an apparent general toxic effect on juxtaglomerular cells since the kidney tissue, which had been preincubated with 10^{-6} M ANP for 90 min and then washed, retained its ability to respond to isoproterenol to an extent similar to that of the control. Specificity of this ANP action on renin secretion was first verified by the pretreatment of ANP solution with anti-ANP antiserum at 4°C overnight, which completely abolished this effect.

Furthermore, we have investigated the structure-activity relationship of this ANP action (Table 4).[49] The effect of ANP disappeared when ANP was pretreated by dithiothreitol, indicating that the ring structure formed by the disulfide linkage between the two cysteine residues in the ANF molecule is essential for biological activity. The activity of hANP(99—126) was equivalent to that of rANP(99—126), whereas hANP(99—126) sulfoxide was devoid of activity. Deletion of amino acids at the amino-terminal end, such as rANP(103—126) and rANP(102—126), only slightly affected the action. In contrast, further removal of amino acids at the carboxy-terminal end, such as rANP(103—123) and rANP(105—121), decreased the inhibitory effect. ANP peptides without ring structure, such as rANP(99—109) and rANP(116—126), were devoid of activity. In addition, inhibition of renin release by hANP(99—126) was attenuated by the concomitant addition of its sulphoxide compound. These structure-activity relationships of ANP in inhibiting renin release are basically well in agreement with those reported for natriuresis and vasorelaxation, which gives further evidence supporting the specificity of this ANP action.

Supporting our findings, Henrich et al.[50,51] demonstrated that ANP inhibits renin release induced by isoproterenol, forskolin, or dibutyril cAMP from rat kidney slices *in vitro*. A

TABLE 3
Effect of ANP on Renin Release *In Vitro*

Species[a]	Methods		ANP		Effects[b]		Ref.
	Sampling	Tissue preparation	Peptide	Dose			
Rat	SD Decapitation	Kidney slice	Atriopeptin	1000 ng	Isop.	→	50
					Forskolin	→	
	W Decapitation	Kidney slice	rANP(99—126)	ID_{50} 5.8 × 10⁻⁸ M	Basal	→	21
	SD Decapitation	Kidney slice	rANP(103—126)	10⁻⁹ to 10⁻⁶ M	Isop.	→	23
					Basal	NC	
					AII	potentiation	
	SD Decapitation	Kidney slice	rANP(103—126)	2.09 × 10⁻⁸ M	Isop.	→	51
					Forskolin	→	
					dbcAMP	→	
	SD Ether	Kidney slice	rANP(102—126)	10⁻⁶ M	Basal	→	22
	SD Ether	Cultured JG cells	rANP(101—126)	10⁻¹³ to 10⁻⁹ M	Basal	←	53
	W Ether	Isolated glomeruli	rANP(101—126)	3 × 10⁻⁶ to 10⁻¹² M	Basal	NC	56
Monkey	CO₂ narcosis	Kidney slice	rANP(103—126)	2 × 10⁻⁸ M	Isop.	→	52

[a]   W, Wistar; SD, Sprague-Dawley rats.

[b]   Isop., isoproterenol; AII, angiotensin II; dbcAMP, dibutyril cAMP; NC, not changed.

TABLE 4
Structure-Activity Relationship of ANP on Renin, cAMP, and cGMP Release

ANP-related peptides	Percent of basal release		
	Renin	cAMP	cGMP
	100	100	100
rANP(99—126)	63 ± 4[a]	57 ± 5[a]	323 ± 18[a]
(102—126)	71 ± 5[a]	67 ± 5[a]	337 ± 25[a]
(103—126)	69 ± 4[a]	62 ± 4[a]	352 ± 15[a]
(103—125)	68 ± 5[a]	62 ± 7[a]	326 ± 25[a]
(103—123)	81 ± 5[b]	58 ± 4[a]	350 ± 23[a]
(105—121)	82 ± 6[b]	65 ± 5[a]	271 ± 25[a]
(99—109)	105 ± 2	100 ± 4	104 ± 3[a]
(116—126)	102 ± 3	104 ± 3	103 ± 2[a]
hANP(99—126)	68 ± 2[a]	61 ± 6[a]	323 ± 17[a]
(99—126) sulfoxide	109 ± 5	76 ± 6[a]	183 ± 27[a]

Note: Values are the mean ± SE.

[a] $p < 0.01$ vs. control.
[b] $p < 0.05$ vs. control.

similar action of ANP on renin release was reported in the primate kidney.[52] This possible direct action of ANP on juxtaglomerular cells was further substantiated by studies using partially purified rat juxtaglomerular cells in culture.[53] Although the reason for the difference in ED_{50} for ANP in the inhibition of renin secretion[21,50,51,53] is not clear, it could be attributed, at least in part, to the varying tissue preparations utilized. The sliced rat kidney tissue contains a large number of tubular and glomerular cells, as well as juxtaglomerular cells. This heterogeneity of cell components and the thickness of the tissues prepared might cause difficulties for ANP in reaching the juxtaglomerular cells, which could result in the requirement for higher concentrations of ANP in order to exhibit its biological activities.

Regardless of the variations in the reported effective dosages of ANP, all these studies suggest that ANP inhibits renin secretion through its direct action on the juxtaglomerular cells. Nevertheless, indirect effects through the coexisting nephron elements cannot be completely excluded since ANP has been shown to produce certain biological actions in the renal tubular cells.[54,55] A lack of inhibitory action of ANP on renin secretion from isolated rat glomeruli[56] may result from the possible involvement of an indirect mechanism of tubular components.

Contrasting results have also been reported using similar rat kidney slice experiments.[22,23] Antonipillai et al.[23] have shown that ANP did not inhibit either basal or isoproterenol-induced renin release, whereas it potentiated angiotensin II-induced inhibition of renin secretion in doses as low as $10^{-9} M$. Furthermore, a rather high concentration of ANP ($10^{-6} M$) increased renin release.[22] Presently, there is no explanation for these conflicting results. Differences in the ANP peptides utilized and/or of rat strains may account, at least in part, for this. Additionally, under certain circumstances the presence of anesthesia will affect the secretory response of the juxtaglomerular cells to various stimuli.[43] Ether anesthesia used during the surgical procedure, therefore, might have affected the mode of renin secretory patterns in response to ANP.[22]

The above-mentioned structure-activity relationship of ANP suggests that ANP acts on renin release through its receptor binding. No definite evidence for the presence of ANP receptor sites has been reported in the juxtaglomerular cells, although specific binding sites for ANP have been found in both the glomeruli and the vascular wall of the kidney.[57,58]

Since immunoreactive ANP has been detected in the kidney tissue by radioimmunoassay,[59] we have applied the immunohistochemical technique (by the avidin-biotin complex method) to investigate ANP binding sites in rat kidney. ANP immunoreactivity was observed in the juxtaglomerular cells and vascular wall of arterioles, including vas afferens and vas efferens, the vascular wall of the interlobular arteries, and arcuate arteries of the rat kidney after administration of synthetic rat ANP.[60] This result suggests possible receptor sites of ANP in the juxtaglomerular cells, although specificity of the finding requires further investigation.

An immunohistochemical study using anti-ANP receptor antiserum raised against purified bovine lung ANP receptor showed immunoreactive materials in the kidney glomeruli and the epithelial cells of the collecting tubules, but failed to show staining in the juxtaglomerular cells and in any of the vascular structure.[61] Further studies concerning the ANP receptor in the juxtaglomerular cells are required to confirm the proposed direct action of ANP on renin release.

V. INTRACELLULAR MECHANISM OF ANP ACTION ON RENIN RELEASE

The intracellular mechanism through which ANP inhibits renin release is also controversial. We have shown that the inhibition of renin release *in vitro* is accompanied by changes in the release of cyclic nucleotides (i.e., a decrease of cAMP and an increase of cGMP) (Table 4).[21] In addition, ANP was shown to inhibit renin release when coupled to cAMP stimuli, such as isoproterenol,[21,51] forskolin, and dibutyryl cAMP.[51] Since cAMP is known to facilitate renin release,[43] it is suggested that the renin-inhibitory effect of ANP is mediated at least in part, by the change in cAMP production.

On the other hand, cyclic GMP has been reported either to stimulate or not to have any influence on renin release.[43] At the same time, sodium nitroprusside, which also increases cGMP levels by activating guanylate cyclase, does not affect renin release.[22] These results suggest that increased cGMP may not have an important role in the inhibition of renin release by ANP. Conversely, Kurtz et al.[53] produced evidence for a causal link between cGMP and inhibition of renin release by ANP: (1) the ANP-induced increase of cGMP levels parallels the inhibition of renin, (2) inhibition of cGMP-phosphodiesterase leads to an increase in cGMP levels and an increase in the ANP sensitivity of the juxtaglomerular cells in the inhibition of renin release, whereas inhibition of guanylate cyclase activity elicits opposite effects, and (3) sodium nitroprusside produces elevated levels of cGMP in juxtaglomerular cells and inhibits renin release simultaneously. These results suggest that ANP also inhibits renin release by a cGMP-dependent mechanism.

ANP has been known to activate guanylate cyclase in the renal tubular cells. Therefore, it cannot be completely dismissed that the cGMP produced by ANP in other nephron segments indirectly affects renin secretion. As shown in Table 4, hANP(99—126) sulfoxide did not affect renin release, although it affected the release of cAMP and cGMP. This discrepancy between renin release and production of the cyclic nucleotides may indicate the involvement of yet unknown additional factors in its intracellular mechanism.

Another important signal of intracellular events is cytosolic calcium. An increase in the cytosolic calcium is a well-known inhibitory signal for renin release from the juxtaglomerular cells.[43] Antonipillai et al.[23] suggested an involvement of the intracellular calcium-calmodulin-mediated steps in the ANP action on renin release, based on the observation that ANP potentiates angiotensin II-induced inhibition in such release. We, however, did not see any potentiation — only an additive effect on the angiotensin II action on the renin release.[24] Furthermore, it was found that ANP inhibits renin release even in a calcium-free medium.[16] This was further supported by the fact that the increase in renin release induced by agents which lower intracellular calcium concentrations was not blocked by the addition of ANP.[51]

Neither the influx of ^{45}Ca into the cells nor the intracellular quin-2 signal (which is a measure for changes of intracellular Ca concentration) was affected by ANP in cultured juxtaglomerular cells.[53] Taken together, these results suggest that the actions of ANP on renin release do not seem to be a calcium-dependent process, as these *in vitro* studies indicate.

VI. PHYSIOLOGIC ASPECTS OF THE INHIBITION OF RENIN RELEASE BY ANP

To date, the physiological significance of the "ANP-induced inhibition of renin release" has not been clarified. However, renin release from partially purified juxtaglomerular cells *in vitro* was inhibited at concentrations as low as 10^{-13} to 10^{-11} M,[53] which is well within the physiological range of reported plasma ANP concentrations. Correspondingly, the infusion of small doses of ANP (1.5 pmol/kg/min, which increases plasma ANP by 8 ± 3 pmol/l) caused a significant fall in plasma renin activity[27] without concomitant changes in blood pressure, heart rate, or urinary sodium excretion in man.[62] A similar dose of ANP (5 ng/kg/min, which increased plasma ANP only by 34.8 pg/ml) was also shown to attenuate elevations in plasma renin activity when renal perfusion pressure is reduced in conscious dogs in the absence of any change of systemic hemodynamics (i.e., blood pressure, heart rate, atrial pressure, or renal perfusion pressure).[8] Based on data obtained at such low levels of ANP, it would appear that inhibition of renin secretion by ANP could occur under such physiological conditions.

One common way to prove the physiological role of a circulating hormone is to block its production and/or action. Since a specific antagonist which would block the ANP action has not been available, we have applied the passive immunization technique for this purpose. The intravenous administration of anti-ANP antiserum caused a significant increase of plasma renin activity (as well as a significant reduction of urine output and urinary sodium excretion in anesthetized rats),[63] whereas no such change was observed following the injection of normal rabbit serum. This increase in plasma renin activity observed by neutralizing the circulating ANP by antibody provides further evidence supporting the physiological significance of the inhibitory action of ANP on renin release.

The inhibition of renin secretion is expected to lead to a diminished formation of angiotensin II. In fact, a decreased plasma angiotensin II concentration and a concomitant reduced plasma renin activity has been observed during ANP infusions.[26] This decreased plasma angiotensin II could be responsible, at least in part, for the suppression of aldosterone secretion,[2,4,7,13-15,18,25,26] in addition to its direct effects on the adrenal cortex and the vascular wall. No definite evidence has been obtained to support the actual function of a renin inhibitory mechanism in the regulation of vascular resistance and aldosterone secretion.

VII. SUMMARY

Conflicting results have been documented in various aspects of the interrelationship between ANP and renin as to whether ANP inhibits renin secretion and as to the mechanisms (intracellular and physiological) of ANP action on renin secretion. Therefore, additional studies are required to give a definite answer to these problems. Yet it seems to be reasonably safe to state that various evidence (which was obtained under well-defined physiological conditions) supports the intriguing thesis that ANP inhibits renin secretion. This ANP action seems to be more enhanced in a high-renin condition. The inhibition of renin secretion (hence, a decrease in plasma angiotensin II concentration) may contribute to a modulation of aldosterone secretion and vascular resistance — an intriguing hypothesis which deserves further evaluation.

It is reasonable to believe that this ANP action is mediated through its renal vascular actions, the *macula densa* mechanism, and the direct action on the juxtaglomerular cells, although effects secondary to the hemodynamic changes by ANP (i.e., reduction of systemic blood pressure and volume contraction) could counterbalance the inhibitory effect. Thus, plasma renin activity could be unchanged or even increased in different settings.

A trend for an inverse correlation has been reported between plasma renin activity and plasma ANP levels within their diurnal rhythm,[64,65] during volume loading,[66] under different sodium intake,[67] and under immersion-induced central hypervolemia.[68] All these findings further support the close and important interrelationship between ANP and the renin-angiotensin-aldosterone system. Studies of the interaction between these two major regulatory systems with counteracting effects are expected to provide good models for further understanding the hierarchy of the endocrine control of electrolytes and blood pressure homeostasis.

REFERENCES

1. **Laragh, J. H.,** Atrial natriuretic hormone, the renin-aldosterone axis, and blood pressure-electrolyte homeostasis, *N. Engl. J. Med.,* 313, 1330, 1985.
2. **Atlas, S. A., Marion, D., Kelinert, H. D., Camarho, M. J., Laragh, J. H., Vaughan, E. D., and Maack, T.,** Inhibition of aldosterone and renin release by synthetic atrial natriuretic factor (ANF), *Circulation,* 70 (Suppl. 2) (Abstr.), 332, 1984.
3. **Burnett, J. C., Jr., Granger, J. P., and Opgenorth, T. J.,** Effects of synthetic atrial natriuretic factor on renal function and renin release, *Am. J. Physiol.,* 247, F863, 1984.
4. **Maack, T., Marion, D. N., Camargo, M. J. F., Kleinert, H. D., Largh, J. H., Vaughan, E. D., Jr., and Atlas, S. A.,** Effects of auriculin (atrial natriuretic factor) on blood pressure, renal function, and the renin-aldosterone system in dogs, *Am. J. Med.,* 77, 1069, 1984.
5. **Scriven, T. A. and Burnett, J. C., Jr.,** Effects of synthetic atrial natriuretic peptide on renal function and renin release in acute experimental heart failure, *Circulation,* 72, 892, 1985.
6. **Seymour, A. A., Smith, S. G., Mazack, E. K., and Blaine, E. H.,** A comparison of synthetic rat and human atrial natriuretic factor in conscious dogs, *Hypertension,* 8, 211, 1986.
7. **Freeman, R. H., Davis, J. O., and Vari, R. C.,** Renal response to atrial natriuretic factor in conscious dogs with caval constriction, *Am. J. Physiol.,* 248, R495, 1985.
8. **Scheuer, D. A., Thrasher, T. N., Quillen, E. W., Jr., Mtzler, C. H., and Ramsay, D. J.,** Atrial natriuretic peptide blocks renin response to renal hypotension, *Am. J. Physiol.,* 251, R423, 1987.
9. **Seymour, A. A., Blaine, E. H., Mazack, E. K., Smith, S. G., Stabilito, I. I., Haley, A. B., Napier, M. A., Whinnery, M. A., and Nutt, R. F.,** Renal and systemic effects of synthetic atrial natriuretic factor, *Life Sci.,* 36, 33, 1985.
10. **Goetz, K. L., Wang, B. C., Geer, P. G., Sundet, W. D., and Needleman, P.,** Effects of atriopeptin infusion versus effects of left atrial stretch in awake dogs, *Am. J. Physiol.,* 250, R221, 1986.
11. **Sosa, R. E., Volpe, M., Marion, D. N., Glorioso, N., Laragh, J. H., Vaughan, E. D., Jr., Maack, T., and Atlas, S. A.,** Effect of atrial natriuretic factor on renin secretion, plasma renin and aldosterone in dogs with acute unilateral renal artery constriction, *J. Hypertens.,* 3 (Suppl. 3), S299, 1985.
12. **Garcia, R., Thibault, G., Gutkowska, J., Hamet, P., Cantin, M., and Genest, J.,** Effect of chronic infusion of synthetic atrial natriuretic factor (ANF 8-33) in conscious two-kidney, one-clip, hypertensive rats, *Proc. Soc. Exp. Biol. Med.,* 178, 155, 1985.
13. **Garcia, R., Thibault, G., Gutkowska, J., and Cantin, M.,** Effect of chronic infusion of atrial natriuretic factor on plasma and urinary aldosterone, plasma renin activity, blood pressure and sodium excretion in 2-K, 1-C hypertensive rats, *Clin. Exp. Hypertens.,* A8(7), 1127, 1986.
14. **Garcia, R., Gutkowska, J., Cantin, M., and Thibault, G.,** Renin dependency of the effect of chronically administered atrial natriuretic factor in two-kidney, one-clip rats, *Hypertension,* 9, 88, 1987.
15. **Volpe, M., Odell, G., Kleinert, H. D., Müller, F., Camargo, M. J., Laragh, J. H., Maack, T., Vaughan, E. D., Jr., and Atlas, S. A.,** Effect of atrial natriuretic factor on blood pressure, renin, and aldosterone in Goldblatt hypertension, *Hypertension,* 7 (Suppl. 1), 43, 1985.
16. **Chartier, L., Schiffrin, E., Thibault, G., and Garcia, R.,** Atrial natriuretic factor inhibits the stimulation of aldosterone secretion by angiotensin II, ACTH and potassium in vitro and angiotensin II, ACTH and potassium in vitro and angiotensin II-induced steroidogenesis in vivo, *Endocrinology,* 115, 2026, 1984.

17. **Volpe, M., Kleinert, H. D., Camargo, M. J., Lewicki, J. A., Laragh, J .H., Maack, T., Vaughan, E. D., Jr., and Atlas, S. A.,** Blood pressure and aldosterone reduction by synthetic atrial natriuretic factor (ANF) in renin-dependent renovascular hypertension, *Hypertension,* 6 (Abstr.), 783, 1984.

18. **Volpe, M., Odell, G., Kleinert, H. D., Camargo, M. J., Laragh, J. H., Lewicki, J. A., Maack, T., Vaughan, E. D., Jr., and Atlas, S. A.,** Antihypertensive and aldosterone-lowering effects of synthetic atrial natriuretic factor in renin-dependent renovascular hypertension, *J. Hypertens.,* 2 (Suppl. 3), 313, 1984.

19. **Hirata, Y., Ishii, M., Matsuoka, H., Sugimoto, T., Ishimitsu, T., Sugimoto, T., Kanagawa, K., and Matsuo, H.,** Effects of α-human natriuretic polypeptide (α-hANP) on plasma renin and aldosterone concentration in rats — comparison with effects of furosemide (Fr)-, *Jpn. Circ. J.,* 49 (Abstr.), 752, 1985.

20. **Flückiger, J. P., Waeber, B., Nussberger, J., Matsueda, G., and Brunner, H. R.,** Effect of indomethacin and propranolol on the blood pressure and renin response to atriopeptin III in conscious rats, *Regul. Peptides,* 17, 277, 1987.

21. **Obana, K., Naruse, M., Naruse, K., Sakurai, H., Demura, H., Inagami, T., and Shizume, K.,** Synthetic rat atrial natriuretic factor inhibits *in vitro* and *in vivo* renin secretion in rats, *Endocrinology,* 117, 1282, 1985.

22. **Hiruma, M., Ikemoto, F., and Yamamoto, R.,** Rat atrial natriuretic factor stimulates renin release from renal cortical slices, *Eur. J. Pharmacol.,* 125, 151, 1986.

23. **Antonipillai, I., Vogelsang, J., and Horton, R.,** Role of atrial natriuretic factor in renin release, *Endocrinology,* 119, 318, 1986.

24. **Naruse, M., Naruse, K., Demura, H., Inagami, T., and Shizume, K.,** unpublished data, 1987.

25. **Cody, R. J., Atlas, S. A., Laragh, J. H., Kubo, S. H., Covit, A. B., Ryman, K. S., Shaknovich, A., Pondolfino, J., Clark, M., Camargo, M. J. F., Scarborough, R. M., and Lewicki, J. A.,** Atrial natriuretic factor in normal subjects and heart failure patients, *J. Clin. Invest.,* 78, 1362, 1986.

26. **Cuneo, R. C., Espiner, E. A., Nicholls, M. G., Yandle, T. G., Joyce, S. L., and Gilchrist, N. L.,** Renal, hemodynamic, and hormonal responses to atrial natriuretic peptide infusions in normal man, and effect of sodium intake, *J. Clin. Endocrinol. Metab.,* 63, 946, 1986.

27. **Struthers, A. D., Anderson, J. V., Payne, N., Causon, R. C., Slater, J. D. H., and Bloom, S. R.,** The effect of atrial natriuretic peptide on plasma renin activity, plasma aldosterone, and urinary dopamine in man, *Eur. J. Clin. Pharmacol.,* 31, 223, 1986.

28. **Espiner, E. A., Crozier, I. G., Nicholls, M. G., Cuneo, R., Yandle, T. G., and Ikram, H.,** Cardiac secretion of atrial natriuretic peptide, *Lancet,* 2, 398, 1985.

29. **Richards, A. M., Nicholls, M. G., Ikram, H., Webster, M. W. I., Yandle, T. G., and Espiner, E. A.,** Renal, hemodynamic, and hormonal effects of human alpha atrial natriuretic peptide in health volunteers, *Lancet,* 1, 545, 1985.

30. **Tikkanen, I., Fyhrquist, F., Metsärinne, K., and Leidenius, R.,** Plasma atrial natriuretic peptide in cardiac diseases and during infusion in healthy volunteers, *Lancet,* 2, 66, 1985.

31. **Biollaz, J., Nussberger, J., Porchet, M., Brunner-Ferber, F., Otterbein, E. S., Gomez, H., Waeber, B., and Brunner, H. R.,** Four-hour infusions of synthetic atrial natriuretic peptide in normal volunteers, *Hypertension,* 8 (Suppl. 2), 96, 1986.

32. **Ohashi, M., Fujio, N., Kato, K., Nawata, N., Ibayashi, H., and Matsuo, H.,** Effect of human α-atrial natriuretic polypeptide on adrenocortical function in man, *J. Endocrinol.,* 110, 287, 1986.

33. **Waldhäusl, W., Vierhapper, H., and Nowotny, P.,** Prolonged administration of human atrial natriuretic peptide in healthy men: evanescent effects on diuresis and natriuresis, *J. Clin. Endocrinol. Metab.,* 62, 956, 1986.

34. **Weidmann, P., Hasler, L., Gnädinger, M. P., Lang, R. E., Uehlinger, D. E., Shaw, S., Rascher, W., and Reubi, F. C.,** Blood levels and renal effects of atrial natriuretic peptide in normal man, *J. Clin. Invest.,* 77, 734, 1986.

35. **Richards, A. M., Nicholls, M. G., Espiner, E. A., Ikram, H., Yandle, T. G., Joyce, S. L., and Cullens, M. M.,** Effects of α-human atrial natriuretic peptide in essential hypertension, *Hypertension,* 7, 812, 1985.

36. **Crozier, I. G., Nicholls, M. G., Ikram, H., Espiner, E. A., Gomez, H. J., and Warner, N. J.,** Hemodynamic effects of atrial peptide infusion in heart failure, *Lancet,* 2, 1242, 1986.

37. **Saito, Y., Nakao, K., Nishimura, K., Sugawara, A., Okumura, K., Obata, K., Sonoda, R., Ban, T., Yasue, H., and Imura, H.,** Clinical application of atrial natriuretic polypeptide in patients with congestive heart failure: beneficial effects on left ventricular function, *Circulation,* 76, 115, 1987.

38. **Ishii, M., Sugimoto, T., Matusoka, H., Ishimitsu, T., Atarashi, K., Hirata, Y., Sugimoto, T., Kangawa, K., and Matsuo, H.,** Hemodynamic, renal and endocrine responses to α-human atrial natriuretic polypeptide (α-hANP) in healthy volunteers, *Circulation,* 72 (Suppl. 3), 294, 1985.

39. **Ishii, M., Sugimoto, T., Matsuoka, H., Ishimitsu, T., Atarashi, K., Hirata, Y., Sugimoto, T., Kangawa, K., and Matsuo, H.,** Blood pressure, renal and endocrine responses to α-human atrial natriuretic polypeptide in healthy volunteers, *Jpn. Heart J.,* 27, 777, 1986.

40. **Weidmann, P., Hellmueller, B., Uehlinger, D. E., Lang, R. E., Gnaedinger, M. P., Hasler, L., Shaw, S., and Backmann, C.,** Plasma levels and cardiovascular, endocrine, and excretory effects of atrial natriuretic peptide during different sodium intakes in man, *J. Clin. Endocrinol. Metab.,* 62, 1027, 1986.

41. **Weidmann, P., Gnädinger, M. P., Ziswiler, H. R., Shaw, S., Bachmann, C., Rascher, W., Uehlinger, D. E., Hasler, L., and Reubi, F. C.,** Cardiovascular, endocrine and renal effects of atrial natriuretic peptide in essential hypertension, *J. Hypertens.,* 4 (Suppl. 2), S71, 1986.

42. **Davis, J. O. and Freeman, R. H.,** Mechanisms regulating renin release, *Physiol. Rev.,* 56, 1, 1976.

43. **Keeton, T. K. and Campbell, W. B.,** The pharmacologic alteration of renin release, *Pharmacol. Rev.,* 31, 81, 1981.

44. **Opgenorth, T. J., Jr., Burnett, J. C., and Granger, J. P.,** Mechanism of inhibition of renin secretion by atrial natriuretic peptide (ANP), *Clin. Res.,* 33, 494A, 1985.

45. **Opgenorth, T. J., Burnett, J. C., Jr., Granger, J. P., and Scriven, T. A.,** Effects of atrial natriuretic peptide on renin secretion in nonfiltering kidney, *Am. J. Physiol.,* 250, F798, 1986.

46. **Deray, G., Branch, R. A., Herzer, W. A., Ohnishi, A., Jackson, E. K.,** Effects of atrial natriuretic factor on hormone-induced renin release, *Hypertension,* 9, 513, 1987.

47. **Villarreal, D., Freeman, R. H., Davis, J. O., Verburg, K. M., and Vari, R. C.,** Renal mechanisms for suppression of renin secretion by atrial natriuretic factor, *Hypertension,* 8 (Suppl. 2), 28, 1986.

48. **Narumi, S., Yasui, T., Yoshizawa, M., Kawamura, M., Suzuki, H., Nakane, H., and Saruta, T.,** Effects of atrial natriuretic peptide on renal function and renin release in the isolated perfused rat kidney, *Jpn. Heart J.,* 28, 221, 1987.

49. **Naruse, M.,** Atrial natriuretic factor and renin, paper presented at the 1st Int. Symp. Atrial Natriuretic Factor, Montreal, March 15 to 17, 1986.

50. **Henrich, W., McAllister, L., Smith, P., Needleman, P., and Campbell, W.,** Direct effects of atriopeptin (AP) on renin release, *Clin. Res.,* 33, 528A, 1985.

51. **Henrich, W. L., Needleman, P., and Campbell, W. B.,** Effect of atriopeptin III on renin release *in vitro, Life Sci.,* 39, 993, 1986.

52. **Henrich, W. L., McAlister, E. A., Smith, P. B., Lipton, J., and Campbell, W. B.,** Direct inhibitory effect of atriopeptin III on renin release in primate kidney, *Life Sci.,* 41, 259, 1987.

53. **Kurtz, A., Bruna, R. D., Pfeilschifter, J., Taugner, R., and Bauer, C.,** Atrial natriuretic peptide inhibits renin release from juxtaglomerular cells by a cGMP-mediated process, *Proc. Natl. Acad. Sci. U.S.A.,* 83, 4769, 1986.

54. **Cantin, M., Garcia, R., Thibault, G., Hamet, P., and Genest, J.,** Atrial natriuretic factor, purification, action on blood vessels and possible mechanism of action, *J. Mol. Cell. Cardiol.,* 15 (Suppl. 1), (Abstr.) 54, 1983.

55. **Hamet, P., Tremblay, J., Pang, S. C., Garcia, R., Thibault, G., Gutkowska, J., Cantin, M., and Genest, J.,** Effect of native and synthetic atrial natriuretic factor on cyclic GMP, *Biochem. Biophys. Res. Commun.,* 13, 515, 1984.

56. **Rodriguez-Puyol, D., Arriba, G., Blanchart, A., Santos, J. C., Caramelo, C., Fernandez-Cruz, A., Hernando, L., and López-Novoa, J. M.,** Lack of a direct regulatory effect of atrial natriuretic factor on prostaglandins and renin release by isolated rat glomeruli, *Biochem. Biophys. Res. Commun.,* 138, 496, 1986.

57. **Bianchi, C., Gutkowska, J., Thibault, G., Garcia, R., Genest, J., and Cantin, M.,** Radioautographic localization of ^{125}I-atrial natriuretic factor (ANF) in rat tissues, *Histochemistry,* 82, 441, 1985.

58. **Cantin, M. and Genest, J.,** The heart and the atrial natriuretic factor, *Endocrine Rev.,* 6, 107, 1985.

59. **Sakamoto, M., Nakao, K., Kihara, M., Morii, N., Sugawara, A., Suda, M., Shimokura, M., Kiso, Y., Yamori, Y., and Imura, H.,** Existence of atrial natriuretic polypeptide in kidney, *Biochem. Biophys. Res. Commun.,* 128, 1281, 1985.

60. **Naruse, M., Mitta, K., Sanaka, T., Naruse, K., Demura, H., Sugino, N., and Shizume, K.,** unpublished data, 1987.

61. **Naruse, K., Naruse, M., Demura, H., and Shizume, K.,** Immunohistochemical localization of ANP receptor sites in bovine kidney, in *Advances in Biologically Active Atrial Peptides,* American Society of Hypertension Symp. Ser. 2, Brenner, B. M. and Laragh, J. H., Eds., Raven Press, New York, in press.

62. **Anderson, J. V., Struthers, A. D., Christofides, N., and Bloom, S. R.,** Atrial natriuretic peptide: an endogenous factor enhancing sodium excretion in man, *Clin. Sci.,* 70, 327, 1986.

63. **Naruse, M., Obana, K., Naruse, K., Sugino, N., Demura, H., Shizume, K., and Inagami, T.,** Antisera to atrial natriuretic factor reduces urinary sodium excretion and increases plasma renin activity in rats, *Biochem. Biophys. Res. Commun.,* 132, 954, 1985.

64. **Donckier, J., Anderson, J. V., Yeo, T., and Bloom, S. R.,** Diurnal rhythm in the plasma concentration of atrial natriuretic peptide, *N. Engl. J. Med.,* 315, 710, 1986.

65. **Halberg, F., Cornelissen, G., and Marte-Sorenson, K.,** Important time, though not causal, relations in atrial natriuretic peptide, cortisol and renin, *Chronobiologia,* 13, 361, 1986.

66. **Andersson, O. K., Persson, B., Wysocki, M., Berglund, G., Towle, A. C., Aurell, M., Hedner, J., and Hedner, T.,** Significant relationships between renin suppression and atrial natriuretic peptide (α-hANP) during volume loading in hypertensive men, *Acta Med. Scand.,* 221, 137, 1987.

67. **Sagnella, G. A., Markandu, N. D., Shore, A. C., Forsling, M. L., and MacGregor, G. A.,** Plasma atrial natriuretic peptide: its relationship to changes in sodium intake, plasma renin activity and aldosterone in man, *Clin. Sci.,* 72, 25, 1987.

68. **Epstein, M., Loutzernhiser, R., Friedland, E., Aceto, R. M., Camargo, M. J. F., and Atlas, S. A.,** Relationship of increased plasma atrial natriuretic factor and renal sodium handling during immersion-induced central hypervolemia in normal humans, *J. Clin. Invest.,* 79, 738, 1987.

Chapter 11

DOES ATRIOPEPTIN REGULATE SODIUM EXCRETION?

Kenneth L. Goetz

TABLE OF CONTENTS

I. INTRODUCTION

Despite an impressive volume of literature on the subject, it is not yet possible to give a precise description of the contribution of the atrial peptides (atriopeptin) to the regulation of renal sodium excretion. Evidence presented in a number of papers implies that atriopeptin is an important regulator of urinary sodium excretion. Indeed, most published data are consistent with the concept that atrial peptides exert important influences on sodium excretion. However, other reports, many published within the past year, provide provocative data that suggest that atriopeptin is of little relevance as a regulator of sodium excretion under day-to-day living conditions. The purpose of this chapter is to review several of these conflicting studies and to attempt to reconcile some of the divergent data. Attention will be focused only on the possible physiological relevance of the natriuretic effects of the atrial peptides. The effects of atriopeptin on other organ systems[1] will not be considered here.

II. NATRIURETIC EFFECTS OF ATRIAL PEPTIDES

A. EARLY EXPERIMENTS

There is no doubt that the atrial peptides can elicit striking natriuretic responses. Indeed, the demonstration that extracts of atrial tissue cause a marked natriuresis when injected into anesthetized rats prompted de Bold et al.[2] to refer to the unidentified substance they had discovered as atrial natriuretic factor. Subsequent chemical identification of the endogenous hormone[3] and the synthesis of peptides that were either identical or closely related to the natural hormone enabled investigators to demonstrate that pharmacological doses of these peptides elicit prompt and substantial increases in renal salt and water excretion in a variety of experimental animals.[1] These early experiments gave rise to the commonly held notion that the atrial peptides are rapidly acting and powerful natriuretic agents and that they are important regulators of renal sodium excretion. It now is recognized, however, that the plasma concentrations of atriopeptin achieved in those earlier experiments must have been hundreds to thousands of times higher than those achieved when endogenous peptide is released under physiological or pathophysiological conditions.

B. EFFECTS OF ATRIAL DISTENSION ON ATRIOPEPTIN SECRETION

The dramatic natriuretic and diuretic effects of large doses of atriopeptin[1,2,4] and the subsequent demonstration that atrial distension increases the rate of secretion of atriopeptin[5,6] provided support for the original hypothesis proposed by de Bold and colleagues. These investigators, recalling the ability of the atria to monitor intravascular volume,[7,8] hypothesized that the natriuretic factor in their atrial extracts might participate in body fluid homeostasis by affecting the volume regulating function of the kidneys.[2]

Given that atrial distension causes an increase in the secretion of atriopeptin, and given that many of the experimental maneuvers known to increase atrial pressure (e.g., blood volume expansion, acute mechanical obstruction of the mitral valve, and water immersion in human subjects) also increase urinary losses of salt and water, it was predictable that many subsequent experiments employing these maneuvers would detect a correlation between circulating atriopeptin and sodium excretion and thereby provide data consistent with the original hypothesis of de Bold and colleagues. A correlation between two variables, of course, is not sufficient to prove that a cause-and-effect relationship exists between them.

C. EVIDENCE SUPPORTING THE CONCEPT THAT ATRIOPEPTIN REGULATES SODIUM EXCRETION

1. Administration of Antiserum

One of the strongest lines of evidence supporting the concept that atrial peptides modulate renal sodium excretion under physiological conditions is derived from experiments in which antibodies raised against atriopeptin were administered to anesthetized rats. In two such investigations, decreases in urinary sodium excretion were detected after administration of the antibody.[9,10] Sasaki et al.[10] reported that urine flow, sodium excretion, and potassium excretion all decreased by about 60% after rats were given an antibody against atrial peptide, even though mean arterial blood pressure increased simultaneously by approximately 10 mmHg. Naruse et al.[9] reported comparable decreases in urinary sodium excretion and also detected increases in plasma renin activity after administration of specific antiserum against atriopeptin, but potassium excretion and arterial blood pressure were unaffected by the antiserum. Each of these studies, therefore, was consistent with the concept that atriopeptin exerts physiological effects on urine flow and sodium excretion. In another study, monoclonal antibodies raised against atriopeptin were injected into anesthetized rats; no decreases in the basal levels of urine flow or sodium excretion occurred, although arterial blood pressure increased transiently.[11] Nevertheless, the antibody prevented the diuretic and natriuretic responses that normally occur following volume expansion. The differences in the effects observed following administration of antibody in the above studies may be attributed to the specificity of the antibody, the amount of antibody administered, or perhaps to direct actions of the antibody itself.[10]

2. Autoimmune Rats

Using a somewhat different approach, Greenwald et al.[12] developed a population of autoimmune rats that were sensitized to their own atriopeptin. High titers of antibody against atriopeptin in these rats made them unresponsive to increases in circulating atriopeptin caused by several experimental conditions. For example, the acute increase in urinary sodium excretion that usually follows intravascular volume expansion was absent in the autoimmune rats, a finding that suggested that atriopeptin is required to elicit the natriuresis induced by acute volume expansion. On the other hand, sodium excretion increased appropriately in the autoimmune rats during chronic oral salt loading. The autoimmune rats also were able to escape from the salt-retaining effects of mineralocorticoids. These latter findings implied that atriopeptin is not required for the long-term regulation of renal sodium excretion.

3. Removal of Atrial Appendages

Evidence implicating the atrial peptides in the renal adaptations to acute volume expansion was obtained from experiments performed on rats after their atrial appendages had been removed surgically. Veress and Sonnenberg[13] removed the right atrial appendage from anesthetized rats and found that the natriuretic response to a subsequent volume expansion with an isotonic-isooncotic solution was attenuated when compared with the response observed in sham-operated rats. Similarly, Kobrin et al.[14] demonstrated that conscious rats with atrial appendages previously excised excreted less urine and sodium following acute volume expansion than did sham-operated control rats. Each of these studies suggested that removal of atrial tissue prevented increases in plasma atriopeptin during intravascular volume expansion. Direct evidence that the rise in circulating atrial peptide levels is attenuated following volume expansion in the rat was obtained after removal of either one[15] or both[16] atrial appendages. Removal of the appendages did not, however, affect basal plasma levels of atriopeptin.[15,16] Results consistent with these data from rats have been obtained following bilateral removal of the atrial appendages from primates. Benjamin and colleagues[17] reported that diuretic and natriuretic responses following volume expansion were significantly attenuated in four conscious monkeys some weeks after their atrial appendages had been excised; plasma atriopeptin did not increase in response to the volume load. Two other identically prepared monkeys demonstrated normal diuretic and natriuretic responses to volume loading and the concentration of atrial peptides increased normally in these two animals. It was not clear why these two animals demonstrated a normal rise in plasma atriopeptin in response to the infusion. On the other hand, bilateral removal of the atrial appendages from the dog does not attenuate the natriuretic response induced by volume expansion,[18,19] thus suggesting that there are species differences in this response.

4. Total Removal of the Heart

In an intriguing preliminary report, Westenfelder et al.[20] described three calves with the cardiac sources of atriopeptin completely removed. The circulation was maintained chronically with implanted artificial atria and ventricles. The calves retained sodium postoperatively, even when cardiac output was increased substantially or when saline was given intravenously. Atriopeptin was detectable in the plasma of these animals (range of 16 to 26 pg/ml) after removal of the cardiac tissue. It appears, therefore, that other organs can contribute to the circulating pool of atriopeptin. It remains to be determined whether the abnormal sodium retention in these preliminary experiments was caused by the relative deficiency of atriopeptin.

5. Other Literature

Many other reports have described the renal effects of atriopeptin, but they are excluded from this chapter because of space limitations. Suffice it to say that there are multiple atriopeptin binding sites in the kidneys. In addition, tubular effects of atriopeptin have been demonstrated, perhaps most impressively in the medullary collecting ducts, and many experiments have detected correlations between plasma concentrations of atriopeptin and sodium excretion. None of these studies, at least none that the author is aware of, appears to have established that atriopeptin plays a major role in the physiological regulation of renal sodium excretion.

D. SUMMARY

The experiments described in this section provide evidence that the atrial peptides serve as physiological regulators of urinary sodium excretion. The data, however, appear to fall short of proving this relationship. The studies in which anesthetized rats were passively immunized against atriopeptin are compelling, but somewhat inconsistent in their results. In a similar vein, data from autoimmune rats imply that the natriuretic response elicited by acute intravascular volume expansion is dependent upon the effects of atriopeptin, whereas the daily adjustments in sodium excretion necessary to balance oral sodium intake are not. Removal of one or both atrial appendages blunts the natriuretic response to volume expansion and the low levels of circulating atriopeptin present following total removal of the heart are associated with sodium retention.

III. ANOTHER ATRIAL COMPONENT THAT INFLUENCES RENAL FUNCTION

A. ATRIAL STRETCH RECEPTORS

In addition to the atrial peptides, the atria also contain neural elements, so-called atrial volume receptors,[7,8] that elicit reflex increases in salt and water excretion when the atria are distended.[21-23] The volume receptors in the left atrium appear to be of greater importance than those in the right atrium, at least in the dog.[7] For example, mild distension of the right atrium in a conscious dog does not elicit a natriuresis or diuresis, whereas distension of the left atrium does.[23] The renal response evoked by left atrial distension is abolished in dogs after their hearts have been denervated surgically.[21,22] This observation indicates that the diuretic and natriuretic responses to this stimulus are dependent upon receptors located within the heart.

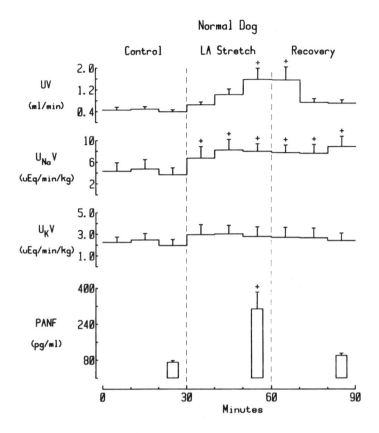

FIGURE 1.   Effect of left atrial (LA) stretch on urine flow (UV), sodium excretion ($U_{Na}V$), potassium excretion (U_KV), and plasma atriopeptin (PANF) in five normal conscious dogs. (From Goetz, K. L., Wang, B. C., Geer, P. G., Leadley, R. J., Jr., and Reinhardt, H. W., *Am. J. Physiol.*, 250, R946, 1986. With permission.)

B. RELATIVE POTENCY OF ATRIAL STRETCH RECEPTORS VS. ATRIOPEPTIN

Plasma levels of atriopeptin were measured during left or right atrial distension in normal dogs and during left atrial distension in dogs with chronic cardiac denervation.[24] Figure 1 illustrates that left atrial distension in normal dogs produced the well-known diuretic and natriuretic responses and also increased plasma atriopeptin. The correlation between the rise in circulating atriopeptin and the increase in salt and water excretion was consistent with the possibility that this peptide caused the renal response. However, when the right atrium was distended in the same dogs on the same day, plasma atriopeptin again increased significantly, but no diuresis or natriuresis occurred (Figure 2). Moreover, when the same experiment was performed in a group of dogs with chronically denervated hearts, urine flow and sodium excretion did not increase during the period of left atrial distension (Figure 3), but plasma atriopeptin levels increased as much as they had during left atrial distension in the normal dogs. In other words, a simple increase in plasma atriopeptin of approximately fourfold was not sufficient to cause natriuresis within 30 min under these conditions.

Data from a study on human subjects are compatible with the above results. Wilkins et al.[25] recently reported that patients with transplanted hearts had higher basal levels of circulating atriopeptin than did healthy volunteers. In the healthy subjects, plasma atriopeptin increased from 7 ± 1 to 12 ± 1 pmol/l during lower body pressure; a small, but significant, increase in sodium excretion occurred in these subjects in the hour after positive pressure was applied. The patients with transplants failed to increase urine flow or sodium excretion

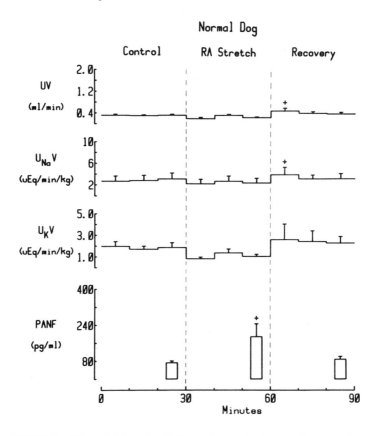

FIGURE 2.   Effect of right atrial (RA) stretch on urine flow, sodium excretion, potassium excretion, and plasma atriopeptin in five normal conscious dogs. (From Goetz, K. L., Wang, B. C., Geer, P. G., Leadley, R. J., Jr., and Reinhardt, H. W., *Am. J. Physiol.*, 250, R946, 1986. With permission.)

during a 1-h period of lower body positive pressure, even though plasma atriopeptin rose from 69 ± 14 to 113 ± 21 pmol/l during this time. Thus, cardiac transplantation, which produces essentially a denervated heart, abolished the renal response to a 1-h period of lower body positive pressure, even though plasma atriopeptin increased during this time.

Under most circumstances atrial distension increases the secretion of atriopeptin and simultaneously elicits reflex responses via atrial stretch receptors. Because each of these changes is capable of increasing urine flow and sodium excretion, it is difficult to determine the relative contributions of these two mechanisms to the renal response evoked by atrial distension. To determine which one of these mechanisms would prevail if they were experimentally forced to oppose each other, we increased left atrial pressure in a conscious dog at a time when plasma atriopeptin was caused to decline.[26] In this situation, distension of the atrial stretch receptors tended to cause a natriuresis, whereas the declining concentration of atriopeptin in plasma tended to cause an antinatriuresis.

An infusion of α-human atrial natriuretic peptide (α-hANP) at 50 ng·kg^{-1}·min^{-1} was given during the control period to elevate control concentrations of plasma atriopeptin to over 1000 pg/ml (Figure 4). The infusion was stopped at the end of the control period and left atrial pressure was increased simultaneously by inflating a balloon positioned above the mitral valve. Atriopeptin declined to about 350 pg/ml during the period of atrial distension. After 40 min of atrial distension, the balloon was deflated to lower atrial pressure to control levels, and the α-hANP infusion was then resumed. The hemodynamic response in these experiments (Figure 4) was similar to the response observed repeatedly during atrial disten-

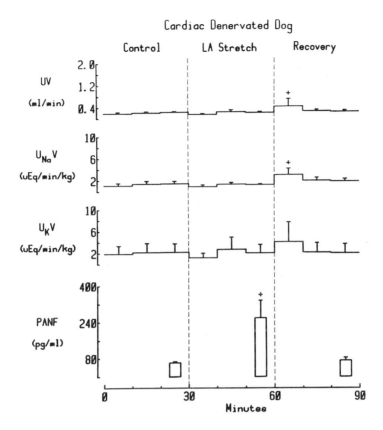

FIGURE 3. Effect of left atrial stretch on urine flow, sodium excretion, potassium excretion, and plasma atriopeptin in four conscious cardiac-denervated dogs. (From Goetz, K. L., Wang, B. C., Geer, P. G., Leadley, R. J., Jr., and Reinhardt, H. W., *Am. J. Physiol.*, 250, R946, 1986. With permission.)

sion in earlier experiments that did not include an infusion of atriopeptin.[21,23] These results indicated that the cardiovascular effects of left atrial distension are evoked by the effects of cardiovascular reflexes, not by the release of atriopeptin, thus confirming earlier experiments.[4] Two variations of this protocol were employed. In one, the control and experimental periods were identical to those described above, but the infusion of α-hANP was not resumed during the recovery period (Figure 4, middle). In the other variation, α-hANP was infused during the control and recovery periods, but the left atrium was not distended during the experimental period (Figure 4, right). Heart rate and pulmonary arterial pressure increased during the experimental period when the atriopeptin infusion was stopped and the left atrium was not distended; these changes were reversed when the atriopeptin infusion was resumed (Figure 4, right).

The renal responses recorded during these experiments are summarized in Figure 5. Despite the decline in plasma atriopeptin, renal sodium excretion increased during the period of atrial distension. Thus, the natriuretic effect of left atrial distension initiated by atrial stretch receptors was sufficient to overcome the antinatriuretic effects of a decline in plasma atriopeptin and elicit the increase in sodium excretion. A decline in plasma atriopeptin was associated with a small decrease in sodium excretion when the left atrium was not distended (Figure 5, right panel); however, the resumption of peptide infusion for 40 min during the recovery period did not cause a natriuresis.

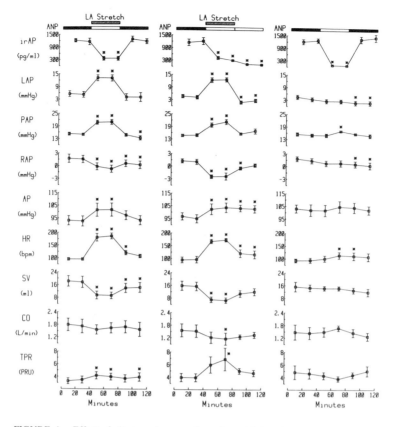

FIGURE 4.   Effect of altering plasma atriopeptin and left atrial pressure on hemodynamics in six conscious dogs. Solid bars (top) represent periods of atriopeptin infusion
at 50 ng·kg^{-1}·min^{-1}. Abbreviations: LA, left atrial; irAP, immunoreactive atriopeptin;
LAP, left atrial pressure; PAP, pulmonary arterial pressure; RAP, right atrial pressure;
AP, aortic pressure; HR, heart rate; SV, stroke volume; CO, cardiac output; TPR, total
peripheral resistance. Asterisks denote values different from control ($p < 0.05$). (From
Goetz, K. L., B. C., Bie, P., Leadley, R. J., Jr., and Geer, P. G., *Am. J. Physiol.*,
255, R259, 1988. With permission.)

IV. RENAL EFFECTS OF LOW-DOSE INFUSIONS OF ATRIOPEPTIN

Several of the above studies implied that relatively small, acute increases in circulating
atriopeptin would elicit neither rapid nor particularly potent natriuretic responses. This has
been confirmed in studies in which α-hANP was infused into conscious dogs[27] or normal
human subjects.[28,29] For example, Bie et al.[27] infused α-hANP into conscious dogs for 1 h
at rates of 12.5, 25, and 50 ng·kg^{-1}·min^{-1} and thereby increased circulating atriopeptin by
3- to 12-fold. Although each infusion caused significant increases in urinary sodium excretion, the changes were quite modest. The increases in sodium excretion caused by the two
lower infusion rates became significant only some 40 to 60 min after the infusion began.
The relatively modest urinary responses in these experiments implied that atrial peptides
may not play a dominant role in the regulation of sodium excretion, although they might
modulate other factors that regulate sodium excretion.

In an investigation conducted on human subjects, the plasma concentration of atriopeptin
was increased over fivefold (from 3.8 to 20.0 pmol/l) by infusing α-hANP at a rate of 1.2
pmol·kg^{-1}·min^{-1}.[28] Although the subjects were very well hydrated throughout the experiment
(average baseline urine flow of 11 ml/min), sodium excretion did not increase during the

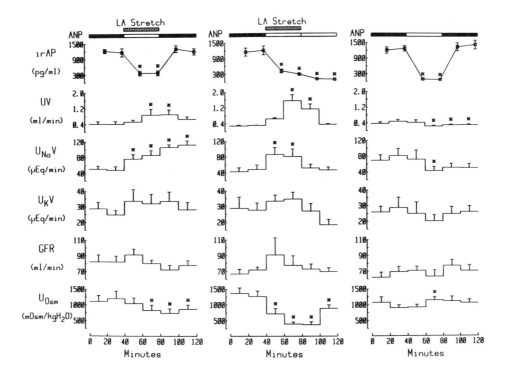

FIGURE 5. Effects of plasma atriopeptin and left atrial pressure on renal function in six conscious dogs. GFR, glomerular filtration rate, Uosm, urine osmolality. Other abbreviations as in previous figures. (From Goetz, K. L., Wang, B. C., Bie, P., Leadley, R. J., Jr., and Geer, P. G., *Am. J. Physiol.*, 255, R259, 1988. With permission.)

first hour of infusion; however, it rose progressively over the second hour and reached a peak increase of 60% over the baseline value during the last 30 min of the 3-h infusion. Other studies in the human employing slightly larger infusion rates have produced corresponding results. For example, infusions that elevated circulating atriopeptin by 11-fold[30] and 25-fold[31] increased renal sodium excretion by only threefold in each study. When a synthetic 25-amino-acid peptide was infused at 100 ng·kg^{-1}·min^{-1} into normal human subjects, plasma atriopeptin increased by 45-fold, but urine sodium excretion increased by only 4.5-fold.[32] Even though the magnitude of the increases in plasma atriopeptin produced by these infusions was higher than has been documented to occur under most normal physiological conditions, the rise in sodium excretion was quite modest when compared to that elicited by a variety of natriuretic stimuli which cause only small increases in plasma atriopeptin.

Richards et al.[29] infused either α-hANP or a 26-amino-acid analog of the human peptide (101—126) at a rate of 2 pmol·kg^{-1}·min^{-1} for 2 h and elevated circulating atriopeptin by eightfold. A small, significant increase in sodium excretion was detectable by the end of the first hour. The maximal sodium excretion attained at the end of the second hour of infusion was about twice that recorded when the same subjects received a placebo infusion. Because the infusion of atrial peptide increased its concentration in plasma to values observed in sodium-replete young men during a brisk intravenous saline challenge, during maximal exercise, or during escape from mineralocorticoid-induced sodium retention, the authors concluded that the plasma levels produced by the infusion were within the normal range.[29] It should be noted, however, that the magnitude of the rise in sodium excretion that follows a brisk intravenous saline challenge is substantially greater and occurs more rapidly than the response obtained during α-hANP infusion. Consequently, one may argue that a major portion of the natriuretic response elicited by the intravenous administration of saline is elicited primarily by other mechanisms. This possibility will be explored in the next section.

V. LACK OF CORRELATION BETWEEN PLASMA ATRIOPEPTIN AND SODIUM EXCRETION

A. EXERCISE

The increase in circulating atriopeptin that occurs during strenuous exercise has been considered by several investigators.[33-35] Although it has been hypothesized[35] that the rise in atriopeptin that occurs during vigorous exercise may contribute to the hyponatremia reported in ultramarathon runners,[36] this hypothesis can be rejected because there is good evidence that renal sodium excretion *decreases* during both acute and chronic strenuous exercise,[37,38] a phenomenon that also has been demonstrated during a marathon race.[39] The decline in sodium excretion that occurs while plasma atrial peptides are elevated is inconsistent with the notion that the rise in plasma atriopeptin reflects a homeostatic mechanism involved in the regulation of salt and water balance during exercise.

B. TACHYCARDIA

Other examples in which the plasma level of atriopeptin does not correlate with renal responses have been reported. In one study of 34 patients with supraventricular tachycardia, plasma atriopeptin was found to be increased during an attack in all but four of the patients.[40] However, only two of the patients reported polyuria during the attack and the plasma concentrations of atriopeptin were not grossly increased in these two subjects. There was no relationship, therefore, between circulating atriopeptin and diuresis in this study. Supraventricular tachycardia appears to consistently elevate atriopeptin in human subjects,[41-43] but only about half of the patients develop an increase in urinary output in response to the tachycardia. In one report, a 60-min period of provoked tachycardia increased plasma atriopeptin by 12- and 24-fold above basal levels in two respective patients with a history of paroxysmal supraventricular tachycardia.[41] Despite the elevated plasma concentration of atrial peptides, sodium excretion declined substantially in each patient during the tachycardia. Nevertheless, urine flow and free water excretion increased in each patient during tachycardia, presumably because of a decrease in vasopressin secretion induced by atrial receptors,[42] or possibly because of a direct inhibitory effect of the elevated plasma atriopeptin on water reabsorption from the renal collecting ducts.[44]

C. WATER IMMERSION

Kurosawa et al.[45] studied six healthy male volunteers after a 14-h overnight dehydration. The subjects were seated for a 1-h control period and then were immersed to the neck in water for 3 h. No food or water was given during the experiment. Urine flow and sodium excretion increased significantly over control values in each of the hourly collections during immersion. However, plasma atriopeptin did not increase during immersion; rather, it gradually declined and was significantly lower than the control value at the end of the immersion period. The natriuretic and diuretic response to immersion, therefore, occurred without any apparent contribution of atriopeptin. These results differ from those obtained from several other investigations in which subjects were well hydrated during immersion.[46,47] In these investigations, immersion caused about a twofold increase in plasma atriopeptin that correlated with an increase in renal sodium excretion. However, the data of Kurosawa et al.[45] demonstrate that an increase in plasma atriopeptin is not required to induce the natriuresis that occurs when a volume of blood is redistributed into the intrathoracic pool during water immersion.

D. INTRAVASCULAR VOLUME EXPANSION WITH SALINE

Singer and colleagues[48] infused 2000 ml of isotonic saline over 1 h into six water-loaded normal male subjects and measured plasma concentrations of atriopeptin, along with urinary sodium excretion. Circulating atriopeptin increased during the infusion and reached a peak value about twofold above basal values 15 min after the infusion had ended. The plasma concentration then declined and reached basal levels by the end of the experiment. Sodium excretion increased early in the experiment and remained significantly elevated throughout the experiment. Thus, the atrial peptides might have been partly responsible for the immediate increase in sodium excretion induced by the saline, but other factors probably were of equal or greater importance in the longer-term adjustments to volume expansion. Several other investigators have concluded that at least a portion of the natriuretic response following saline administration is mediated by the atrial peptides.[49,50] When Kojima et al.[51] infused 1500 ml of saline into human hypertensive subjects, the resulting increases in sodium excretion did not correlate with the increases in plasma atrial peptide induced by the saline, thus suggesting that other mechanisms were responsible for the natriuretic response. We have demonstrated that infusion of saline is able to produce a fourfold increase in renal sodium excretion at a time when the plasma concentration of atriopeptin is decreasing.[26]

E. INFERIOR CAVAL CONSTRICTION

Paganelli and co-workers[52] measured circulating atriopeptin and renal function before, during, and after a period of chronic constriction of the thoracic inferior cava in conscious dogs. Right and left atrial pressures declined in response to caval constriction and remained depressed for 2 to 3 d after the constriction. Atrial pressures then increased toward the control level as the dogs retained fluid and progressively expanded their extracellular volume; nevertheless, plasma atriopeptin remained depressed. Consequently, the sodium retention that occurred during this time period could have been caused, at least in part, by the reduced concentration of circulating atriopeptin. When the constriction was removed, however, sodium excretion increased markedly, even though plasma atriopeptin levels increased only to control levels. The authors suggested that atriopeptin plays only a modulatory role in sodium and water homeostasis.

VI. EFFECTS OF SODIUM INTAKE ON CIRCULATING ATRIOPEPTIN

A. ACUTE EFFECTS

As mentioned earlier, intravenous administration of low doses of α-hANP to normal humans produces significant, but delayed, increases in urinary sodium excretion.[28,29] It therefore is pertinent to ask whether physiological events normally elicit increases in plasma atriopeptin comparable to the five- to eightfold increases that were produced by infusions of the peptide. Maximal exercise may increase plasma levels by this amount, but as mentioned above, natriuresis does not occur during exercise, so the increase in circulating atriopeptin would appear to be unrelated to sodium regulation in this situation.

Under physiological conditions, essentially all sodium taken into the body enters via the oral route. We therefore investigated the effects of a single high-salt meal on plasma atrial peptide levels and simultaneously measured renal sodium excretion. The ingestion of a meal containing 100 mmol of sodium by eight normal human subjects caused an increase in urinary sodium excretion of 346% above control pre-meal values.[53] Plasma atriopeptin, however, did not increase at all following the meal, thus allowing the conclusion that atriopeptin was not responsible for the postprandial increase in sodium excretion in these experiments. Compatible data have been reported by Solhaug et al.[54]

B. CHRONIC EFFECTS

Chronic intravenous infusions of small amounts of atrial peptides to conscious rats,[55,56] dogs,[57] and sheep[58] have been found to produce significant decreases in arterial blood pressure, but undetectable[55-57] or trivial[58] effects on sodium excretion, even though plasma atriopeptin was increased by nine- to tenfold in the two studies in which plasma values were reported.[57,58] The lack of a natriuretic effect during chronic atriopeptin administration was of particular interest in the study of Granger and colleagues[57] because they controlled sodium intake by feeding their animals a low sodium diet and providing sodium via an intravenous infusion of isotonic saline at a constant rate. Consequently, the possibility of changes in sodium intake affecting urinary sodium excretion in these experiments was eliminated. Overall, the long-term infusion experiments provide rather convincing evidence that chronic elevations of circulating atrial peptides of up to tenfold above basal values have no appreciable effect on sodium excretion, but do significantly lower arterial blood pressure.

The data obtained during chronic infusions of atriopeptin appear to be relevant to results from experiments in which plasma atriopeptin concentrations were measured after several days of either low- or high-sodium diets. Although Weidmann and colleagues[59] were unable to detect significant alterations in the concentration of plasma atriopeptin when normal subjects consumed diets containing sodium in the range from 10 to 310 mmol/d, other investigators have reported that subjects on a high-sodium diet developed elevated circulating levels of atrial peptides that were 1.4- to 3.5-fold higher than values obtained when the subjects consumed a low salt diet.[31,60,61] Although it is conceivable that the modest changes in plasma atriopeptin contributed to the adjustments in renal sodium excretion that were necessary to balance sodium intake in these studies, one should recall that a tenfold increase in plasma atrial peptides produced by chronic intravenous infusion of atriopeptin caused essentially no alterations in renal sodium excretion. Accordingly, the considerably smaller elevations in circulating atrial peptides that may be induced by dietary changes appear to indicate that the atrial peptides contribute little to the long-term adjustments of renal sodium excretion.

VII. SUMMARY

As this brief and incomplete review of the literature indicates, one can marshall evidence both for and against the hypothesis that atriopeptin is a physiological regulator of sodium excretion. The studies employing antibodies raised against atriopeptin generally have provided evidence for this hypothesis, as have the investigations that demonstrated that volume expansion in rats or monkeys after removal of one or both atrial appendages produces an attenuated natriuresis after removal. On the other hand, there are plentiful examples of conditions in which circulating levels of atriopeptin do not correlate with concomitant measures of renal sodium excretion. The plasma concentration of atriopeptin may increase with either no change or a simultaneous decrease in sodium excretion. In addition, oral sodium intake, the physiological route by which essentially all salt enters the body, does not appear to increase plasma atriopeptin concentrations acutely, although it may cause small increases chronically. The rather small increases in renal sodium excretion caused by infusions of atrial peptide, which increase circulating levels of the peptide several fold, suggest that atriopeptin may not play a dominant role in acute adjustments of sodium excretion. Similarly, because chronic elevations of circulating atriopeptin do not produce chronic increases in sodium excretion, the peptide appears to be of minimal importance as a regulator of sodium excretion over the long term.

Is there any way to reconcile the positive results obtained with antibodies and removal of the atrial appendages with the negative data? Species differences may account for some of the differences. For example, the antibody studies and most of the studies in which the atrial appendages were removed were performed on rats. Most of the negative data have been derived from dogs and humans. Most of the data would appear to be compatible if one postulates that atriopeptin acts as a permissive agent that enables other regulators of renal sodium excretion to exert their influence more effectively. For example, effective blockade of a permissive or modulating role of atriopeptin by employing antibodies or atrial resection might be sufficient to lower basal sodium excretion and attenuate renal responses to acute volume expansion. On the other hand, the lack of a rise in plasma atriopeptin in response to ingestion of a sodium-containing meal, for example, could be interpreted as indicating that the presence of a normal amount of circulating atriopeptin enabled other sodium regulators to appropriately excrete the ingested sodium. These possibilities remain largely speculative. For the present, it seems prudent to delay a final judgment concerning the physiological effects of atriopeptin on renal sodium excretion.

REFERENCES

1. **Goetz, K. L.,** Physiology and pathophysiology of atrial peptides, *Am. J. Physiol.*, *(Endocrinol. Metab. 17)*, 254, E1, 1988.
2. **deBold, A. J., Borenstein, H. B., Veress, A. T., and Sonnenberg, H.,** A rapid and potent natriuretic response to intravenous injection of atrial myocardial extract in rats, *Life Sci.*, 28, 89, 1981.
3. **Kangawa, K. and Matsuo, H.,** Purification and complete amino acid sequence of α-human atrial natriuretic polypeptide (α-hANP), *Biochem. Biophys. Res. Commun.*, 118, 131, 1984.
4. **Goetz, K. L., Wang, B. C., Geer, P. G., Sundet, W. D., and Needleman, P.,** Effects of atriopeptin infusion versus effects of left atrial stretch in awake dogs, *Am. J. Physiol.*, *(Regul. Integrative Comp. Physiol. 19)*, 250, R221, 1986.
5. **Lang, R. E., Thölken, H., Ganten, D., Luft, F. C., Ruskoaho, H., and Unger, T.,** Atrial natriuretic factor — a circulating hormone stimulated by volume loading, *Nature (London)*, 314, 264, 1985.
6. **Ledsome, J. R., Wilson, N., Courneya, C. A., and Rankin, A. J.,** Release of atrial natriuretic peptide by atrial distension, *Can. J. Physiol. Pharmacol.*, 63, 739, 1985.
7. **Henry, J. P., Gauer, O. H., and Reeves, J. L.,** Evidence of the atrial location of receptors influencing urine flow, *Circ. Res.*, 4, 85, 1956.
8. **Goetz, K. L., Bond, G. C., and Bloxham, D. D.,** Atrial receptors and renal function, *Physiol. Rev.*, 55, 157, 1975.
9. **Naruse, M., Obana, K., Naruse, K., Sugino, N., Demura, H., Shizume, K., and Inagami, T.,** Antisera to atrial natriuretic factor reduces urinary sodium excretion and increases plasma renin activity in rats, *Biochem. Biophys. Res. Commun.*, 132, 954, 1985.
10. **Sasaki, A., Kida, O., Kato, J., Nakamura, S., Kodama, K., Miyata, A., Kangawa, K., Matsuo, H., and Tanaka, K.,** Effects of antiserum against α-rat atrial natriuretic peptide in anesthetized rats, *Hypertension*, 10, 308, 1987.
11. **Hirth, C., Stasch, J.-P., John, A., Kazda, S., Morich, F., Neuser, D., and Wohlfeil, S.,** The renal response to acute hypervolemia is caused by atrial natriuretic peptides, *J. Cardiovasc. Pharmacol.*, 8, 268, 1986.
12. **Greenwald, J. E., Sakata, M., Michener, M. L., Sides, S. D., and Needleman, P.,** Is atriopeptin a physiological or pathophysiological substance?, *J. Clin. Invest.*, 81, 1036, 1988.
13. **Veress, A. T. and Sonnenberg, H.,** Right atrial appendectomy reduces the renal response to acute hypervolemia in the rat, *Am. J. Physiol.*, *(Regul. Integrative Comp. Physiol. 16)*, 247, R610, 1984.
14. **Kobrin, I., Kardon, M. B., Trippodo, N. C., Pegram, B. L., and Frohlich, E. D.,** Renal responses to acute volume overload in conscious rats with atrial appendectomy, *J. Hypertens.*, 3, 145, 1985.
15. **Schwab, T. R., Edwards, B. S., Heublein, D. M., and Burnett, J. C., Jr.,** Role of atrial natriuretic peptide in volume-expansion natriuresis, *Am. J. Physiol.*, *(Regul. Integrative Comp. Physiol. 20)*, 251, R310, 1986.
16. **Villarreal, D., Freeman, R. H., Davis, J. O., Verburg, K. M., and Vari, R. C.,** Effects of atrial appendectomy on circulating atrial natriuretic factor during volume expansion in the rat, *Proc. Soc. Exp. Biol. Med.*, 183, 54, 1986.
17. **Benjamin, B. A., Metzler, C. H., and Peterson, T. V.,** Chronic atrial appendectomy alters sodium excretion in conscious monkeys, *Am. J. Physiol.*, *(Regul. Integrative Comp. Physiol. 23)*, 254, R699, 1988.

18. **Benjamin, B. A., Metzler, C. H., and Peterson, T. V.,** Renal response to volume expansion in atrial-appendectomized dogs, *Am. J. Physiol., (Regul. Integrative Comp. Physiol. 22),* 253, R786, 1987.

19. **Kinter, L. B., Kopia, G., DePalma, D., Brennan, F., Landi, M., and Inagami, T.,** Chronic bilateral atrial appendectomy does not affect salt excretion in dogs, *J. Hypertens.,* 4 (Suppl. 5), S80, 1986.

20. **Westenfelder, C., Baranowski, R. L., Riebman, J. B., Olsen, D. B., Burns, G. L., and Kablitz, C.,** The lack of cardiac atrial natriuretic factor (ANF) prevents salt excretion in calves when cardiac-output (CO) is increased, *Clin. Res.,* 36, A529, 1988.

21. **Fater, D. C., Schultz, H. D., Sundet, W. D., Mapes, J. S., and Goetz, K. L.,** Effects of left atrial stretch in cardiac-denervated and intact conscious dogs, *Am. J. Physiol., (Heart Circ. Physiol. 11),* 242, H1056, 1982.

22. **Kaczmarczyk, G., Drake, A., Eisele, R., Mohnhaupt, R., Noble, M. I. M., Simgen, B., Stubbs, J., and Reinhardt, H. W.,** The role of the cardiac nerves in the regulation of sodium excretion in conscious dogs, *Pfluegers Arch.,* 390, 125, 1981.

23. **Schultz, H. D., Fater, D. C., Sundet, W. D., Geer, P. G., and Goetz, K. L.,** Reflexes elicited by acute stretch of atrial vs. pulmonary receptors in conscious dogs, *Am. J. Physiol., (Heart Circ. Physiol. 11),* 242, H1065, 1982.

24. **Goetz, K. L., Wang, B. C., Geer, P. G., Leadley, R. J., Jr., and Reinhardt, H. W.,** Atrial stretch increases sodium excretion independently of release of atrial peptides, *Am. J. Physiol., (Regul. Integrative Comp. Physiol. 19),* 250, R946, 1986.

25. **Wilkins, M. R., Gammage, M. D., Lewis, H. M., Tan, L. B., and Weissberg, P. L.,** Effect of lower body positive pressure on blood pressure, plasma atrial natriuretic factor concentration, and sodium and water excretion in healthy volunteers and cardiac transplant recipients, *Cardiovasc. Res.,* 22, 231, 1988.

26. **Goetz, K. L., Wang, B. C., Bie, P., Leadley, R. J., Jr., and Geer, P. G.,** Natriuresis during atrial distension and a concurrent decline in plasma atriopeptin, *Am. J. Physiol., (Regul. Integrative Comp. Physiol. 24),* 255, R259, 1988.

27. **Bie, P., Wang, B. C., Leadley, R. J., Jr., and Goetz, K. L.,** Hemodynamic and renal effects of low-dose infusions of atrial peptide in awake dogs, *Am. J. Physiol., (Regul. Integrative Comp. Physiol. 23),* 254, R161, 1988.

28. **Anderson, J. V., Donckier, J., Payne, N. N., Beacham, J., Slater, J. D. H., and Bloom, S. R.,** Atrial natriuretic peptide: evidence of action as a natriuretic hormone at physiological plasma concentrations in man, *Clin. Sci.,* 72, 305, 1987.

29. **Richards, A. M., Tonolo, G., Montorsi, P., Finlayson, J., Fraser, R., Inglis, G., Towrie, A., and Morton, J. J.,** Low dose infusions of 26- and 28-amino acid human atrial natriuretic peptides in normal man, *J. Clin. Endocrinol. Metab.,* 66, 465, 1988.

30. **Weidmann, P., Hasler, L., Gnädinger, M. P., Lang, R. E., Uehlinger, D. E., Shaw, S., Rascher, W., and Reubi, F. C.,** Blood levels and renal effects of atrial natriuretic peptide in normal man, *J. Clin. Invest.,* 77, 734, 1986.

31. **Cuneo, R. C., Espiner, E. A., Nicholls, M. G., Yandle, T. G., Joyce, S. L., and Gilchrist, N. L.,** Renal, hemodynamic, and hormonal responses to atrial natriuretic peptide infusions in normal man, and effect of sodium intake, *J. Clin. Endocrinol. Metab.,* 63, 946, 1986.

32. **Cody, R. J., Atlas, S. A., Laragh, J. H., Kubo, S. H., Covit, A. B., Ryman, K. S., Shaknovich, A., Pondolfino, K., Clark, M., Camargo, M. J. F., Scarborough, R. M., and Lewicki, J. A.,** Atrial natriuretic factor in normal subjects and heart failure patients, *J. Clin. Invest.,* 78, 1362, 1986.

33. **Nishikimi, T., Kohno, M., Matsuura, T., Akioka, K., Teragaki, M., Yasuda, M., Oku, H., Takeuchi, K., and Takeda, T.,** Effect of exercise on circulating atrial natriuretic polypeptide in valvular heart disease, *Am. J. Cardiol.,* 58, 1119, 1986.

34. **Tanaka, H., Shindo, M., Gutkowska, J., Kinoshita, A., Urata, H., Ikeda, M., and Arakawa, K.,** Effect of acute exercise on plasma immunoreactive atrial natriuretic factor, *Life Sci.,* 39, 1685, 1986.

35. **Anderson, J. V., Bloom, S. R., Somers, V. K., Conway, J., and Sleight, P.,** Letter to the editor, *JAMA,* 256, 213, 1986.

36. **Lathan, S. R., Lowance, D. C., and Frizzell, R. T.,** Letter to the editor, *JAMA,* 256, 214, 1986.

37. **Lijnen, P., Hespel, P., Vanden Eynde, E., and Amery, A.,** Urinary excretion of electrolytes during prolonged physical activity in normal man, *Eur. J. Appl. Physiol.,* 53, 317, 1985.

38. **Prashad, D. N., Fletcher, P. A., and Cooper, M.,** Exercise-induced changes in urinary water and mineral output during the menstrual cycle, *Br. J. Sports Med.,* 21, 9, 1987.

39. **Irving, R. A., Noakes, T. D., Irving, G. A., and Van Zyl-Smit, R.,** The immediate and delayed effects of marathon running on renal function, *J. Urol.,* 136, 1176, 1986.

40. **Crozier, I. G., Ikram, H., Nicholls, M. G., Espiner, E. A., and Yandle, T. G.,** Atrial natriuretic peptide in spontaneous tachycardias, *Br. Heart J.,* 58, 96, 1987.

41. **Kojima, S., Akabane, S., Ohe, T., Tsuchihashi, K., Yamamoto, K., Kuramochi, M., Shimomura, K., Ito, K., and Omae, T.,** Plasma atrial natriuretic polypeptide and polyuria during paroxysmal tachycardia in Wolff-Parkinson-White syndrome patients, *Nephron,* 44, 249, 1986.

42. **Nicklas, J. M., DiCarlo, L. A., Koller, P. T., Morady, F., Diltz, E. A., Shenker, Y., and Grekin, R. J.,** Plasma levels of immunoreactive atrial natriuretic factor increase during supraventricular tachycardia, *Am. Heart J.,* 112, 923, 1986.

43. **Nilsson, G., Pettersson, A., Hedner, J., and Hedner, T.,** Increased plasma levels of atrial natriuretic peptide (ANP) in patients with paroxysmal supraventricular tachyarrhythmias, *Acta Med. Scand.,* 221, 15, 1987.

44. **Dillingham, M. A. and Anderson, R. J.,** Inhibition of vasopressin action by atrial natriuretic factor, *Science,* 231, 1572, 1986.

45. **Kurosawa, T., Sakamoto, H., Katoh, Y., and Marumo, F.,** Atrial natriuretic peptide is only a minor diuretic factor in dehydrated subjects immersed to the neck in water, *Eur. J. Appl. Physiol.,* 57, 10, 1988.

46. **Epstein, M., Loutzenhiser, R., Friedland, E., Aceto, R. M., Camargo, M. J. F., and Atlas, S. A.,** Relationship of increased plasma atrial natriuretic factor and renal sodium handling during immersion-induced central hypervolemia in normal humans, *J. Clin. Invest.,* 79, 738, 1987.

47. **Leung, W. M., Logan, A. G., Campbell, P. J., Debowski, T. E., Bull, S. B., Wong, P. Y., Blendis, L. M., and Skorecki, K. L.,** Role of atrial natriuretic peptide and urinary cGMP in the natriuretic and diuretic response to central hypervolemia in normal human subjects, *Can. J. Physiol. Pharmacol.,* 65, 2076, 1987.

48. **Singer, D. R., Shore, A. C., Markandu, N. D., Buckley, M. G., Sagnella, G. A., and MacGregor, G. A.,** Dissociation between plasma atrial natriuretic peptide levels and urinary sodium excretion after intravenous saline infusion in normal man, *Clin. Sci.,* 73, 285, 1987.

49. **Barbee, R. W. and Trippodo, N. C.,** The contribution of atrial natriuretic factor to acute volume natriuresis in rats, *Am. J. Physiol., (Renal Fluid Electrolyte Physiol.* 22), 253, F1129, 1987.

50. **Kaneko, K., Okada, K., Ishikawa, S., Kuzuya, T., and Saito, T.,** Role of atrial natriuretic peptide in natriuresis in volume-expanded rats, *Am. J. Physiol., (Regul. Integrative Comp. Physiol.* 22), 253, R877, 1987.

51. **Kojima, S., Inoue, I., Hirata, Y., Saito, F., Yoshida, K., Abe, H., Deguchi, F., Kawano, Y., Kimura, G., Yoshimi, H., Yokouchi, M., Kuramochi, M., Ito, K., and Omae, T.,** Effects of changes in dietary sodium intake and saline infusion on plasma atrial natriuretic peptide in hypertensive patients, *Clin. Exp. Hypertens. A,* 9, 1243, 1987.

52. **Paganelli, W. C., Cant, J. R., Pintal, R. R., Kifor, I., Barger, A. C., and Dzau, V. J.,** Plasma atrial natriuretic factor during chronic thoracic inferior vena caval constriction, *Circ. Res.,* 62, 279, 1988.

53. **Saville, M. A., Geer, P. G., Wang, B. C., Leadley, R. J., Jr., and Goetz, K. L.,** A high-salt meal produces natriuresis in humans without elevating plasma atriopeptin, *Proc. Soc. Exp. Biol. Med.,* 188, 387, 1988.

54. **Solhaug, M. J., Stacy, D. L., Scott, J. W., and Granger, J. P.,** Effect of sodium intake on postprandial and fasting plasma atrial natriuretic factor levels in normal humans, *FASEB J.,* 2 (Abstr.), A308, 1988.

55. **Garcia, R., Gutkowska, J., Genest, J., Cantin, M., and Thibault, G.,** Reduction of blood pressure and increased diuresis and natriuresis during chronic infusion of atrial natriuretic factor (ANF Arg[101]-Tyr[126]) in conscious one-kidney, one-clip hypertensive rats, *Proc. Soc. Exp. Biol. Med.,* 179, 539, 1985.

56. **Garcia, R., Thibault, G., Gutkowska, J., and Cantin, M.,** Effect of chronic infusion of atrial natriuretic factor on plasma and urinary aldosterone, plasma renin activity, blood pressure and sodium excretion in 2-K, 1-C hypertensive rats, *Clin. Exp. Hypertens. A,* 8, 1127, 1986.

57. **Granger, J. P., Opgenorth, T. J., Salazar, J., Romero, J. C., and Burnett, J. C., Jr.,** Long-term hypotensive and renal effects of atrial natriuretic peptide, *Hypertension,* 8 (Suppl. 2), 112, 1986.

58. **Parkes, D. G., Coghlan, J. P., McDougall, J. G., and Scoggins, B. A.,** Long-term hemodynamic actions of atrial natriuretic factor (99—126) in conscious sheep, *Am. J. Physiol., (Heart Circ. Physiol.* 23), 254, H811, 1988.

59. **Weidmann, P., Hellmueller, B., Uehlinger, D. E., Lang, R. E., Gnaedinger, M. P., Hasler, L., Shaw, S., and Bachmann, C.,** Plasma levels and cardiovascular, endocrine, and excretory effects of atrial natriuretic peptide during different sodium intakes in man, *J. Clin. Endocrinol. Metab.,* 62, 1027, 1986.

60. **Gutkowska, J., Schiffrin, E. L., Cantin, M., and Genest, J.,** Effect of dietary sodium on plasma concentration of immunoreactive atrial natriuretic factor in normal humans, *Clin. Invest. Med.,* 9, 222, 1986.

61. **Sagnella, G. A., Markandu, N. D., Shore, A. C., and MacGregor, G. A.,** Plasma immunoreactive atrial natriuretic peptide and changes in dietary sodium intake in man, *Life Sci.,* 40, 139, 1987.

Chapter 12

LOCALIZATION OF ATRIAL NATRIURETIC POLYPEPTIDE IN THE BRAIN

Mitsuhiro Kawata and Yutaka Sano

TABLE OF CONTENTS

I. INTRODUCTION

Over the past decades, tremendous progress has been made in identifying a number of peptides. Immunological techniques such as radioimmunoassay and immunohistochemistry have shown that a large number of peptides are found simultaneously in both the endocrine organs and central nervous system, and special attention has been paid to the functional significance between their peripheral and central actions. Recently, the heart was identified as an endocrine organ, as well as a cardiovascular organ, due to the fact that the atria synthesize and release a family of peptides, atrial natriuretic polypeptides, into the blood.[1] It has been shown by radioimmunoassay and immunohistochemistry that, like the other peptides, ANP occurs in the central nervous system and its receptor binding sites have been demonstrated, suggesting a potential function as a central neuromodulator.[6,7,9,10,13,17,18,20,21,24-27] The purpose of this chapter is to focus on a detailed description of the distribution of ANP-containing neurons via the use of an immunohistochemical technique. Thus far, three independent groups besides ours have described the detailed neuroanatomical distribution of ANP-immunoreactive neurons in rat and frog brain.[6,7,17,24-26] A description of the similarities and discrepancies in the distributional pattern of these neurons is another subject of the present chapter, and we will discuss a few functional possibilities of the ANP in the brain.

II. ASPECTS OF METHODOLOGY

A. IMMUNOHISTOCHEMISTRY

A detailed description of the variations of the immunostaining procedure which we have used, as well as the production of the antisera, have been published previously.[7,13] In this study, adult male Wistar rats were used. For the purpose of mapping the ANP-containing neurons in rat brain, two experimental groups were studied: (1) normal, untreated animals and (2) colchicine-treated animals (60 to 80 μg in 25 μl of saline was injected into the lateral ventricle 48 h before sacrifice). Antisera to synthetic alpha-human ANP which were raised in rabbits were used for the immunohistochemical investigation. Antisera interacted with both alpha-rat ANP and alpha-human ANP equally well.[13] The specificity for the antisera was checked by the following protocol: (1) preabsorption of the antisera overnight with 5 to 10 μg of rat and human alpha-ANP and bovine thyroglobulin, (2) omission of the primary and secondary antisera, and (3) incubation with normal rabbit serum instead of the primary antiserum. The possible cross-reactivities of the primary antiserum were tested on adjacent sections stained after absorption with each of the following antigens: [Arg]-vasopressin, oxytocin, thyrotropin-releasing hormone, luteinizing hormone-releasing hormone, somatostatin, corticotropin-releasing factor, growth hormone-releasing factor, angiotensin I and II, substance P, adrenocorticotropin, and [Met]-enkephalin.

B. RADIOIMMUNOASSAY

Although radioimmunoassay does not allow the precise location of peptides, it does provide a quantitative comparison of peptides in various brain regions. In this context, radioimmunoassay and immunohistochemistry complement each other. Therefore, we tried to compare the results from two different techniques. Brain sampling was performed according to the Glowinski and Iversen method.[2] A detailed account of the radioimmunoassay is provided in the previous papers.[13,14]

III. ANP-CONTAINING PERIKARYA

Alpha-ANP immunoreactivity was present in the neuronal perikarya of different regions of the rat brain, but not in glial cells, blood vessels, or the choroidal plexus. Immunoreactive perikarya were found in the brains of both normal and colchicine-treated rats. In normal rats, ANP-immunoreactive perikarya were observed only in the periventricular preoptic nucleus, bed nucleus of the stria terminalis, and the endopiriform nucleus. In colchicine-treated rats, however, the number of immunoreactive cell bodies and the intensity of the immunoreaction were greater than in normal rats.

The regional distribution of ANP-immunoreactive perikarya is schematically illustrated in the rostrocaudal sequence on the frontal planes (Figures 1 to 17). The atlas used in the mapping was from Paximos and Watson.[19]

A. TELENCEPHALON

The first rostral regions where ANP-immunoreactive perikarya were found were the lateral septal nucleus and the bed nucleus of the stria terminalis (Figure 18). The anterior part of the cingulate cortex and the endopiriform nucleus ventral to the claustrum and lateral to the external capsule contained a number of immunoreactive perikarya.

The amygdala contained ANP-immunoreactive perikarya, particularly in the medial amygdaloid nucleus. No immunoreactive cells were found in the striatum and the hippocampal formation.

In addition to these areas, Standaert et al.[26] found ANP-immunoreactive cells in the olfactory tubercle associated with the island of Calleja.

B. DIENCEPHALON

The most numerous population of the ANP-immunoreactive perikarya was present in the periventricular preoptic nucleus (Figure 19). This nucleus had one of the largest concentrations of immunoreactive neurons in the brain. The neurons in this nucleus were observed without treatment of colchicine, but colchicine treatment increased the number of immunoreactive perikarya. These immunoreactive perikarya were of various shapes and their average diameter on the long axis was 15 to 18 μm.

A considerable number of ANP-containing perikarya were also seen in the medial-preoptic nucleus. In other regions of the diencephalon, immunoreactive perikarya were found in the preoptic suprachiasmatic nucleus, periventricular and dorsal parts of the paraventricular nucleus (parvocellular division), anterior commissural nucleus, perifornical area, arcuate nucleus (Figure 20), ventrolateral portion of the ventromedial nucleus, dorsomedial nucleus, medial habenular nucleus, zona incerta, median part of the medial mamillary nucleus, supramamillary nucleus, and dorsal and lateral hypothalamic nuclei.

Besides these regions, Skofitsch et al.[25] and Standaert et al.[26] found ANP-immunoreactive perikarya in the organum vasculosum laminae terminalis, suprachiasmatic nucleus, premamillary nucleus, lateral mamillary nucleus, posterior hypothalamic area, central gray, and the fasciculus retroflexus (Meynert).

C. MESENCEPHALON

The mesencephalon contained several groups of immunoreactive perikarya, which were located in the ventral surface of the interpeduncular nucleus, periaqueductal gray (Figure 21) and the pretectal mesencephalic area.

Skofitsch et al.[25] found immunoreactive perikarya in the substantia nigra pars lateralis and the lateral aspects of the dorsal raphe nucleus, whereas Standaert et al.[26] observed the immunoreactive cell bodies in the ventral tegmental area.

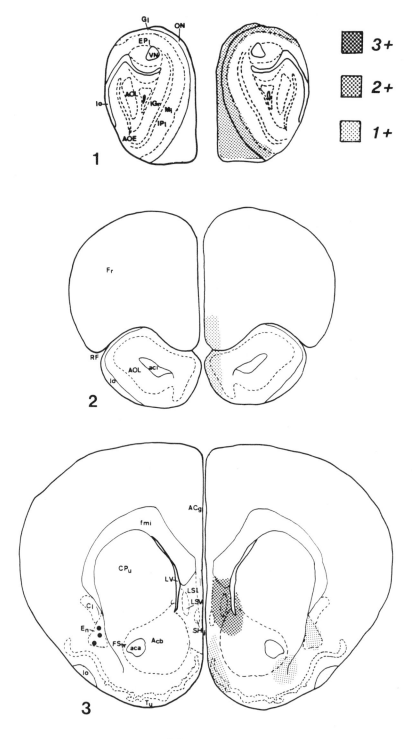

FIGURES 1 TO 3.

FIGURES 1 TO 17.   An atlas of schematic drawings of frontal sections through the rat brain depicting the distribution of ANP-immunoreactive perikarya and nerve fibers. ANP-immunoreactive perikarya are illustrated in dots. Densities of ANP-immunoreactive nerve fibers are represented according to the three-graded scale given beside Figure 1.

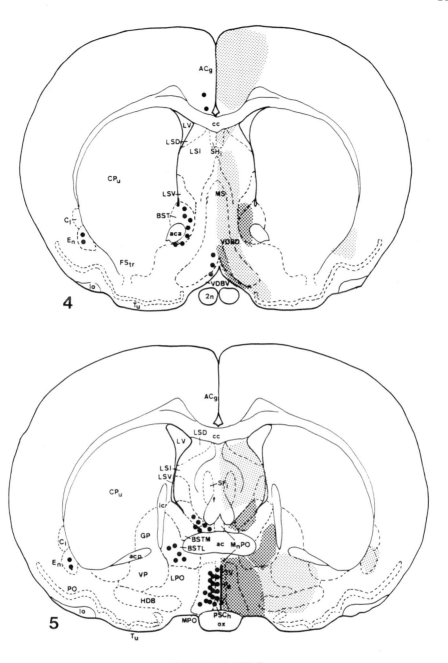

FIGURES 4 AND 5.

D. METENCEPHALON

Neurons with ANP immunoreactivity were scattered in the dorsal parabrachial nucleus and the nucleus of the spinal tract of the trigeminal nerve. Some cells above the nucleus tegmenti dorsalis and in the locus coeruleus were shown to possess ANP immunoreactivity.[25] The metencephalon also contained immunoreactive cells in the pedunculopontoine tegmental nucleus, laterodorsal tegmental nucleus, and Barrington's nucleus.[26]

E. MYELENCEPHALON

It was shown by Skofitsch et al.[25] and Standaert et al.[26] that ANP-immunoreactive

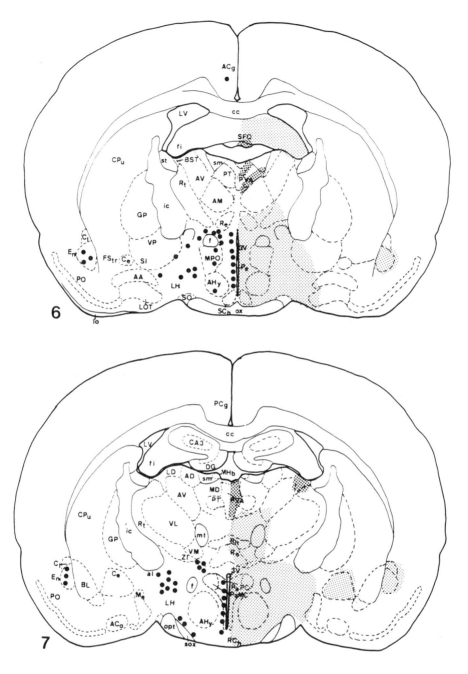

FIGURES 6 AND 7.

perikarya are present in the nucleus prepositus hypoglossi, medial vestibular nucleus, nucleus tractus solitarius, and the substantia gelatinosa.

F. SPINAL CORD

No immunoreactive perikarya were found in the spinal cord.

G. CIRCUMVENTRICULAR ORGAN

There was no immunoreactive perikarya in any regions of the circumventricular organs, except for the organum vasculosum laminae terminalis.[25,26]

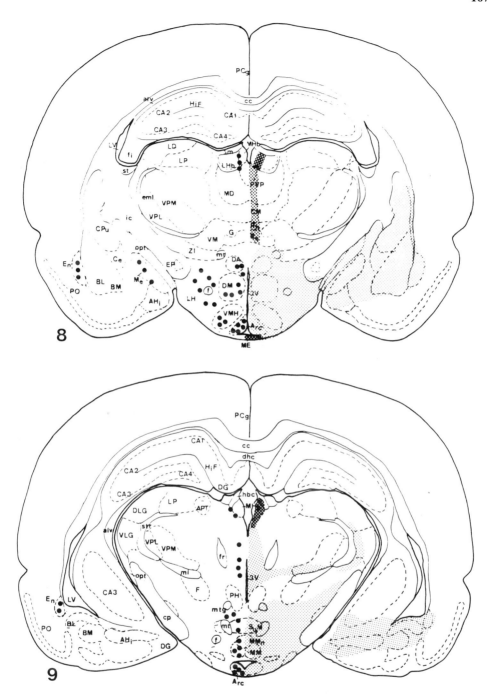

FIGURES 8 AND 9.

H. PITUITARY GLAND

Interestingly, ANP immunoreactivity was detected in the anterior pituitary gland and within the gonadotrophs, corticotrophs, and some lactotrophs.[3,11,12]

IV. ANP-CONTAINING NERVE FIBERS

The widespread distribution of varicose ANP-immunoreactive nerve fibers was observed

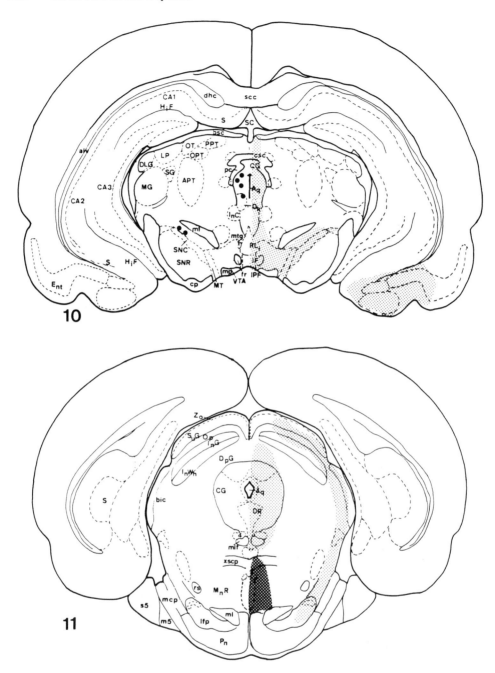

FIGURES 10 AND 11.

in the rat brain (Figures 1 to 17). Colchicine treatment did not substantially change the staining of varicose fibers in most regions of the brain.

In general, it is always difficult to distinguish between a terminal innervation area and a region where immunoreactive nerve fibers course *en route* to other regions. However, in the median eminence, interpeduncular nucleus, and the medial habenular nucleus, immunoreactive punctates were observed, indicating the terminal fields of nerve fibers.

A. TELENCEPHALON

Olfactory bulb, particularly the olfactory nerve layer and glomerular layer, contained a

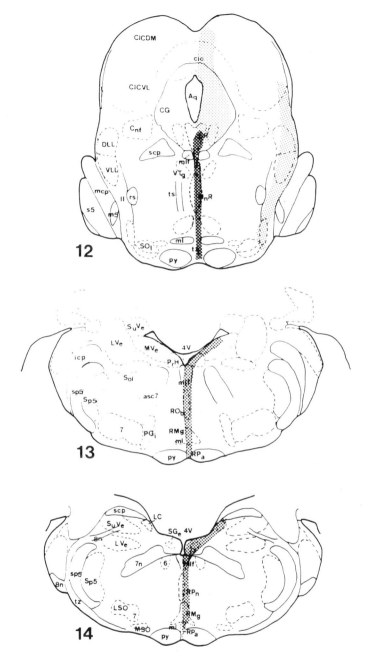

FIGURES 12 TO 14.

light accumulation of immunoreactive nerve fibers. A large number of immunoreactive varicose fibers were observed in the central part of the nucleus accumbens and the bed nucleus of the stria terminalis (Figure 22). The lateral septal nucleus, ventral limb of the diagonal band of Broca, and three central and basolateral amygdaloid nuclei, as well as the medial amygdaloid nucleus, hippocampus, and dentate gyrus, globus pallidus, caudate putamen, and endopiriform nucleus, showed a moderate number of varicose fibers. Sparse immunoreactive fibers were seen in the cingulate cortex, medial septal nucleus, and septohippocampal nucleus.

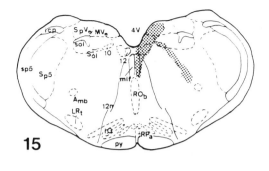

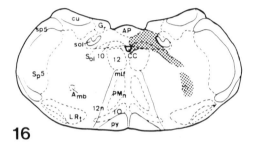

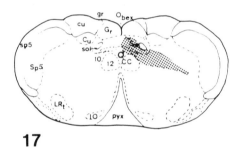

FIGURES 15 TO 17.

B. DIENCEPHALON

There was a dense innervation of immunoreactive fibers in the periventricular preoptic nucleus. A moderate number of immunoreactive fibers were observed in the medial preoptic nucleus, periventricular and peripheral aspects of the paraventricular nucleus (Figure 23), anterior commissural nucleus, supraoptic decussation, arcuate nucleus, ventromedial nucleus, dorsomedial nucleus, perifornical area, and mamillary complex (median, medial, lateral, and supramamillary nuclei). In the median eminence, profuse fibers terminated in the vicinity of capillary loops of the hypophysial portal system in its external layer (Figure 24). In addition to these areas, a dense accumulation of immunoreactive fibers was observed in the area between the medial and lateral habenular nuclei (Figure 25), zona incerta, paraventricular thalamic nucleus, nucleus reuniens, central and medial nuclei of the thalamus, the area ventromedial to the fasciculus retroflexus (Meynert), and along the medial lemniscus. A moderate number of immunoreactive fibers were seen in the suprachiasmatic nucleus, anterior and lateral hypothalamic areas, globus pallidus, medial preoptic nucleus, and interstitial nucleus of the stria terminalis. Few nerve fibers were found in the supraoptic nucleus.

C. MESENCEPHALON

The interpeduncular nucleus, particularly its dorsal and lateral subdivisions, was densely innervated by ANP-immunoreactive fibers (Figure 26). The nonimmunoreactive perikarya were surrounded by varicose dots. This interpeduncular nucleus was the densest area supplied by immunoreactive dots seen anywhere in the brain. A dense accumulation of ANP-immunoreactive nerve fibers was observed at the medial side to the medial longitudinal fasciculus (Figure 27). A moderate number of immunoreactive fibers were also seen along the medial side to the brachium colliculus inferior, cerebral peduncle, and in all areas of the periaqueductal grey matter. Skofitsch et al.[25] observed a moderate innervation of immunoreactive fibers in the nucleus centralis superior, nucleus reticularis tegmenti pontis, and the ventral parabrachial nucleus.

D. METENCEPHALON

A moderate innervation of ANP-immunoreactive nerve fibers was observed in the central gray matter, predominantly beneath the fourth ventricle, dorsal part of the parabrachial nucleus, locus coeruleus, and the dorsal tegmental nucleus. There were no immunoreactive fibers in the cerebellum.

E. MYELENCEPHALON

The solitary nucleus and the dorsal motor nucleus of the vagus nerve contained a dense accumulation of immunoreactive fibers. The nucleus of the spinal tract of the trigeminal nerve, the nucleus ambiguus, and the central gray matter showed a moderate number of immunoreactive fibers.

F. SPINAL CORD

A small number of immunoreactive fibers were found by Standaert et al.[26] around the central canal of the spinal chord and Skofitsch et al.[25] also observed immunoreactive fibers in the dorsal and ventral horns.

G. CIRCUMVENTRICULAR ORGAN

A large number of immunoreactive fibers was distributed around the organum vasculosum laminae terminalis, where profuse nerve fibers terminated in the vicinity of the blood vessels. A moderate number of immunoreactive fibers were observed in the subfornical organ, where varicose fibers also terminated in the perivascular areas. In the pineal organ, subcommissural organ, and the area postrema, no immunoreactive materials were found.

H. PITUITARY GLAND

Skofitsch et al.[25] found a moderate number of immunoreactive fibers in the posterior lobe, whereas the anterior and intermediate lobes were devoid of varicose fibers.

V. ANP FIBER PROJECTION SYSTEM

Standaert et al.,[26] using retrograde fluorescent tracers in combination with immunohistochemistry, demonstrated that a majority of ANP-immunoreactive fibers in the hypothalamic paraventricular nucleus originate in the anteroventral periventricular nucleus, whereas some neurons in the bed nucleus of the stria terminalis, the nucleus of the solitary tract, and the laterodorsal and pedunculopontine tegmental nuclei contribute to the innervation of ANP-immunoreactive fibers in the paraventricular nucleus.

Since the median eminence, particularly its external layer, showed a dense accumulation of ANP-immunoreactive fibers by immunohistochemistry and a high concentration of ANP immunoreactivity by radioimmunoassay, experiments were done for the bilateral lesioning

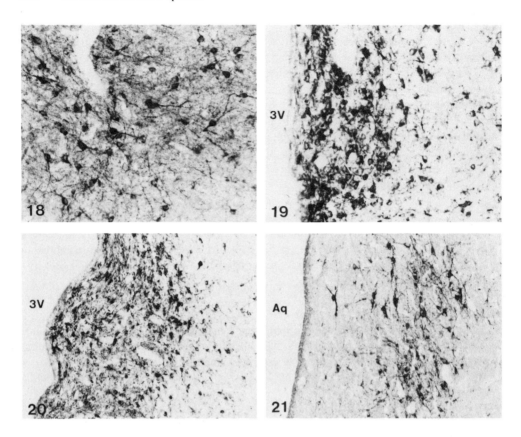

FIGURE 18. Bed nucleus of the stria terminalis. FIGURE 19. Periventricular preoptic nucleus. FIGURE 20. Arcuate nucleus. FIGURE 21. Periaqueductal gray.

of the paraventricular nucleus.[27] It was demonstrated that after lesioning, immunoreactive ANP disappeared almost completely from the median eminence, indicating that ANP-containing neurons in the paraventricular nucleus are the major source of nerve terminals in the median eminence.

The interpeduncular nucleus was the densest area where ANP-immunoreactive fibers were distributed in the rat brain. According to the observations of Standaert and Saper, the neurons in the laterodorsal and pedunculopontine tegmental nuclei might supply a substantial portion of ANP-immunoreactive nerve fibers in the interpeduncular nucleus.

ANP-immunoreactive fibers were generally seen where immunoreactive perikarya were observed. Except for the area above that three regions, where a high concentration of immunoreactive fibers was seen in the brain, it is still unknown whether fibers in these regions are intrinsic or represent descending or ascending projections.

VI. COMMENTS ON THE DISTRIBUTION OF ANP IMMUNOREACTIVITY

It is a fundamental problem that ANP in the brain is similar or identical to the peptide present in the heart. Lewicki et al.[8] have found, using a specific DNA probe, that messenger RNA from hypothalamic extracts was identical to that found in the atria of the heart. Immunoreactive materials were observed in the perinuclear region of the myocytes in the atria, not in the ventricle, with the use of the same antisera which displayed the immunopositive reaction products in the brain. Therefore, it is reasonably safe to say that immu-

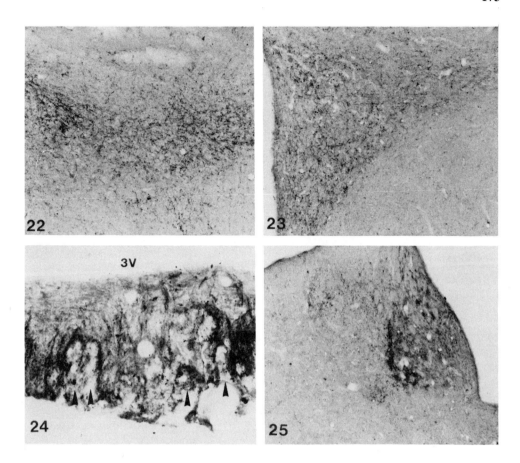

FIGURE 22. Bed nucleus of the stria terminalis. FIGURE 23. Paraventricular hypothalamic nucleus. FIGURE 24. Median eminence; arrowhead indicates the capillary plexus of the hypophyseal portal vessels. FIGURE 25. Medial habenular nucleus.

noreactive products observed in the brain could be identical to those found in the atria, as indicated by Standaert et al.[26]

Thus far, three independent groups have described the distribution of ANP-immuno-reactive cell bodies and nerve fibers in the rat brain.[6,7,17,24-26] There were several discrepancies among the descriptions of the distribution of immunoreactive perikarya, whereas there were fewer discrepancies regarding the distribution of immunoreactive nerve fibers. The discrepant descriptions of the distribution of the ANP-immunoreactive perikarya may have been caused by the different antisera used in the mapping study. Standaert et al.[26] have found some additional groups of ANP-immunoreactive neurons in the rat brain, compared to results from Skofitsch et al.[25] and Kawata et al.[7] The antisera used by Standaert et al.[26] was raised against a 92-amino-acid fragment of the high molecular weight precursor of atriopeptin. This might lead to the hypothesis that antisera raised to a large fragment of the precursor might be more sensitive than small fragments. A second explanation for the differences in the distribution of immunoreactive perikarya involves the amount of colchicine. All groups studying the immunohistochemical localization of the ANP-immunoreactive neuron system in the rat brain used colchicine to increase the number of immunopositive neurons. Without pretreatment with colchicine, the periventricular preoptic nucleus was the only site showing the immunoreactive perikarya.

Netchitailo et al.[17] have recently demonstrated the distribution of ANP-like immuno-reactivity in frog brain with the use of antiserum raised to synthetic ANP (Arg_{101}-Tyr_{126}).

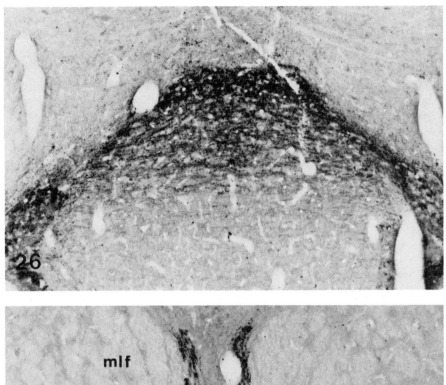

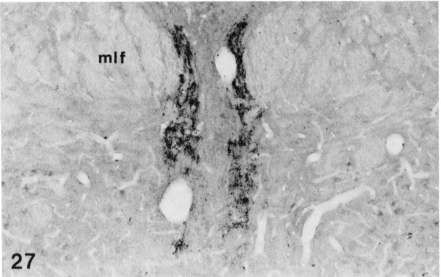

FIGURE 26.   Interpeduncular nucleus.   FIGURE 27.   Area medial to the medial longitudinal fasciculus.

This antiserum has been used to show immunoreactive materials in frog atrial myocytes. In addition to the brain regions reported to be enriched with ANP-immunoreactive materials in the rat, it has been shown that various thalamic nuclei and many mesencephalic areas contained ANP-immunoreactive perikarya in frog brain, suggesting the species-dependent distributional pattern of the ANP-immunoreactive neuron system.

We have found by radioimmunoassay that the highest concentration of ANP immunoreactivity was in the hypothalamus (23.2 ng/mg of wet tissue) and septum (20.7 ng/mg), followed by the mesencephalon, cerebral cortex, olfactory bulb, and thalamus, as dissected by the method of Glowinski and Iversen.[2,7,13] A more detailed radioimmunoassay study was done by Zamir et al.,[27] using Palkovits' punch-out method. According to their data, high concentrations of ANP immunoreactivity were found in the nucleus of the diagonal band, bed nucleus of the stria terminalis, periventricular nucleus, medial preoptic nucleus, suprachiasmatic nucleus, paraventricular nucleus, medial forebrain bundle, anterior hypothalamic nucleus, dorsomedial nucleus, ventromedial nucleus, arcuate nucleus, median eminence, posterior hypothalamic nucleus, periventricular thalamic nucleus, habenula, interpeduncular nucleus, periaqueductal gray, dorsal raphe nucleus, locus coeruleus, dorsolateral tegmental nucleus, and organum vasculosum laminae terminalis. These quantitative distributions of immunoreactive ANP materials in rat brain by radioimmunoassay is well in agreement with the localization of ANP-immunoreactive neurons and nerve fibers detected by immunohistochemistry.

Localization of binding sites for ANP in the rat brain was demonstrated by receptor autoradiography, in conjunction with ^{125}I-ANF(1—28), ^{125}I-ANF, and ^{3}H-atriopeptin, and these studies were reviewed in this volume.[9,10,20,21] These autoradiographic studies performed by various groups have shown quite similar results. In the rat brain, high densities of binding sites were found in the olfactory bulb, subfornical organ, habenular nucleus, area postrema, and ventricular lining. There was a good correlation between the distribution of ANP-immunoreactive materials and receptor binding sites such as olfactory bulb, cortical areas, habenula, hippocampus, striatum, thalamus, and most brainstem areas. However, there were apparent mismatches between them, as frequently observed in many neuropeptides and transmitters.

VII. BRIEF COMMENTS ON THE FUNCTIONAL SIGNIFICANCE OF ANP IN BRAIN FROM A NEUROANATOMICAL VIEWPOINT

Widespread distribution of ANP-immunoreactive perikarya and nerve fibers in the rat brain indicates that these peptides might have a role in diverse physiological actions. Several possible functional roles of ANP in brain should be considered. Immunohistochemical investigations have clearly shown that the high concentrations of immunoreactive perikarya are in the periventricular preoptic nucleus and immunoreactive nerve fibers in the medial preoptic nucleus, bed nucleus of the stria terminalis, and around the organum vasculosum laminae terminalis. This area, the so-called anteroventral third ventricle (AV3V), has been known to integrate humoral homeostatic systems such as those associated with body fluid, electrolyte balance, and cardiovascular regulation.[4,16,22]

ANP may also have a possible role in regulating the neuroendocrine hypothalamohypophysial system since high concentrations of immunoreactive nerve fibers terminated in the vicinity of the hypophysial portal system.[5,23]

ANP-immunoreactive materials are extensively distributed in various regions of the brain. Injections of ANP into the brain induce a range of biological effects, indicating that these peptides should be considered as a new family of heart-brain peptides acting as neurotransmitters of neuromodulators.[15,16]

APPENDIX

ABBREVIATIONS IN FIGURES

2n	Optic nerve
3	Principal oculomotor nucleus
3V	Third ventricle
4	Trochlear nucleus
4V	Fourth ventricle

6	Abducens nucleus
7	Facial nucleus
7n	Facial nerve
8n	Vestibulocochlear nerve
10	Dorsal motor nucleus of vagus
12	Hypoglossal nucleus
12n	Hypoglossal nerve
AA	Anterior amygdaloid area
ac	Anterior commissure
aca	Anterior commissure, anterior part
Acb	Accumbens nucleus
ACg	Anterior cingulate cortex
aci	Anterior commissure, intrabulbar part
ACo	Anterior cortical amygdaloid nucleus
acp	Anterior commissure, posterior part
AD	Anterodorsal thalamic nucleus
AHi	Amygdalohippocampal area
AHy	Anterior hypothalamic area
al	Ansa lenticularis
alv	Alveus of the hippocampus
AM	Anteromedial thalamic nucleus
Amb	Ambiguus nucleus
AOB	Accessory olfactory bulb
AOE	Anterior olfactory nucleus, external part
AOL	Anterior olfactory nucleus, lateral part
AOP	Anterior olfactory nucleus, posterior part
AP	Area postrema
APT	Anterior pretectal area
Aq	Cerebral aqueduct
Arc	Arcuate hypothalamic nucleus
asc7	Ascending fibers of the facial nerve
AV	Anteroventral thalamic nucleus
B	Cells of the basal nucleus of Meynert
bic	Brachium of the inferior colliculus
BL	Basolateral amygdaloid nucleus
BM	Basomedial amygdaloid nucleus
bsc	Brachium of the superior colliculus
BST	Bed nucleus of the stria terminalis
BSTL	Bed nucleus of the stria terminalis, lateral part
BSTM	Bed nucleus of the stria terminalis, medial part
CA1	Field of CA1 of Ammon's horn
CA2	Field CA2 of Ammon's horn
CA3	Field CA3 of Ammon's horn
CA4	Field CA4 of Ammon's horn
CC	Central canal
Ce	Central amygdaloid nucleus
CG	Central grey
cic	Commissure of the inferior colliculus
CICDM	Central nucleus of the inferior colliculus, dorsomedial part
CICVL	Central nucleus of the inferior colliculus, ventromedial part
Cl	Claustrum

CM	Central medial thalamic nucleus
Cnf	Cuneiform nucleus
cp	Cerebral peduncle
CPu	Caudate putamen
csc	Commissure of the superior colliculus
Cu	Cuneate nucleus
cu	Cuneate fasciculus
DA	Dorsal hypothalamic nucleus
DG	Dentate gyrus
dhc	Dorsal hippocampal commissure
Dk	Nucleus of Darkschewitsch
DLG	Dorsal lateral geniculate nucleus
DLL	Dorsal nucleus of the lateral lamniscus
DM	Dorsomedial hypothalamic nucleus
DPB	Dorsal parabrachial nucleus
DpG	Deep gray layer of the superior colliculus
DR	Dorsal raphe nucleus
DTg	Dorsal tegmental nucleus (Gudden)
dtgx	Dorsal tegmental decussation
eml	External medullary lamina
En	Endopiriform nucleus
Ent	Entorhinal cortex
EP	Entopeduncular nucleus
EP1	External plexiform layer of the olfactory bulb
F	Nucleus of the field of Forel
f	Fornix
fi	Fimbria of the hippocampus
fmi	Forceps minor of the corpus callosum
fmj	Forceps major of the corpus callosum
Fr	Frontal cortex
fr	Fasciculus retroflexus
FStr	Fundus striati
G	Gelatinosus nucleus of the thalamus
gcc	Genu of the corpus callosum
Gl	Glomerular layer of the olfactory bulb
GP	Globus pallidus
Gr	Gracile nucleus
gr	Gracile fasciculus
hbc	Habenular commissure
HBD	Nucleus of the horizontal limb of the diagonal band (Broca)
HiF	Hippocampal fissure
ic	Internal capsule
icp	Inferior cerebellar peduncle
IF	Interfascicular nucleus
IGr	Internal granular layer of the olfactory bulb
InC	Interstitial nucleus of Cajal
InfS	Infundibular stem
InG	Intermediate grey matter of the superior colliculus
InWh	Intermediate white matter of the superior colliculus
IO	Inferior olive
IPC	Interpeduncular nucleus, central part

IPF	Interpeduncular fossa
IPIP	Interpeduncular nucleus, inner part of the posterior subnucleus
IPl	Internal plexiform layer of the olfactory bulb
IPP	Interpeduncular nucleus, paramedian part
La	Lateral amygdaloid nucleus
LC	Locus coeruleus
LD	Laterodorsal thalamic nucleus
LDTg	Laterodorsal tegmental nucleus
lfp	Longitudinal fasciculus of the pons
LH	Lateral hypothalamic area
LHb	Lateral habenular nucleus
ll	Lateral lemniscus
LM	Lateral mamillary nucleus
lo	Lateral olfactory tract
LOT	Nucleus of the lateral olfactory nucleus
LP	Lateral posterior thalamic nucleus (pulvinar)
LPO	Lateral preoptic area
LRt	Lateral reticular nucleus
LSD	Lateral septal nucleus, dorsal part
LSI	Lateral septal nucleus, intermediate part
LSO	Lateral superior olive
LSV	Lateral septal nucleus, ventral part
LV	Lateral ventricle
LVe	Lateral vestibular nucleus
m5	Motor root of the trigeminal nerve
mcp	Middle cerebellar peduncle
MD	Mediodorsal thalamic nucleus
ME	Median eminence
Me	Medial amygdaloid nucleus
me5	Mesencephalic tract of the trigeminal nerve
MG	Medial geniculate nucleus
MHb	Medial habenular nucleus
Mi	Mitral cell layer of the olfactory bulb
ML	Medial mamillary nucleus, lateral part
ml	Medial lemniscus
mlf	Medial longitudinal fasciculus
MM	Medial mamillary nucleus, medial part
MMn	Medial mamillary nucleus, median part
MnPO	Medial preoptic nucleus
MnR	Median raphe nucleus
Mo5	Motor trigeminal nerve
mp	Mamillary peduncle
MPO	Medial preoptic area
MS	Medial septal nucleus
MSO	Medial superior olive
mt	Mamillothalamic tract
MY	Medial terminal nucleus of the accessory optic tract
mtg	Mamillotegmental tract
MVe	Medial vestibular nucleus
Obex	Obex
ON	Olfactory nerve layer

Op	Optic nerve layer of the superior colliculus
OPT	Olivary pretectal nucleus
opt	Optic nerve
OT	Nucleus of the optic tract
ox	Optic chiasm
PaMC	Paraventricular hypothalamic nucleus, magnocellular part
PaPC	Paraventricular hypothalamic nucleus, parvocellular part
pc	Posterior commissure
PCg	Posterior cingulate cortex
Pe	Periventricular hypothalamic nucleus
PGi	Paragigantocellular reticular nucleus
PH	Posterior hypothalamic nucleus
PMn	Paramedian reticular nucleus
Pn	Pontine nuclei
PO	Primary olfactory cortex
PPT	Posterior pretectal nucleus
Pr5	Principal sensory trigeminal nucleus
PrH	Prepositus hypoglossal nucleus
PSCh	Preoptic suprachiasmatic nucleus
PT	Parataenial thalamic nucleus
PV	Paraventricular thalamic nucleus
PVa	Paraventricular thalamic nucleus, anterior part
PVP	Paraventricular thalamic nucleus, posterior part
py	Pyramidal tract
pyx	Pyramidal decussation
PMV	Premamillary nucleus, ventral part
RCh	Retrochiasmatic area
Re	Reuniens thalamic nucleus
RF	Rhinal fissure
Rh	Rhomboid thalamic nucleus
RLi	Rostral linear nucleus of the raphe
RMC	Red nucleus, magnocellular part
RMg	Raphe magnus nucleus
ROb	Raphe obscurus nucleus
RPa	Raphe pallidus nucleus
RPn	Raphe pontis nucleus
RRF	Retrorubal field
rs	Rubospinal tract
Rt	Reticular thalamic nucleus
S	Subiculum
s5	Sensory root of the trigeminal nerve
SC	Superior colliculus
scc	Splenium of the corpus callosum
SCh	Suprachiasmatic nucleus
SCO	Subcommissural organ
scp	Superior cerebellar peduncle
SFi	Septofimbrial nucleus
SFO	Subfornical organ
SG	Suprageniculate thalamic nucleus
SGe	Suprageniculate nucleus of the pons
SHi	Septohippocampal nucleus

SI	Substantia innominata
sm	Stria medullaris of the thalamus
SNC	Substantia nigra, compact part
SNR	Substantia nigra, reticular part
SO	Supraoptic hypothalamic nucleus
SOl	Superior olive
Sol	Nucleus of the solitary tract
sol	Solitary tract
sox	Suraoptic decussation
Sp5	Nucleus of the spinal tract of the trigeminal nerve
sp5	Spinal tract of the trigeminal nerve
SpVe	Spinal vestibular nucleus
st	Stria terminalis
STh	Subthalamic nucleus (Luys)
str	Superior thalamic radiation
SuG	Superficial grey layer of the superior colliculus
SuM	Supramimillary nucleus
SuVe	Superior vestibular nucleus
tfp	Transverse fibers of the pons
ts	Tectospinal tract
TT	Taenia tecta
Tu	Olfactory tubercle
TuPo	Olfactory tubercle, polymorphic layer
tz	Trapezoid body
VDBD	Nucleus of the vertical limb of the diagonal band, dorsal part
VDBV	Nucleus of the vertical limb of the diagonal band, ventral part
VL	Ventrolateral thalamic nucleus
VLG	Ventral lateral geniculate nucleus
VLL	Ventral nucleus of the lateral lemniscus
VM	Ventromedial thalamic nucleus
VMH	Ventromedial hypothalamic nucleus
VN	Vomeronasal nerve
VP	Ventral pallidum
VPL	Ventroposterior thalamic nucleus, lateral part
VPM	Ventroposterior thalamic nucleus, medial part
VTA	Ventral tegmental area (Tsai)
VTg	Ventral tegmental nucleus (Gudden)
xscp	Decussation of the superior cerebellar peduncle
ZI	Zona incerta
ZO	Zone layer of the superior colliculus

REFERENCES

1. **de Bold, A. J.,** Atrial natriuretic factor: an overview, *Fed. Proc.,* 45, 2081, 1986.
2. **Glowinski, J. and Iversen, L. L.,** Regional studies of catecholamines in the rat brain, *J. Neurochem.,* 13, 655, 1969.
3. **Inagaki, S., Kubota, Y., Kito, S., Kangawa, T., and Matsuo, H.,** Atrial natriuretic polypeptide-like immunoreactivity in the rat pituitary: light and electron microscopic studies, *Regul. Peptides,* 14, 101, 1986.

4. **Itoh, H., Nakao, K., Katsuura, G., Morii, N., Shiono, S., Sakamoto, M., Sugawara, A., Yamada, T., Saito, Y., Matsushita, A., and Imura, H.,** Centrally infused atrial natriuretic polypeptide attenuates exaggerated salt appetite in spontaneously hypertensive rats, *Circ. Res.,* 59, 342, 1986.

5. **Itoh, H., Nakao, K., Katsuura, G., Morii, N., Yamada, T., Shiono, S., Sakamoto, M., Sugawara, A., Saito, Y., Eigyo, M., Matsushita, A., and Imura, H.,** Possible involvement of central atrial natriuretic polypeptide in regulation of hypothalamo-pituitary-adrenal axis in conscious rat, *Neurosci. Lett.,* 69, 254, 1986.

6. **Jacobowitz, D. M., Skofitsch, G., Keiser, H. R., Eskay, R. L., and Zamir, N.,** Evidence for the existence of atrial natriuretic factor-containing neurons in the rat brain, *Neuroendocrinology,* 40, 92, 1985.

7. **Kawata, M., Nakao, K., Morii, N., Kiso, Y., Yamashita, H., Imura, H., and Sano, Y.,** Atrial natriuretic polypeptide: topographical distribution in the rat brain by radioimmunoassay and immunohistochemistry, *Neuroscience,* 16, 521, 1985.

8. **Lewicki, J. A., Greenberg, B., Yamanaka, M., Vlasuk, G., Brewer, M., Gardner, D., Baxter, J., Johnson, L. K., and Fiddes, J. C.,** Cloning, sequence analysis, and processing of the rat and human atrial natriuretic peptide precursors, *Fed. Proc.,* 45, 2086, 1986.

9. **Mantyh, C. R., Kruger, L., Brecha, N. C., and Mantyh, P. W.,** Localization of specific binding sites for atrial natriuretic factor in the central nervous system of rat, guinea pig, cat and human, *Brain Res.,* 412, 329, 1987.

10. **McCarty, R. and Plunkett, L. M.,** Binding sites for atrial natriuretic factor (ANF) in brain: alteration in Brattleboro rats, *Brain Res. Bull.,* 17, 767, 1986.

11. **McKensie, J. C., Tanaka, I., Misono, K. S., and Inagami, T.,** Immunocytochemical localization of atrial natriuretic factor in the kidney, adrenal medulla, pituitary, and atrium of rat, *J. Histochem. Cytochem.,* 33, 828, 1985.

12. **Morel, G., Chabot, J.-G., Belles-Isles, M., and Heisler, S.,** Synthesis and internalization of atrial natriuretic factor in anterior pituitary cell, *Mol. Cell. Endocrinol.,* 55, 219, 1988.

13. **Morii, N., Nakao, K., Sugawara, A., Sakamoto, M., Suda, M., Shimokura, M., Kiso, Y., Kihara, M., Yamori, Y., and Imura, H.,** Occurrence of atrial natriuretic polypeptide in brain, *Biochem. Biophys. Res. Commun.,* 127, 413, 1985.

14. **Nakao, K., Sugawara, A., Morii, N., Sakamoto, M., Suda, Y., Soneda, J., Ban, T., Kihara, M., Yamori, Y., Shimokura, M., Kiso, Y., and Imura, H.,** Radioimmunoassay of alpha-human and rat atrial natriuretic polypeptide, *Biochem. Biophys. Res. Commun.,* 124, 815, 1984.

15. **Nakao, K., Katsuura, G., Morii, N., Itoh, H., Shiono, S., Yamada, T., Sugawara, A., Sakamoto, M., Saito, Y., Eigyo, M., Matsushita, A., and Imura, H.,** Inhibitory effect of centrally administered atrial natriuretic polypeptide on brain dopaminergic system in rats, *Eur. J. Pharmacol.,* 131, 171, 1986.

16. **Nakao, K., Morii, N., Itoh, H., Sugawara, A., Sakamoto, M., Yamada, T., Shiono, S., Saito, Y., and Imura, H.,** Atrial natriuretic polypeptide in brain: implication in water and electrolyte balance and blood pressure control, in *Brain and Blood Pressure Control,* Nakamura, K., Ed., Elsevier, Amsterdam, 1986, 195.

17. **Netchitailo, P., Feuilloley, M., Pelletier, G., Leboulengen, F., Cantin, M., Gutkowska, J., and Vaudry, H.,** Atrial natriuretic factor-like immunoreactivity in the central nervous system of the frog, *Neuroscience,* 22, 341, 1987.

18. **Palkovits, M., Eskay, R. L., and Antoni, F. A.,** Atrial natriuretic peptide in the median eminence is of paraventricular nucleus origin, *Neuroendocrinology,* 46, 542, 1987.

19. **Paxinos, G. and Watson, G.,** *The Rat Brain in Stereotaxic Coordinates,* Academic Press, Sydney, 1982.

20. **Quirion, R., Dalpe, M., DeLean, A., Gutdowka, J., Cantin, M. M., and Genest, J.,** Atrial natriuretic factor (ANF) binding sites in brain and related structures, *Peptides,* 5, 1167, 1984.

21. **Quirion, R., Dalpe, M., and Dam, T. V.,** Characterization and distribution of receptors for the atrial natriuretic peptides in mammalian brain, *Proc. Natl. Acad. Sci. U.S.A.,* 83, 174, 1986.

22. **Samson, W. K.,** Atrial natriuretic factor inhibits dehydration and hemorrhage-induced vasopressin release, *Neuroendocrinology,* 8, 509, 1985.

23. **Samson, W. K. and Eskay, R. L.,** Endocrine and neuroendocrine actions of cardiac peptides, in *Neural and Endocrine Peptides and Receptors,* Moody, T. W., Ed., Plenum Press, New York, 1986, 521.

24. **Saper, C. B., Standaert, D. G., Currie, M. G., Schwartz, D., Geller, D. M., and Needleman, P.,** Atriopeptin-immunoreactive neurons in the brain: presence in cardiovascular regulatory areas, *Science,* 227, 1047, 1985.

25. **Skofitsch, G., Jacobowitz, D. W., Eskay, R. L., and Zamir, N.,** Distribution of atrial natriuretic factor-like immunoreactive neurons in the rat brain, *Neuroscience,* 16, 917, 1985.

26. **Standaert, D. G., Needleman, P., and Saper, C. B.,** Organization of atriopeptin-like immunoreactive neurons in the central nervous system of the rat, *J. Comp. Neurol.,* 253, 315, 1986.

27. **Zamir, N., Skofitsch, G., Eskay, R. L., and Jacowobitz, D. M.,** Distribution of immunoreactive atrial natriuretic peptides in the central nervous system of the rat, *Brain Res.,* 365, 105, 1986.

Chapter 13

BRAIN RECEPTOR SITES FOR ATRIAL NATRIURETIC POLYPEPTIDES

Jean-Guy Chabot and Rémi Quirion

TABLE OF CONTENTS

I. INTRODUCTION

Atrial natriuretic factors and/or polypeptides (ANP) are a recently discovered group of peptide hormones isolated from atrial extracts and localized in the electron-dense granules of mammalian atrial myocardium.[1-4] Many of the established actions of ANP were first described using crude atrial extracts or partially purified preparations and these actions have now been confirmed with pure synthetic peptides. It is well known that ANP-related peptides induce a variety of biological effects in target tissues.[1-4] In addition to natriuresis, diuresis, and vasorelaxation, ANP-related substances modulate aldosterone production, as well as vasopressin and androgen release.[1-7] It is now clear that these ANP actions are mediated by highly selective and specific ANP receptor sites localized on plasma membranes, as well as inside the cells of target tissues.[8-10] Moreover, many ANP effects in target tissues are accompanied by the production of guanosine $3',5'$-monophosphate (cGMP) since it appears that one class of ANP receptor sites is coupled to particulate guanylate cyclase (see Section II.D).[11]

Over the past few years, it became evident that ANP-like peptides and receptor sites discovered in peripheral tissues can also be identified in the central nervous system (CNS) and may represent a new family of brain/heart peptides.[12-27] In fact, the presence and detailed neuroanatomical distribution of ANP-like immunoreactive substances have been recently reported in rat, dog, and frog brain using specific radioimmunoassays and immunohisto-chemical techniques.[12-18] The release of ANP-like peptides from hypothalamic slice preparations is Ca^{2+}-dependent[28,29] and recent data suggest that ANP brain peptides are derived from a large prohormone expressed by a specific ANP gene.[30] Moreover, Sudoh et al.[31] have just reported the existence in porcine brain of a new peptide having around 60% sequence homology with ANP. Thus, it appears that two different groups of ANP-like peptides exist in brain tissues. This may be highly relevant in terms of the existence of brain ANP receptor subtypes, although we do not have much information concerning this aspect at the present time. In this chapter, we review the current information related to the presence of brain ANP receptor sites in mammals.

II. CHARACTERIZATION OF BRAIN ANP RECEPTORS

A. RECEPTOR BINDING PARAMETERS

The pharmacological characterization of ANP binding sites has been recently performed in guinea pig and rat brain.[21,22,24,26,27,32-34] In guinea pig thalamus/hypothalamus and cerebellum membrane preparations, radiolabeled ANP-related peptides apparently bind to a single class of sites.[21,22] The apparent affinity (K_d) of these sites is in the low picomolar range (20 to 60 pM), as reported in various peripheral tissues.[8,9] However, the capacities (Bmax) are much lower in these two guinea pig brain regions than in other tissues, such as kidney, adrenal gland, blood vessels, and lung.[8,9,35] In the rat brain, determinations of these binding kinetic parameters have been possible mostly using quantitative *in vitro* receptor autoradiography because of the limited distribution of ANP sites in rat brain.[24,26,33,34] In these various studies, K_d values in the high picomolar range and B_{max} around 30 to 60 fmol/mg protein have been observed in the rat subfornical organ,[26,33,34] area postrema,[26,33] olfactory bulb,[24] and choroid plexus.[33,34] These discrepancies are most likely due to the techniques used since autoradiographic methods can focus on very discrete brain areas where binding is concentrated, whereas membrane-binding techniques utilized much larger brain regions not uniformly labeled.

B. LIGAND SELECTIVITY PATTERNS

Competitive studies of ANP binding in guinea pig brain membrane preparations have been performed using various ANP-related peptides and other neuropeptides and drugs.[21,22]

The ligand selectivity pattern shows that ANP(101—126) is the most potent competitor against [^{125}I]ANP binding, whereas ANP(99—126) and ANP(103—125) are weaker and ANP(103—123) is almost inactive. Similar results have also been reported using rat olfactory bulb.[24,32] In this assay, ANP(99—126) and ANP(103—126) are the most potent analogs tested, whereas ANP(103—124) is weaker and ANP(111—126) is almost inactive. Various other neuropeptides and drugs such as angiotensin II, β-endorphin, cholescytokinin-8, substance P, somatostatin, ACTH, TRH, α-MSH, insulin, haloperidol, muscinol, atropine, isoproterenol, clonidine, carbachol, phentolamine, propanolol, and prazonin are not able to compete for the [^{125}I]ANP binding in these preparations.[21,22,24] This reveals the selectivity of brain ANP sites and indicates that an extension of the NH$_2$ terminus by two amino acids (serine and leucine) (ANF[99—126]) diminishes the affinity of this ANP-like peptide for its receptor sites, as compared to ANP(101—126). Moreover, the deletion of the two arginine residues in positions 101 and 102 and the COOH-terminal arginine (124) and tyrosine (125) residues markedly decreases the activity of these peptides in binding assays, as shown by ANP(103—125) and ANP(103—124). Thus, it is likely that these residues are most important to maintain the affinity of ANP-like peptides to brain ANP receptor sites. Similar data have been obtained in various peripheral tissue bioassays.[36-38] This indicates that the structural requirements of central and peripheral ANP receptors are fairly similar (at least for the B-ANP receptor type, see below) and that it seems that the COOH-terminal portion of the molecule is more important than the NH$_2$-terminal one for the binding of ANP-like peptides to their receptors.

C. RECEPTOR COUPLING TO cGMP PRODUCTION

Since it is well known that ANP receptors are coupled to the particulate guanylate cyclase system in peripheral tissues,[11] the possibility of a similar association in the brain has recently been investigated. It has been shown that ANP-like peptides stimulates cGMP production in rat and guinea pig brain areas which are enriched in specific ANP binding sites.[22,39] In addition, ANP-related peptides also increase cGMP production in neural cell lines.[40] Thus, brain ANP receptor sites also appear to be coupled to the particulate guanylate cyclase system and may thus represent physiologically relevant receptors.

D. ANP RECEPTOR SUBTYPES

The existence of two different peripheral ANP receptor subtypes with apparent M_rs of 60 to 70 kDa (C-type) and 120 to 140 kDa (B-type) has recently been proposed.[41-46] This is based on differential binding characteristics and the ability to generate cGMP in response to various ANP-related peptides truncated at the amino and/or carboxy termini. The B-ANP receptor subtype possesses the binding characteristic observed with guanylate cyclase-coupled ANP binding sites and an apparent molecular weight of 120 kDa, and has been proposed as the physiologically relevant subtype.[44,46,47] On the other hand, the C-ANP receptor subtype is most likely not coupled to cGMP production, possesses lower affinity and larger capacity, and binds with high affinity both cyclic and linear forms of ANP-like peptides.[44-47] This latter subtype may serve as a specific "storage clearance" binding site for ANP-related peptides in order to appropriately control circulating levels of these peptides.[45]

Recently, the biochemical characteristics of rat brain ANP receptor sites have been investigated. Chemical cross-linking and subsequent purification of [^{125}I]ANP binding sites in rat olfactory bulb membrane preparations have revealed the presence of a single band with an apparent molecular weight of 116 kDa.[32] Thus, based on the classification of receptor subtypes proposed for peripheral tissues, these brain ANP brain receptor sites can be considered to be of the B-ANP subtype since they are linked to cGMP production, possess stringent structural requirements, and represent the high molecular weight entity, at least in olfactory bulb.[32] However, the presence of the C-ANP receptor type in some brain tissues cannot be ruled out, especially in circumventricular organs which are exposed to circulating levels of ANP-like peptides and where ANP binding sites have been observed (see Section III). Finally, the recent isolation of a new ANP-like peptide in porcine brain (see Section I) may suggest the existence of an additional subtype of ANP receptor sites in the CNS.

III. DISTRIBUTION OF BRAIN ANP RECEPTORS

Autoradiographic studies performed in various laboratories have clearly demonstrated the discrete and heterogeneous distribution of ANP binding sites in mammalian brain of different species. However, some discrepancies have been reported in the distribution and densities of ANP receptor sites in rat[20-23,25,26] and guinea pig brain (see Table 1).[21-23] These observed differences may be related to the use of different protocols and assay systems (for example, type and concentration of ligands, incubation conditions, washing conditions, etc.).

In rat brain, most studies have shown that the highest densities of ANP binding sites are concentrated in the circumventricular organs (subfornical organ, area postrema, vascular organ of the lamina terminalis) and the olfactory bulb.[20-23,25,26] Moderate levels of sites are also seen in the nuclei of the hypothalamus and various midbrain and brainstem structures, while low levels are seen throughout the forebrain, diencephalon, basal ganglia, cortex, and cerebellum.[20-23,25,26] In addition, high levels of ANP binding sites have been observed in the linings of ventricles, choroid plexus, and leptomeninges, whereas low levels have been found in the pineal gland (see Table 1, Figure 1A).[20-23]

In the guinea pig, the localization of specific brain ANP receptor sites is broader than that found in the rat. Quirion and co-workers[21,22] have shown that in addition to areas associated with the regulation of cardiovascular parameters (for example, the subfornical organ, area postrema, and nucleus of the solitary tract), various other areas such as the hippocampus, thalamus, amygdala, and cerebellum are enriched with high densities of specific ANP binding sites (see Table 1, Figure 1B).

In monkey brain, high levels of ANP receptor sites are found in the cerebellum (Figure 1C), while other brain areas such as the cortex, striatum, and midbrain are mostly devoid of specific binding sites.[21,22] Moreover, high amounts of ANP binding sites have been observed in the subfornical organ, area postrema, and olfactory bulb of the hamster brain, whereas low levels were seen in the striatum.[22] Thus far, we have been unable to obtain clear evidence for the existence of specific ANP binding sites in human brain.[105] These preliminary negative results could be related to various factors, such as long post-mortem delays (10 to 12 h), incubation conditions, etc. Recently, Mantyh et al.[23] have reported that in the cat brainstem and in the spinal cord of the rat, guinea pig, cat, and human, specific ANP binding sites were only in the pia/arachnoid tissues.

Thus, the distribution of brain ANP binding sites appears to be highly species dependent. Similar results have been reported for various classes of neurotransmitter and neuropeptide receptors, the opioid being one of the most prominent examples.[48] This demonstrates that results obtained in one animal species cannot necessarily be extrapolated to others. It would be of interest to study the localization of brain ANP binding sites in other mammals, as well as in lower species, in order to determine the phylogenic appearance and distribution of this new class of brain receptor site.

Finally, the present section only provides some information concerning the distribution of brain ANP binding sites. However, immunohistochemical and radioimmunochemical data have revealed that ANP-like immunoreactive material is also present and selectively distributed in certain brain areas,[12-16] although current data are limited to localization in rat, dog, and frog brain. Other species will have to be studied in order to adequately compare the distribution of the receptor and its putative endogenous ligands. Already, it can be said that some disparities between the localization of ANP-like peptides and its receptor site can

TABLE 1
Distribution of ANF Receptor Sites in Rat Brain

Structure	ANF receptor sites apparent density			
	A[24]	B[20-22]	C[26]	D[23]
Olfactory apparatus				
Olfactory bulb				
Plexiform layer	+ + + +	+ + + +	+ + + +	+ + + +
Granular layer	+ +	—	—	+ + + +
Glomerular layer	+ +	—	—	—
Olfactory nerve	+ +	—	—	—
Accessory olfactory bulb	+ + + +	—	—	—
Olfactory nuclei	+	—	—	—
Lateral olfactory tract	+ + +	+	+ +	+ + + +
Primary olfactory pathway	—	—	—	—
Cortex				
Frontal cortex	+	—	—	—
Primary olfactory cortex	+	—	—	—
Anterior cingulate cortex	+	—	—	—
Posterior cingulate cortex	+	—	—	—
Striate cortex	+ +	—	—	—
Parietal cortex	—	+	—	0
Limbic system				
Olfactory tubercle	+	—	—	—
Lateral septum				
Dorsal	+	+	—	—
Intermediate	+	+	—	—
Ventral	+ +	—	—	
Medial septum	+	+	—	—
Diagonal band of Broca	+	—	—	—
Bed nucleus of the stria terminalis	+	—	—	—
Ventral hippocampal commissure	+ +	—	—	—
Hippocampus				
CA1	+	+	—	0
CA2	+	+	—	0
CA3	+	+	—	0
Dentate gyrus	+	+	—	0
Fimbria hippocampi	—	—	+ +	—
Amygdala				
Central nucleus	+	—	—	—
Lateral nucleus	+	—	—	—
Fasciculus retroflexus	—	—	+ +	+
Basal ganglia				
Caudate-Putamen	+	+	0	0
Nucleus accumbens	+	—	—	+
Ventral palladum	+	—	—	—
Globus pallidus	+	+	—	0
Circumventricular organs				
Subfornical organ	+ + + +	+ + + +	+ + + +	+ +
Area postrema	+ + + +	+ + +	+ + + +	0
Ependyma	—	+ + +	—	+ + +
Linings of ventricles	—	+ + + +	–	+ + +
Median eminence	+	+ +	+	—
Vascular organ of the lamina terminalis	—	—	+ + + +	—
Hypothalamus				
Periventricular nucleus	+	—	—	—

TABLE 1 (continued)
Distribution of ANF Receptor Sites in Rat Brain

Structure	ANF receptor sites apparent density			
	A[24]	B[20-22]	C[26]	D[23]
Medial preoptic area	+	+ +	+ + +	—
Lateral preoptic area	+	—	—	—
Anterior hypothalamic area	+	—	—	—
Lateral hypothalamic area	+	—	—	—
Supraoptic nucleus	+	—	+ + + +	+
Paraventricular nucleus	+	—	+ + +	—
Arcuate nucleus	+	—	—	—
Ventromedial nucleus	+	—	—	—
Dorsomedial nucleus	+	—	—	+
Posterior nucleus	+	—	—	—
Mammillary nuclei	+	—	—	—
Thalamus				
Paraventricular nucleus	+ +	+	—	+
Anterioventral nucleus	+	+	—	—
Anteromedial nucleus	+	+	—	—
Ventrolateral nucleus	+	+	—	—
Ventroposterolateral nucleus	+	+	—	—
Lateral dorsal thalamus	+	+	—	—
Lateral posterior thalamus	+	+	—	—
Habenular nucleus	+ +	+	+ +	+ +
Midbrain				
Substantia nigra	+	+	0	0
Central gray	+	—	—	—
Superior colliculus	+ +	0	—	—
Interpenduncular nucleus	+ +	—	—	+ +
Brainstem				
Nucleus tractus solitarius	—	+ +	—	0
Pontine nucleus	+ +	—	—	—
Inferior colliculus	+ +	0	—	—
Dorsal raphe	+ +	—	—	—
Medial raphe	+ +	—	—	—
Pontine caudal reticular nucleus	+ +	—	—	—
Superior olive	+	—	—	—
Inferior olive	+	—	—	—
Parvocellular reticular nucleus	+ +	—	—	—
Paragigantocellular nucleus	+ +	—	—	—
Lateral reticular nucleus	+	—	—	—
Medullary reticular nucleus	+	—	—	—
Locus coeruleus	—	+	0	—
Cerebellum	+	+	—	0
Spinal cord	—	0	—	—
Others				
Anterior commissure	+ +	—	—	—
Choroid plexus	—	+ + +	+ + + +	+ + + +
Corpus callosum		+	—	0
Medial	+ +			
Lateral	+ +			

Note: + + + +, high to very high; + + +, moderate to high; + +, low to moderate; +, low; 0, very low densities; — , not determined.

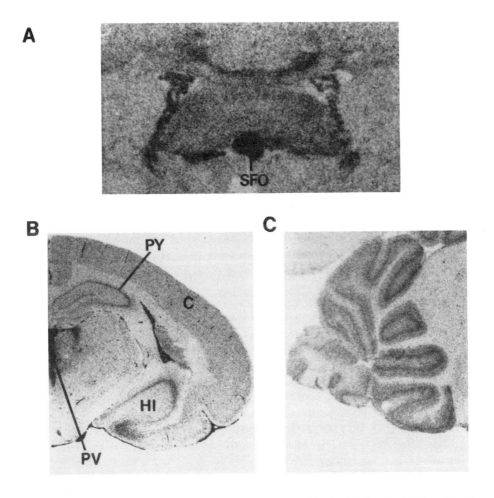

FIGURE 1. Photomicrographs of the autoradiographic distribution of [^{125}I]ANP binding sites in (A) rat, (B) guinea pig, and (C) monkey brain. High densities of binding are seen in the subfornical organ (A), certain thalamic nuclei (B), hippocampus (B), and cerebellum (C). Abbreviations used: C, cortex; HI, hippocampus; PV, periventricular nucleus of the thalamus; PY, pyramidal cell layers of the hippocampus; SFO, subfornical organ.

be found in the rat brain. Such apparent discordance has been observed previously for a wide variety of neurotransmitter systems and several explanations have been proposed for these "mismatches", which may constitute the rule rather than the exception.[49-51] It is also possible that certain ANP receptor sites found in some brain regions could be associated with the newly discovered ANP-like peptide.[31]

IV. PLASTICITY OF BRAIN ANP RECEPTORS

A. ANIMAL MODELS OF CARDIOVASCULAR DISORDERS

Modification in the densities of ANP receptor sites have been reported in various animal models of cardiovascular dysfunctions. Saavedra and co-workers[52] were the first to observe a significant decrease in the number of ANP binding sites in certain brain areas such as the subfornical organ, area postrema, nucleus of the solitary tract, and choroid plexus in spontaneously hypertensive rats (SHR). Similar results have been obtained by two other groups.[22,53] However, we have not found significant alterations in the capacity of ANP binding sites in the subfornical organ of SHR animals, although we have seen changes in the brainstem.[22]

This discrepancy can be related to assay conditions, use of animals obtained from different sources, and animal age. Nevertheless, it clearly shows that the density of ANP receptor sites is altered in certain brain regions in SHR rats. Moreover, an up-regulation in ANP binding sites has been observed in the subfornical organ of acutely and chronically dehydrated rats[33,34,54] and in the area postrema and subfornical organ of 6- to 7-month-old cardiomyopathic hamsters.[22] However, ANP binding was not affected in other brain regions such as the olfactory bulb and striatum.[22,34] Since the subfornical organ and area postrema are located outside the blood-brain barrier, ANP receptor sites in these areas could be sensitive to alterations in circulating levels of ANP-like substances.[27,54] Finally, these results clearly demonstrate the plasticity of ANP binding sites in mammalian brains — important information revealing the physiological relevance of these sites.

B. ONTOGENIC DEVELOPMENT OF BRAIN ANP BINDING SITES

The ontogenic development of ANP receptor sites has recently been reported in rat brain.[55] it is apparent that ANF binding sites undergo major redistribution during postnatal ontogeny. While most structures labeled in the adult brain (subfornical organ, choroid plexus) were shown to contain ANF binding sites before birth, certain regions demonstrated significant differences. For example, high levels of ANP binding sites are seen in the cerebral cortex to postnatal day 14, but rapidly decrease thereafter to become almost undetectable in the adult brain. Thus, the ontogenic appearance and expression of ANF receptor sites varies between brain regions, suggesting a possible involvement of ANF-like peptides in brain development, especially in cortical structures. Moreover, the ANP receptor gene appears to be turned on during the first 2 weeks after birth and to be subsequently repressed during adult life. This would be a good model to study the control of the expression of ANP receptor sites in brain tissues.

C. INTERACTIONS WITH OTHER NEUROTRANSMITTER SYSTEMS

To date, relatively few studies have been done to determine the possible effects of ANP-like peptides on well-established neurotransmitter systems. An inhibitory effect of ANP has been reported on the cholinergically stimulated synthesis of dopamine in rat superior cervical ganglia[56] and ANP-like peptides may inhibit certain brain dopaminergic pathways.[57] It has been shown that ANP decreases the level of dopamine and its metabolites in the septum and hypothalamus, but not in other areas such as the striatum and olfactory tubercule.[57] No changes in the concentration of noradrenaline and serotonin were seen throughout the brain following ANP injection, demonstrating some selectivity for the dopaminergic system.[57] However, a 3-week treatment with haloperidol, a dopamine D_2 receptor antagonist, did not alter [^{125}I]ANP binding parameters in various regions of the rat brain, including the striatum, cortex, subfornical organ, and area postrema.[22] This may suggest that dopamine probably does not reciprocally modulate the activity of the brain ANF system, at least through manipulation of the D_2 receptor subtype.

Multiple central and peripheral actions of ANP-like peptides are opposite to those induced by angiotensin II and vasopressin. For example, ANP-like substances antagonize the ability of angiotensin II to stimulate aldosterone secretion from cells of the adrenal glomerulosa[58] and have opposite effects on diuresis and vascular tone.[59] ANP apparently also antagonizes numerous biological effects of angiotensin II in the CNS.[60] Moreover, Itoh and co-workers[61] have recently reported that the brain renin-angiotensin system modulates the secretion of ANP-like substances from the heart and that direct injection of ANP in the brain attenuates this antagonistic effect of brain angiotensin II. Consequently, it seems likely that renin-angiotensin and ANP systems could act as physiological antagonists in the CNS and in the periphery to modulate the integration of various cardiovascular parameters.

V. RELEVANCE OF BRAIN AND RECEPTOR TO FUNCTION

The presence and widespread distribution of ANP-like peptides and receptors in the brain strongly suggest that this new family of peptides could act as putative neuromodulators/ neurotransmitters. Already, various biological effects have been noted following direct injections of ANP-related peptides into the brain.

Most studies have focused on the possible effect of ANP-like substances on the control of cardiovascular parameters. This is most likely based on the known biological actions of ANP-related peptides in the peripheral cardiovascular system, as well as on the presence of ANP-like immunoreactivity and receptor sites in various circumventricular organs and other brain areas involved in the central regulation of cardiovascular parameters.[2,19,22,27,54,60] It has been shown that discrete injections of ANP-like peptides into the brain markedly increase blood pressure and heart rate,[62] modify diuresis and salt appetite,[63-67] and modulate vasopressin secretion[68-70] and angiotensin-II-induced drinking responses.[71,72] Thus, it appears that ANP-like peptides, through their specific receptors, act as an important regulator of cardiovascular functions in the organism.

Additionally, ANP binding sites have been localized in several other brain regions not necessarily or directly involved in the control of cardiovascular parameters. For example, the choroid plexus, a structure involved in the secretion of cerebrospinal fluid, possesses high densities of ANP binding sites[22,23,26,33,34,52,73] which may be altered in SHR rats.[52,74] These sites are apparently coupled to a guanylate cyclase system since ANP stimulates cGMP production in this structure.[75] Thus, it is possible that ANP-related peptides could be involved in the production of cerebrospinal fluids. In the guinea pig, the presence of ANP binding sites in the amygdala and hippocampus could suggest a possible role for these peptides in these structures. Additionally, ANP-like peptides could be involved in the control of certain sensory pathways and in the coordination of movements since high densities of ANF sites are found in the thalamus and cerebellum in guinea pig and monkey brain. ANP-related peptides may also play a role in the regulation of the functions of the anterior pituitary through binding sites located in the adenohypophyseal lobe itself (see Section IV), as well as through receptor sites present in the median eminence and related hypothalamic nuclei.[20-22,24,26] For example, ANP-like peptides inhibit angiotensin II-induced ACTH secretion[76] and ANP injections into the third ventricle provoke inhibition of prolactin release.[77] This suggests that ANP-like peptides can act centrally to modulate the release of the neural factor responsible for hypothalamic control of the anterior pituitary function. Finally, specific ANP binding sites have recently been demonstrated to be present on brain microvessels.[78] These sites are specifically seen on brain capillaries which constitute the blood-brain barrier and, thus, participate in the constant exchange of fluid between the blood and the brain. This is of great interest since it has been shown that ANP-like peptides alter the rate of cerebrospinal fluid production.[79] Hence, the possible role(s) of ANP-like peptides on the permeability of the blood-brain barrier and brain circulation should be carefully investigated.

VI. ANF RECEPTOR SITES IN BRAIN CLOSELY RELATED STRUCTURES

A. EYE

High levels of ANP-like materials have recently been reported in the anterior uvea of the eye[80] and high densities of ANP binding sites have been identified on the pigmented epithelium of the ciliary body of rat and guinea pig eye.[20,22,81-83] Additionally, these binding sites are moderately concentrated in the choriocapillaris.[81] Interestingly, the ciliary body of the eye is involved in the production of the vitreous fluid and it has been shown that ANP lowers intraocular pressure in rabbit eye.[84] Since ANP-like peptides modulate fluid production in various tissues, further studies on the role of these peptides on the physiology of the eye are certainly warranted.

B. PITUITARY GLAND

ANP-like immunoreactive materials and receptor sites have also been detected in the anterior and posterior lobe of the pituitary gland.[10,15,20,26,81,85-88] ANP-like immunoreactivity is especially found in adenohypophyseal gonadotrophs.[10,86,87] The presence of an ANP messenger RNA has also been reported in these cells.[89] However, the biological significance of ANP-like peptides in the anterior pituitary gland is not clear. Although ANP stimulates cGMP production in gonadotroph-enriched cell populations,[90] controversial results have been reported on the physiological relevance of this effect. In fact, ANP-like peptides have been shown to either increase[91] or have no effect[92] on LH secretion. Similarly, ANP does not significantly modify ACTH secretion from either normal or clonal corticotrophs,[85,92,93] even though cGMP production is stimulated in these preparations.[94] Controversies also exist about ANP effects on the release of prolactin from the adenohypophysis.[77,93] The presence of ANP binding sites in the posterior lobe of the pituitary gland have been demonstrated.[10,20,26,81] However, the role of ANP-like peptides in this tissue is not clear. It has been shown that these peptides could either induce[95] or inhibit[96,97] vasopressin secretion from the posterior lobe. Thus, further studies are urgently needed to elucidate the possible role of ANP-like peptides and receptor sites in the pituitary gland.

C. ADRENAL MEDULLA

Finally, most recent studies have demonstrated the presence of ANP-like peptides and binding sites in the adrenal medulla[83,87,98-102] and it seems that nicotine can induce ANP secretion from bovine adrenal cells.[103] This is of interest, especially since cultured chromaffin cells derived from the adrenal medulla are widely used as models of nondifferentiated brain neurons. Morel et al.[101] have recently reported (using *in situ* hybridization and immuno-cytochemical and ultrastructural autoradiographic techniques) that ANP is most likely synthesized in the noradrenaline-containing cell types from which it is released to act in a paracrine fashion on adrenalin-containing cells through the interaction with specific ANP binding sites localized on this cell type. If this is the case, it would constitute a unique model system to study interactions between peptides and "classical" neurotransmitters. Moreover, Heisler and Morrier[102] have shown that ANP apparently binds to a single class of high-affinity, low-capacity sites in bovine adrenal chromaffin cell membrane preparations. These sites are apparently coupled to cGMP production.[102,104] Thus, the adrenal medulla may constitute a good model with which to study the action of ANF-like peptides on CNS-like structures.

VII. CONCLUSION

In summary, ANP-like peptides and highly specific receptor binding sites are broadly distributed in the brain of various mammalian species. Their presence in multiple brain areas suggests that the biological effects of these peptides may extend beyond the strict control of cardiovascular parameters. Thus, these peptides should be considered as a new family of brain-heart peptides acting as neurotransmitter/neuromodulators in the CNS.

REFERENCES

1. **de Bold, A. J.**, Atrial natriuretic factor: a hormone produced by the heart, *Science*, 230, 767, 1985.
2. **Cantin, M. and Genest, J.**, The heart and the atrial natriuretic factor, *Endocrine Rev.*, 6, 107, 1985.
3. **Anderson, J. V. and Bloom, S. R.**, Atrial natriuretic peptide: what is the excitement all about?, *J. Endocrinol.*, 110, 7, 1986.
4. **Atlas, S. A.**, Atrial natriuretic factor: a new hormone of cardiac origin, in *Recent Progress in Hormone Research*, Vol. 42, Greep, R. O., Ed., Academic Press, New York, 1987, 207.
5. **Pandey, K. N., Pavlou, S. M., Kovacs, W. J., and Inagami, T.**, Atrial natriuretic factor regulates steroidogenic responsiveness and cyclic nucleotide levels in mouse Leydig cells *in vitro*, *Biochem. Biophys. Res. Commun.*, 138, 399, 1986.
6. **Mukhopadhyay, A. K., Bohnet, H. G., and Leidenberger, F. A.**, Testosterone production by mouse Leydig cells is stimulated in vitro by atrial natriuretic factor, *FEBS Lett.*, 202, 111, 1986.
7. **Bex, F. and Corbin, A.**, Atrial natriuretic factor stimulates testosterone production by mouse interstitial cells, *Eur. J. Pharmacol.*, 115, 126, 1985.
8. **De Léan, A., Gutkowska, J., McNicoll, N., Schiller, P. W., Cantin, M., and Genest, J.**, Characterization of specific receptors for atrial natriuretic factor in bovine adrenal zona glomerulosa, *Life Sci.*, 35, 2311, 1984.
9. **Napier, M. A., Vandlen, R. L., Albers-Schomberg, G., Nutt, R. F., Brady, S., Lyle, T., Winquist, R., Faison, E. P., Heinel, L. A., and Blaine, E. H.**, Specific membrane receptors for atrial natriuretic factor in renal and vascular tissues, *Proc. Natl. Acad. Sci. U.S.A.*, 81, 5946, 1984.
10. **Morel, G., Chabot, J. G., Belles-Isles, M., and Heisler, S.**, Synthesis and internalization of atrial natriuretic factor in anterior pituitary cells, *Mol. Cell. Endocrinol.*, 55, 219, 1988.
11. **Hamet, P., Tremblay, J., Pang, S. C., Skuherska, R., Schiffin, E. L., Garcia, R., Cantin, M., Genest, J., Palmour, R., Ervin, F. R., Martin, S., and Goldwater, R.**, Cyclic GMP as mediator and biological marker of atrial natriuretic factor, *J. Hypertens.*, 4, S49, 1986.
12. **Saper, C. B., Standaert, D. G., Currie, M. G., Schwartz, D., Geller, D. M., and Needleman, P.**, Atriopeptin-immunoreactive neurons in the brain: presence in cardiovascular regulatory areas, *Science*, 227, 1047, 1985.
13. **Skofitsch, G., Jacobowitz, D. M., Eskay, R. L., and Zamir, N.**, Distribution of atrial natriuretic factor-like immunoreactive neurons in the rat brain, *Neuroscience*, 16, 917, 1985.
14. **Zamir, N., Skofitsch, G., Eskay, R. L., and Jacobowitz, D. M.**, Distribution of immunoreactive atrial natriuretic peptides in the central nervous system of the rat, *Brain Res.*, 365, 105, 1986.
15. **Netchitailo, P., Feuilloley, M., Pelletier, G., Leboulenger, F., Cantin, M., Gutkowska, J., and Vaudry, H.**, Atrial natriuretic factor-like immunoreactivity in the central nervous system of the frog, *Neuroscience*, 22, 341, 1987.
16. **Kawata, M., Nakao, K., Morii, N., Kiso, Y., Yamashita, H., Imura, H., and Sano, Y.**, Atrial natriuretic polypeptide: topographical distribution in the rat brain by radioimmunoassay and immunohistochemistry, *Neuroscience*, 16, 521, 1985.
17. **Standaert, D. G., Needleman, P., and Saper, C. G.**, Organization of atriopeptin-like immunoreactive neurons in the central nervous system of the rat, *J. Comp. Neurol.*, 253, 315, 1986.
18. **Fujio, N., Ohashi, M., Nawata, H., Kato, K.-I., Tateishi, J., Matsuo, H., and Ibayashi, H.**, Unique distribution of atrial hormones in dog brain, *Regul. Peptides*, 18, 131, 1987.
19. **Quirion, R.**, Atrial natriuretic factors: the brain-heart peptides, in *Neural and Endocrine Peptides and Receptors*, Moody, T. W., Ed., Plenum Press, New York, 1986, 299.
20. **Quirion, R., Dalpé, M., De Léan, A., Gutkowska, J., Cantin, M., and Genest, J.**, Atrial natriuretic factor (ANF) binding sites in brain and related structures, *Peptides*, 5, 1167, 1984.
21. **Quirion, R., Dalpé, M., and Dam, T. V.**, Characterization and distribution of receptors for the atrial natriuretic peptides in mammalian brain, *Proc. Natl. Acad. Sci. U.S.A.*, 83, 174, 1986.
22. **Quirion, R., Dalpé, M., and De Léan, A.**, Characterization, distribution and plasticity of atrial natriuretic factor binding sites in brain, *Can. J. Physiol. Pharmacol.*, 66, 280, 1988.
23. **Mantyh, C. R., Kruger, L., Brecha, N. C., and Mantyh, P. W.**, Localization of specific binding sites for atrial natriuretic factor in the central nervous system of rat, guinea pig, cat and human, *Brain Res.*, 412, 329, 1987.
24. **Gibson, T. R., Wildey, G. M., Manaker, S., and Glembotski, C. C.**, Autoradiographic localization and characterization of atrial natriuretic peptide binding sites in the rat central nervous system and adrenal gland, *J. Neurosci.*, 6, 2004, 1986.
25. **Lynch, D. R., Braas, K. M., and Snyder, S. H.**, Atrial natriuretic factor receptors in rat kidney, adrenal gland, and brain: autoradiographic localization and fluid balance dependent changes, *Proc. Natl. Acad. Sci. U.S.A.*, 83, 3357, 1986.

26. **Kurihara, M., Saavedra, J. M., and Shigematsu, K.,** Localization and characterization of atrial natriuretic peptide binding sites in discrete areas of rat brain and pituitary gland by quantitative autoradiography, *Brain Res.*, 408, 31, 1987.

27. **Quirion, R.,** Receptor sites for atrial natriuretic factors in brain and associated structures: an overview, *Cell Mol. Neurobiol.*, 9, 45, 1989.

28. **Shibasaki, T., Naruse, M., Naruse, K., Masuda, A., Kim, Y. S., Imaki, T., Yamauchi, N., Demura, H., Inagami, T., and Shizune, K.,** Atrial natriuretic factor is released from rat hypothalamus in vitro, *Biochem. Biophys. Res. Commun.*, 136, 590, 1986.

29. **Tanaka, I. and Inagami, T.,** Release of immunoreactive atrial natriuretic factor from rat hypothalamus in vitro, *Eur. J. Pharmacol.*, 122, 353, 1986.

30. **Gardner, D. G., Viasuk, G. P., Baxter, J. D., Fiddes, J. C., and Lewicki, J. A.,** Identification of atrial natriuretic factor gene transcripts in the central nervous system of the rat, *Proc. Natl. Acad. Sci. U.S.A.*, 84, 2175, 1987.

31. **Sudoh, T., Kangawa, K., Minamino, N., and Matsuo, H.,** A new natriuretic peptide in porcine brain, *Nature (London)*, 332, 78, 1988.

32. **Wildey, G. M. and Glembotski, C. C.,** Cross-linking of atrial natriuretic peptide to binding sites in rat olfactory bulb membranes, *J. Neurosci.*, 6, 3767, 1986.

33. **McCarty, R. and Plunkett, L. M.,** Binding sites for atrial natriuretic factor (ANF) in brain: alterations in Brattleboro rats, *Brain Res. Bull.*, 17, 767, 1986.

34. **Saavedra, J. M., Israel, A., and Kurihara, M.,** Increased atrial natriuretic peptide binding sites in the rat subfornical organ after water deprivation, *Endocrinology*, 120, 426, 1987.

35. **Olins, G. M., Patton, D. R., Tjoeng, F. S., and Blehm, D. J.,** Specific receptors for atriopeptin III in rabbit lung, *Biochem. Biophys. Res. Commun.*, 140, 302, 1986.

36. **Sugiyama, M., Fukumi, H., Grammer, R. T., Misono, K. S., Yabe, Y., Morisawa, Y., and Inagami, T.,** Synthesis of atrial natriuretic peptides and studies on structural factors in tissue specificity, *Biochem. Biophys. Res. Commun.*, 123, 338, 1984.

37. **Tang, J., Webber, R. J., Chang, D., Chang, J. K., Klang, J., and Wei, E. T.,** Depressor and natriuretic activities of several atrial peptides, *Regul. Peptides*, 9, 53, 1984.

38. **Cantin, M., Thibault, G., Garcia, R., Gutkowska, J., De Léan, A., Schiffrin, E., Seidah, N., Lazure, C., and Chrétien, M.,** Structure-activity relationships of atrial natriuretic factors on renal function and renin release, *Clin. Res.*, 33, 607A, 1985.

39. **Takayanagi, R., Grammer, R. T., and Inagami, T.,** Regional increase of cyclic GMP by atrial natriuretic factor in rat brain: markedly elevated response in spontaneously hypertensive rats, *Life Sci.*, 39, 573, 1986.

40. **Friedl, A., Harmening, B., nad Hamprecht, B.,** Atrial natriuretic hormones raise the level of cyclic GMP in neural cell lines, *J. Neurochem.*, 46, 1522, 1986.

41. **Leitman, D. C., Andresen, J. W., Kuno, T., Kaminski, Y., Chang, J. K., and Murad, F.,** Identification of multiple binding sites for atrial natriuretic factor by affinity cross-linking in cultured endothelial cells, *J. Biol. Chem.*, 261, 11650, 1986.

42. **Scarborough, R. M., Schenk, D. B., McEnroe, G. A., Arfsten, A., Kang, L.-L., Schwartz, K., and Lewicki, J. A.,** Truncated atrial natriuretic peptide analogs: comparison between receptor binding and stimulation of cyclic GMP accumulation in cultured vascular smooth muscle cells, *J. Biol. Chem.*, 261, 12960, 1986.

43. **Budzik, G. P., Firestone, S. L., Bush, B. N., Connolly, P. J., Rockway, T. W., Sarine, V. K., and Holleman, W. H.,** Divergence of ANF analogs in smooth muscle cGMP response and aorta vasorelaxation: evidence for receptor subtypes, *Biochem. Biophys. Res. Commun.*, 144, 422, 1987.

44. **Pandey, K., Inagami, T., and Misono, K. S.,** Three distinct forms of atrial natriuretic factor receptors: kidney tubular epithelium cells and vascular smooth muscle cells contain different types of receptors, *Biochem. Biophys. Res. Commun.*, 147, 1146, 1987.

45. **Maack, T., Suzuki, M., Almeida, F. A., Nussenzveig, D., Scarborough, R. M., McEnroe, G. A., and Lewicki, J. A.,** Physiological role of silent receptors for atrial natriuretic factor, *Science*, 238, 675, 1987.

46. **Glembotski, C. C.,** in 1st Int. Symp. Atrial Natriuretic Factors and the Brain, Margarita Island, Venezuela, June 1987.

47. **Quirion, R.,** Atrial natriuretic peptides and the brain: an update, *Trends Neurosci.*, 11, 58, 1988.

48. **Quirion, R., Weiss, A. S., and Pert, C. B.,** Comparative pharmacological properties and autoradiographic distribution of [^{3}H]ethylketocyclazocine binding sites in rat and guinea pig brain, *Life Sci.*, 33, 183, 1983.

49. **Goedert, M., Mantyh, P. W., Emson, P. C., and Hunt, S. P.,** Inverse relationship between neurotensin receptors and neurotensin-like immunoreactivity in the cat striatum, *Nature (London)*, 307, 543, 1984.

50. **Mantyh, P. W., Maggio, J. E., and Hunt, S. P.,** The autoradiographic distribution of kassinin and substance K binding sites is different from the distribution of substance P binding sites in the rat brain, *Eur. J. Pharmacol.*, 102, 361, 1984.

51. **Kuhar, M. J. and Unnerstall, J. R.,** Quantitative receptor mapping by autoradiography. Some current technical problems, *Trends Neurosci.,* 8, 49, 1985.

52. **Saavedra, J. M., Correa, F. M. A., Plunkett, L. M., Israel, A., Kurihara, M., and Shigematsu, K.,** Binding of angiotensin and atrial natriuretic peptide in brain of hypertensive rats, *Nature (London),* 320, 758, 1986.

53. **McCarty, R. and Plunkett, L. M.,** Binding sites for atrial natriuretic factor (ANF) in brain: alterations in spontaneously hypertensive rats, *Neurochem. Int.,* 9, 177, 1986.

54. **Saavedra, J. M.,** Regulation of atrial natriuretic peptide receptors in the rat brain, *Cell. Mol. Neurobiol.,* 7, 151, 1987.

55. **Tong, Y. and Pelletier, G.,** Ontogenesis of atrial natriuretic factor (ANF) receptors in the rat brain, in *Symp. Molecular Biology of Brain and Endocrine Peptidergic Systems,* Montreal, October 1987.

56. **Debinski, W., Kuchel, O., Buu, N. T., Cantin, M., and Genest, J.,** Atrial natriuretic factor partially inhibits the stimulated catecholamine synthesis in superior cervical ganglia of rat, *Neurosci. Lett.,* 77, 92, 1987.

57. **Nakao, K., Katsuura, G., Morii, N., Itoh, H., Shiono, S., Yamada, T., Sugawara, A., Sakamoto, M., Saito, Y., Eigyo, M., Matsushita, A., and Imura, H.,** Inhibitory effect of centrally administered atrial natriuretic polypeptide on the brain dopaminergic system in rats, *Eur. J. Pharmacol.,* 131, 171, 1986.

58. **Goodfriend, T. L., Elliot, M. E., and Atlas, S. A.,** Action of synthetic atrial natriuretic factor on bovine adrenal glomerulosa, *Life Sci.,* 35, 1675, 1984.

59. **Ballermann, B. J. and Brenner, B. N.,** Role of atrial peptides in body fluid homeostasis, *Circ. Res.,* 58, 619, 1986.

60. **Nakao, K., Morii, N., Itoh, H., Yamada, T., Shiono, S., Sugawara, A., Saito, Y., Mukoyama, M., Arai, H., Sakamoto, M., and Imura, H.,** Atrial natriuretic polypeptide in the brain: implication of central cardiovascular control, *J. Hypertens.,* 4, S492, 1986.

61. **Itoh, H., Nakao, K., Yamada, T., Morii, N., Shiono, S., Sugawara, A., Saito, Y., Mukoyama, M., Arai, H., and Imura, H.,** Central interaction of brain atrial natriuretic polypeptide (ANP) system and brain renin-angiotensin system in ANP secretion from heart. Evidence for possible brain-heart axis, *Can. J. Physiol. Pharmacol.,* 66, 255, 1988.

62. **Sills, M. A., Nguyen, K. Q., and Jacobowitz, D. M.,** Increases in heart rate and blood pressure produced by microinjections of atrial natriuretic factor into the AV3V region of rat brain, *Peptides,* 6, 1037, 1985.

63. **Antunes-Rodrigues, J., McCann, S. M., Rogers, L. C., and Samson, W. K.,** Atrial natriuretic factor inhibits dehydration- and angiotensin II-induced water intake in the conscious, unrestrained rat, *Proc. Natl. Acad. Sci. U.S.A.,* 82, 8720, 1985.

64. **Fitts, D. A., Thunhorst, R. L., and Simpson, J. B.,** Diuresis and reduction of salt appetite by lateral ventricular infusions of atriopeptin II, *Brain Res.,* 348, 118, 1985.

65. **Itoh, H., Nakao, K., Katsuura, G., Morii, N., Shiono, S., Yamada, T., Sugawara, A., Saito, Y., Watanabe, K., Igano, K., Inouye, K., and Imura, H.,** Atrial natriuretic polypeptides: structure-activity relationship in the central action — a comparison of their antidipsogenic actions, *Neurosci. Lett.,* 74, 102, 1987.

66. **Katsuura, G., Nakamura, M., Inouye, K., Kono, M., Nakao, K., and Imura, H.,** Regulatory role of atrial natriuretic polypeptide in water drinking in rats, *Eur. J. Pharmacol.,* 121, 285, 1986.

67. **Lee, J., Feng, J. Q., Malvin, R. L., Huang, B.-S., and Grekin, R. J.,** Centrally administered atrial natriuretic factor increases water excretion, *Am. J. Physiol.,* 252, F1011, 1987.

68. **Crandall, M. E. and Gregg, C. M.,** In vitro evidence for an inhibitory effect of atrial natriuretic peptide on vasopressin release, *Neuroendocrinology,* 4, 439, 1986.

69. **Samson, W. K.,** Atrial natriuretic factor inhibits dehydration and hemorrhage-induced vasopressin release, *Neuroendocrinology,* 40, 277, 1985.

70. **Samson, W. K.,** Dehydration-induced alterations in rat brain vasopressin and atrial natriuretic factor immunoreactivity, *Endocrinology,* 117, 1279, 1985.

71. **Lappe, R. W., Dinish, J. L., Bex, F., Michalak, K., and Wendt, R. L.,** Effects of atrial natriuretic factor on drinking responses to central angiotensin II, *Pharmacol. Biochem. Behav.,* 24, 1573, 1986.

72. **Nakamura, M., Takayanagi, R., and Inagami, T.,** Effect of atrial natriuretic factor on central angiotensin II-induced responses in rat, *Peptides,* 7, 373, 1986.

73. **Von Schroeder, H. P., Nishimura, E., McIntosh, C. H. S., Buchan, A. M. J., Wilson, N., and Ledsome, J. R.,** Autoradiographic localization of binding sites for atrial natriuretic factor, *Can. J. Physiol. Pharmacol.,* 63, 1373, 1985.

74. **Saavedra, J. M., Israel, A., Kurihara, M., and Fuchs, E.,** Decreased number and affinity of rat atrial natriuretic peptide$_{o-33}$ in the subfornical organ of spontaneously hypertensive rats, *Circ. Res.,* 58, 389, 1986.

75. **Tsutsumi, K., Niwa, M., Kawano, T., Ibaragi, M., Ozaki, M., and Mori, K.,** Atrial natriuretic polypeptides elevate the level of cyclic GMP in the rat choroid plexus, *Neurosci. Lett.,* 79, 174, 1987.

76. **Itoh, H., Nakao, K., Katsuura, G., Morii, N., Yamada, T., Shiono, S., Sakamoto, M., Sugawara, A., Saito, Y., Eigyo, M., Matsushita, A., and Imura, H.,** Possible involvement of central atrial natriuretic polypeptide in regulation of hypothalamic-pituitary-adrenal axis in conscious rats, *Neurosci. Lett.,* 69, 254, 1986.

77. **Samson, W. K. and Bianchi, B. R.,** Further evidence for a hypothalamic site of action of atrial natriuretic factor: inhibition of prolactin secretion in the conscious rat, *Can. J. Physiol. Pharmacol.,* 66, 301, 1988.

78. **Chabrier, P. E., Roubert, P., and Braquet, P.,** ANF-receptors on brain microvessels, *Proc. Natl. Acad. Sci. U.S.A.,* 84, 2078, 1987.

79. **Steardo, L. and Nathanson, J. A.,** Brain barrier tissues: end organs for atriopeptins, *Science,* 235, 470, 1987.

80. **Stone, R. A. and Glembotski, C. C.,** Immunoreactive atrial natriuretic peptide in the rat eye: molecular forms in anterior uvea and retina, *Biochem. Biophys. Res. Commun.,* 134, 1022, 1986.

81. **Mantyh, C. R., Kruger, L., Brecha, N. C., and Mantyh, P. W.,** Localization of specific binding sites for atrial natriuretic factor in peripheral tissues of the guinea pig, rat, and human, *Hypertension,* 8, 712, 1986.

82. **Bianchi, C., Anand-Srivastava, M. B., De Léan, G., Gutkowska, J., Forthomme, D., Genest, J., and Cantin, M.,** Localization and characterization of specific receptors for atrial natriuretic factor in ciliary processes of the eye, *Curr. Eye Res.,* 5, 283, 1986.

83. **Bianchi, C., Gutkowska, J., Thibault, G., Garcia, R., Genest, J., and Cantin, M.,** Radioautographic localization of ^{125}I-atrial natriuretic factor (ANF) in rat tissues, *Histochemistry,* 82, 441, 1985.

84. **Sugrue, M. F. and Viader, M.-P.,** Synthetic atrial natriuretic factor lowers rabbit intraocular pressure, *Eur. J. Pharmacol.,* 130, 349, 1986.

85. **Gutkowska, J. and Cantin, M.,** Bioactive ANF-like peptides in rat anterior pituitary, *Can. J. Physiol. Pharmacol.,* 66, 270, 1988.

86. **Inagami, S., Kobuta, Y., Kito, S., Kangwah, T., and Matsuo, M.,** Atrial natriuretic polypeptide-like immunoreactivity in the rat pituitary: light and electron microscopic studies, *Regul. Peptides,* 14, 101, 1986.

87. **McKenzie, J. C., Tanaka, I., Misono, K. S., and Inagami, T.,** Immunocytochemical localization of atrial natriuretic factor in the kidney, adrenal medulla, pituitary and atrium of rat, *J. Histochem. Cytochem.,* 8, 828, 1985.

88. **Gutkowska, J., Racz, K., Debinski, W., Thibault, G., Garcia, R., Kuchel, O., Cantin, M., and Genest, J.,** An atrial natriuretic factor-like activity in rat posterior hypophysis, *Peptides,* 8, 461, 1987.

89. **Gardner, D. G., Deschepper, C. F., Ganong, W. F., Hane, S., Fiddes, J., Baxter, J. D., and Lewicki, J.,** Extra-atrial expression of the gene for atrial natriuretic factor, *Proc. Natl. Acad. Sci. U.S.A.,* 83, 6697, 1986.

90. **Horvath, J., Ertl, T., and Schally, A. V.,** Effect of atrial natriuretic peptide on gonadotropin release in superfused rat anterior pituitary cells, *Proc. Natl. Acad. Sci. U.S.A.,* 83, 3444, 1986.

91. **Samson, W. K., Aguila, M. C., Norris, M., and Bianchi, R.,** Anterior pituitary hormone response to atrial natriuretic factor, *Soc. Neurosci.,* 12, 1027, 1986.

92. **Simard, J., Hubert, F. F., Labrie, F., Assayag, E., and Heisler, S.,** Atrial natriuretic factor-induced cGMP accumulation in rat anterior pituitary cells in culture is not coupled to hormonal secretion, *Regul. Peptides,* 15, 269, 1986.

93. **Hashimoto, K., Hattori, T., Suemaro, S., Sugawara, M., Takao, T., Kageyama, J., and Ota, Z.,** Atrial natriuretic peptide does not affect corticotropin-releasing factor-, arginine vasopressin- and angiotensin II-induced andrenocorticotropic hormone release in vivo and in vitro, *Regul. Peptides,* 17, 53, 1987.

94. **Heisler, S., Simard, J., Assayag, E., Mehri, Y., and Labrie, F.,** Atrial natriuretic factor does not affect basal, forskolin- and CRF-stimulated adenylate cyclase activity, cAMP formation or ACTH secretion but does stimulate cGMP synthesis in anterior pituitary, *Mol. Cell. Endocrinol.,* 44, 125, 1986.

95. **Januszewicz, F., Gutkowska, J., De Léan, A., Thibault, G., Garcia, R., Genest, J., and Cantin, M.,** Synthetic atrial natriuretic factor induces release (possibly receptor mediated) of vasopressin from rat posterior pituitary, *Proc. Soc. Exp. Biol. Med.,* 178, 321, 1985.

96. **Januszewicz, F., Thibault, G., Garcia, R., Gutkowska, J., Genest, J., and Cantin, M.,** Effect of synthetic atrial natriuretic factor on arginine vasopressin release by the rat hypothalamo-neurohypophyseal complex in organ culture, *Biochem. Biophys. Res. Commun.,* 134, 652, 1986.

97. **Obana, K., Naruse, M., Inagami, T., Brown, A. B., Naruse, K., Kurimoto, F., Sakurai, H., Demura, H., and Shizume, K.,** Atrial natriuretic factor inhibits vasopressin secretion from rat posterior pituitary, *Biochem. Biophys. Res. Commun.,* 132, 1088, 1985.

98. **Inagaki, S., Kubota, Y., Kito, S., Kangawa, K., and Matsuo, H.,** Immunoreactive atrial natriuretic polypeptides in the adrenal medulla and sympathetic ganglia, *Regul. Peptides,* 15, 249, 1986.

99. **Fuchs, E., Shigematsu, K., and Saavedra, J.,** Binding sites of atrial natriuretic peptide in tree shrew adrenal gland, *Peptides,* 7, 873, 1986.

100. **Ong, H., Lazure, C., Nguyen, T. T., McNicoll, N., Seidah, N., Chrétien, M., and De Léan, A.,** Bovine adrenal chromaffin granules are a site of synthesis of atrial natriuretic factor, *Biochem. Biophys. Res. Commun.*, 147, 957, 1987.

101. **Morel, C., Chabot, J.-G., Garcia-Caballero, T., Gossard, F., Dihl, F., Belles-Isles, M., and Heisler, S.,** Synthesis, internalization and localization of atrial natriuretic peptide in rat adrenal medulla, *Endocrinology,* 123, 149, 1988.

102. **Heisler, S. and Morrier, E.,** Bovine adrenal medullary cells contain functional atrial natriuretic peptide receptors, *Biochem. Biophys. Res. Commun.*, 150, 781, 1988.

103. **Nguyen, T. T., Ong, H., and De Léan, A.,** Aldosterone secretion inhibitor factor is an endogenous neuropeptide secreted by cultured chromaffin cells, *Fed. Proc.,* 46, 1451, 1987.

104. **Waldman, S. A., Rapoport, R. M., and Murad, F.,** Atrial natriuretic factor selectively activates particulate guanylate cyclase and elevates cyclic CMP in rat tissues, *J. Biol. Chem.,* 259, 14332, 1984.

105. **Chabot, J.-G. and Quirion, R.,** unpublished data.

Chapter 14

ELECTROPHYSIOLOGY OF ANP

Bernd Hamprecht and Georg Reiser

TABLE OF CONTENTS

I. INTRODUCTION

One of the physiologically most prominent characteristics of nervous tissue is the communication between excitable cells, the neurons. The transfer of information from one neuron to its target, which may be another neuron, is mediated by neurohormones released from the cells that emit information. Such neurohormones bind to specific receptors at the surface of the target cell, which eventually will open (or close) special receptor-regulated ion channels. The resulting change in ion permeability, in turn, will alter the membrane potential and electrical activity of the cell. Besides influencing the electrical activity of their target neurons, neurohormones may also regulate other neuronal properties. In fact, their action may not at all be restricted to neurons, but may also influence other neural cells, e.g., astroglia.

This chapter deals with electrophysiological effects evoked by ANP in cultured cells and the living animal. It is meant to emphasize the complementary nature of the two experimental systems, which might eventually clarify the functions and mechanisms of action of ANP in the nervous system.

The facts about ANP which are needed as a basis for the subsequent discussions are extensively covered in the preceding chapters and a number of review articles that have been published in recent years.[1-12]

II. ACTION OF ANP ON NEURAL CELLS IN CULTURE

A. CULTURE SYSTEMS

Early experiments reported from several laboratories, including our own, had indicated that cultured cells of the nervous system may be useful in elucidating basic biochemical mechanisms underlying the functioning of the nervous system.[13-22] Several reviews and monographs[23-28] comprehensively cover those culture systems[13,25,29-36] which have been successfully used as models for studying neural mechanisms at the cellular and molecular level. These culture systems comprise two classes; (1) cell lines that mostly originate from tumors of the nervous system and (2) primary cultures derived from normal nervous tissue.

In the authors' laboratory, both classes of cell culture systems are used for studying the mechanism of ANP action. Within each class, the cultures can be categorized according to the cell types, which are most frequently neurons or glial cells. The clonal neuroblastoma × glioma hybrid cell lines 108CC15[25,27,28,37] and 108CC25[38] were used in our investigations on ANP action. The two clonal glioma lines involved in these experiments, both derived from the C6 rat glioma line,[13] are a bromodeoxyuridine resistant variant, C6-BU-1,[39] and the polyploid line C6-4-2.[40] The latter was prepared by multiple cell fusions in order to generate a big cell that would be easily amenable to electrophysiological studies.

The glial primary cultures we employed in the studies on ANP action are derived from the brains of newborn mice[41,42] and rats.[43] Besides the prominent population of astroglial cells, these cultures also contain minor populations of oligodendroglia,[44-46] ependymal cells,[31,42,47] phagocytes,[48,49] and, among others, presumably also capillary endothelial cells,[50] pericytes, and meningeal cells. The neuronal primary cultures introduced into our work on ANP were prepared from the brains of 16-day-old rat embryos. They are neuron rich, which essentially means that the cultures contain a few astroglial cells besides the prevalent neurons.[43]

B. BIOCHEMICAL EFFECTS
1. Cyclic GMP

The influence of vasoactive peptide hormones on cultured neural cells was investigated. Vasoactive intestinal peptide (VIP) raised the level of cyclic AMP in astroglia-rich primary cultures from brain[52] and bradykinin, that of cyclic GMP in neuroblastoma × glioma hybrid cells.[53] We had been searching for a hormone that would elevate the level of cyclic GMP in astroglia-rich brain cell cultures in order to study the targets of this second messenger in glial cells. Whereas none of the vasoactive peptides mentioned above changed the concentration of cyclic GMP,[54] several of the ANPs raised the level of cyclic GMP at least 100-fold in astroglia-rich cultures from rat brain.[54-56] Atriopeptin III (rat ANF[103—126]) was about 1.5 orders of magnitude more potent than rat cardionatrin I (rat ANF[99—126]). None of the concentration-response curves for the ANPs tried reached a plateau at a range of concentrations up to 1 μM. Thus, for EC_{50} only a minimal value could be estimated, which was approximately 50 nM.[57] Similar responses to ANP were also observed in the glioma cells C6-BU-1 and C6-4-2 and in the hybrid cell 108CC15.[56]

In all the cell systems mentioned above that were susceptible to ANP, the concentration-response curve for atriopeptin I (rat ANF[103—123]) appeared to be biphasic,[54,56,57] indicating the involvement of two different species of receptors. Indeed, at least two kinds of ANP receptors have been discovered (see Chapters 1 and 7). The relationship of these results to those of other research groups in other, mostly nonneural cell systems and tissues are discussed elsewhere.[56,57]

2. Cytosolic Calcium Ions

In a nonneural system, the elevation by bradykinin of the tissue level of cyclic GMP was strictly dependent on the presence of Ca^{2+} in the incubation medium.[58] This is also the case for the cyclic GMP response of neuroblastoma × glioma hybrid cells 108CC15 to bradykinin.[54] In contrast, in the same cell line, ANPs raise the cellular concentration of cyclic GMP, regardless of whether Ca^{2+} is present or not.[56] This difference in Ca^{2+} dependence becomes intelligible in view of the following facts: (1) the ANP receptors are tightly coupled to membrane-bound guanylate cyclase,[59] and (2) the bradykinin receptors regulate the soluble guanylate cyclase via a chain of reactions requiring Ca^{2+} and involving an eicosanoid.[54,60]

Compatible with these facts are the observations that in the hybrid cell 108CC15, bradykinin raises the Ca^{2+} concentration in the cytosol[61,62] and activates the transport of $^{45}Ca^{2+}$ across the plasma membrane,[63] whereas atriopeptin III does not.[63,64]

C. ELECTROPHYSIOLOGICAL EFFECTS

Membrane potential was recorded from single cells in culture by intracellular microelectrodes.[38] From micropipets filled with a concentrated solution of the peptide, the peptides to be studied were applied iontophoretically or by pressure pulses to the surface of the cell investigated.

In cells of the clonal tumor lines neuroblastoma × glioma hybrid cells 108CC25[66,67] and polyploid glioma cells C6-4-2,[66] bradykinin administered iontophoretically caused a slow hyperpolarization (10 to 30 s; maximally 20 mV), followed by a slow depolarization (30 to 180 s; amplitude 5 to 10 mV).

Several lines of evidence suggest that activation of K^+ channels is the underlying mechanism of the hyperpolarization induced by bradykinin. The hyperpolarization effect vanishes reversibly if the cell is superfused with Ca^{2+} free medium. Furthermore, it is inhibited by divalent cations, known as Ca^{2+} antagonists, such as Mn^{2+} or Co^{2+}, or by the Ca^{2+} chelator EGTA, iontophoretically injected into the cell.[68] The effect of bradykinin could be mimicked to some extent by intracellular injection of inositol-1,4,5-trisphosphate,[69,70] pointing to the release of intracellularly stored Ca^{2+} in the chain of events triggered by binding of the peptide to its receptor. Clearly, bradykinin regulates a Ca^{2+}-dependent K^+ channel.

A very similar sequence of hyperpolarization and depolarization was observed,[71] if

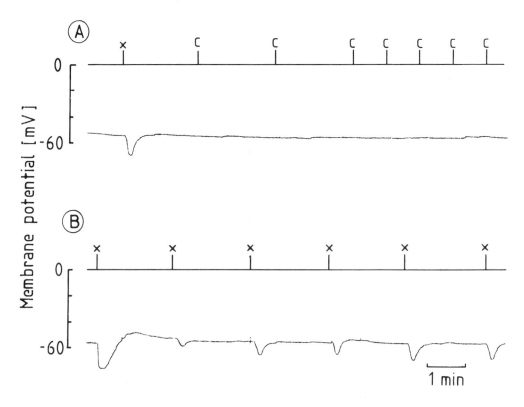

FIGURE 1.   The effect of atriopeptin III on the membrane potential of a polyploid rat glioma cell C6-4-2. The time points of the onset of pressure pulses are indicated on the zero potential line. (A) Atriopeptin pulse (x) of 0.3 bar, 0.3 s, followed by control pulses (c) of 1 bar, 0.3 s; 1 bar, 1 s; 1.5 bar, 1 s (3 pulses); and 2 bar, 1 s. (B) atriopeptin pulse (x) 0.3 bar, 1 s, followed by pulses of 0.3 bar, 0.3 s each. Membrane potential and response to atriopeptin were stable for 130 min. (From Reiser, G., Höpp, H.-P., and Hamprecht, B., *Brain Res.*, 402, 164, 1987. With permission.)

angiotensin II instead of bradykinin was applied to glioma cells C6-4-2. These glioma cells proved to be sensitive to ANP as well.[64,65] If atriopeptin III — or α-hANP (human ANF[98—126]) — was administered to the cell surface by a pressure pulse, a hyperpolarization-depolarization response similar to that seen on application of bradykinin[66] or angiotensin[71] was induced (Figure 1). Again, the hyperpolarization appears to be due to the activation of a K^+ channel. Evidence for this is provided by the facts that (1) the membrane resistance is decreased during hyperpolarization and (2) the reversal potential of the response, derived from a current-voltage analysis, lies at -87 mV, i.e., close to the equilibrium potential of K^+ under the experimental conditions.[65]

As outlined above, both the bradykinin-induced accumulation of cellular cyclic GMP and the hyperpolarization were strictly dependent on Ca^{2+} and, indeed, were accompanied by a rise in the cytosolic activity of Ca^{2+}. Since the ANP-evoked increase in the level of cyclic GMP was not accompanied by a change in the activity of cytosolic Ca^{2+}, one might have expected that the hyperpolarization due to ANP was independent of Ca^{2+}. Surprisingly, the Ca^{2+}-dependent hyperpolarization caused by ANP could be blocked by removal of Ca^{2+} from the medium.[92] Since the cytosolic activity of Ca^{2+} did not change upon addition of ANP, the K^+ channel involved in this case might be activated by Ca^{2+} from the extracellular side. Nevertheless, the possibility has not been excluded that ANP would cause an increase in cytosolic Ca^{2+} only in cells attached to their substratum. So far, cytosolic Ca^{2+} activity has only been measured in cells in suspension.

What would be the sequence of events from ANP binding to its receptor to hyperpolarization? A possibility is that the cyclic GMP formed concomitantly would open a K^+ channel by direct interaction or indirectly via cyclic GMP-dependent protein kinase. This would imply that any means of raising the level of cyclic GMP should cause a comparable hyperpolarization. However, several lines of evidence clearly rule out this possibility. (1) Nitroprusside, an agent that activates the soluble guanylate cyclase by direct interaction[72] and thus raises the concentration of cyclic GMP in the cell, does not exert any effect on the membrane potential. (2) Bradykinin hyperpolarizes C6-4-2 glioma cells, but does not change the level of cyclic GMP,[54] whereas in the hybrid cells, bradykinin evokes both effects. (3) Angiotensin II hyperpolarizes the polyploid glioma cells C6-4-2, but leaves the cyclic GMP concentration in the cells unchanged.[54] At present, the role of cyclic GMP in the receptor-mediated signal transduction process is still largely unknown; studies of patterns of protein phosphorylation[73] might help locate possible targets of this second messenger.

Two different ANP receptors coupled to the particulate guanylate cyclase seem to exist in neural cells, as deduced from the biphasic concentration-response curves mentioned.[56,57] Still another receptor type not coupled to guanylate cyclase might be responsible for the ANP-induced hyperpolarization. Certainly, there is good evidence for the existence of two or three types of ANP receptors (see Chapters 1 and 7).

Another phenomenon represented in Figure 1 is cellular desensitization. On a large dose of ANP, the hybrid cells or the glioma cells became desensitized and recovered in the course of minutes. A similar desensitization has been observed with the hyperpolarization elicited by the two other vasoactive peptides investigated, bradykinin[66] and angiotensin II.[71] There is also cross-desensitization between these two peptides.[71] The question as to the mechanism of this desensitization is open. So far, we can only state that cyclic GMP is again not involved since nitroprusside does not render the cells insensitive to the hyperpolarizing peptides.

III. ACTION OF ANP ON NEURONS IN BRAIN

Some years ago, we had observed that secretin, a gut peptide at that time not known to occur in the brain, stimulated the formation of cyclic AMP in neuroblastoma × glioma hybrids and astroglia-rich primary cultures.[74,75] Subsequently, this peptide was found to occur in all regions of the brain.[76] A similar situation was encountered in the case of ANP.

Several groups reported the presence and localization of ANP in rat brain[80-87] (for details, see Chapter 12). These histochemical studies were the more important ones since ANP was found in paraventricular areas of the hypothalamus, regions known to be involved in the central control of blood volume and electrolyte balance (for details, see Chapter 17). Also, ANP receptors have been localized in these areas.[85,86]

The paraventricular nucleus of the hypothalamus contains the cell bodies of neurons which extend their axons into the posterior hypophysis, where they secrete vasopressin into the circulation. Three laboratories studied (by extracellular recordings) the influence of ANP, applied iontophoretically or by pressure ejection, on the activity of paraventricular hypothalamic neurons.[87-89] Generally, ANP was found to inhibit the spontaneous electrical activity of the neurons. In some cases, the depression of neuronal action potentials could by far outlast the duration of the pulse of application. As expected, increasing the blood pressure by inducing peripheral vasoconstriction also inhibited the firing of neurons, which subsequently were immunocytochemically identified by their vasopressin-containing somata.[89] These data are in agreement with the results of experiments in which ANP was infused into the lateral ventricle or the third ventricle of conscious rats in order to inhibit vasopressin release.[90,91] ANP inhibited at the somata of the hypothalamic neurons the hemorrhage-induced hypophyseal release of vasopressin into the blood. By using neurohypophyseal or neuro-hypophyseal-hypothalamic explants, it could be shown that ANP would have to act on the somata of the hypothalamic neurons in order to inhibit vasopressin release.[91]

IV. DISCUSSION

Of course, only physiological experiments in the animal, such as were described above,[89,90] can establish the feedback of information on the level of blood pressure into the neurons, which release vasopressin into the circulation and, thus, elevate blood pressure. Only investigations in the animal could establish that ANP is involved in the regulation of blood pressure and the homeostasis of body fluid at the two levels possible, i.e., in the periphery and in the central nervous system.

Culture techniques turned out to be most helpful in clarifying at which cellular (soma vs. axon) and anatomical (hypothalamus vs. hypophysis) locus ANP stimulates the vasopressin neurons. In order to unravel the molecular mechanisms of this action of ANP, one would eventually have to employ cell culture techniques. Indeed, it would be most interesting to study vasopressin release in hypothalamic neurons in cultures.

When the action of ANP in the brain was studied *in vivo*, neuronal functions were investigated. Since the frequency of action potentials and release of neurohormones can be measured rather easily, it is already from a technical point of view well justified to first focus research on neuronal functions. Glial cells in the brain might also express ANP receptors, as they do in culture. However, the physiological functions of ANP receptors on glial cells are still unclear. Thus, electrophysiological studies on normal cultured glial cells would be most desirable in order to see if the phenomena encountered in the tumor cell lines described here reflect possible cell-physiological functions. Thus, cell culture studies might help to elucidate ANP functions in the nervous system.

REFERENCES

1. **Needleman, P., Currie, M. G., Geller, D. M., Cole, R. J., and Adams, S. P.,** Atriopeptins: potential mediators of an endocrine relationship between heart and kidney, *Trends Pharmacol. Sci.*, 5, 506, 1984.
2. **Cantin, M. and Genest, J.,** The heart and the atrial natriuretic factor, *Endocrine Rev.*, 6, 107, 1985.
3. **Turner, A. J.,** Hormone from the heart, *Trends Biochem. Sci.*, 10, 2, 1985.
4. **Atlas, S. A.,** Atrial natriuretic factor — a new hormone of cardiac origin, *Rec. Progress Horm. Res.*, 42, 207, 1986.
5. **Atlas, S. A. and Laragh, J. H.,** Atrial natriuretic peptide — a new factor in hormonal control of blood pressure and electrolyte homeostasis, *Annu. Rev. Med.*, 37, 397, 1986.
6. **Cantin, M. and Genest, J.,** The heart as an endocrine organ, *Clin. Invest. Med.*, 9, 319, 1986.
7. **de Bold, A. J.,** Atrial natriuretic factor — an overview, *Fed. Proc.*, 45, 2081, 1986.
8. **Thibault, G., Garcia, R., Gutkowska, J., Genest, J., and Cantin, M.,** Atrial natriuretic factor — a newly discovered hormone with significant clinical implication, *Drugs*, 31, 369, 1986.
9. **Genest, J. and Cantin, M.,** Atrial natriuretic factor, *Circulation*, 75, 118, 1987.
10. **Lang, R. E., Unger, T., and Ganten, D.,** Atrial natriuretic peptide — a new factor in blood pressure control, *J. Hypertens.*, 5, 255, 1987.
11. **Trippodo, N. C., Cole, F. E., Macphee, A. A., and Pegram, B. L.,** Biological mechanisms of atrial natriuretic factor, *J. Lab. Clin. Med.*, 109, 112, 1987.
12. **Vantyghem, M. C. and Lefebvre, J.,** Facteurs natriuretiques, *Pathol. Biol.*, 35, 405, 1987.
13. **Benda, P., Lightbody, J., Sato, G., Levine, L., and Sweet, W.,** Differentiated rat glial cell-strain in tissue culture, *Science*, 161, 370, 1968.
14. **Augusti-Tocco, G. and Sato, G.,** Establishment of functional clonal lines of neurons from mouse neuroblastoma, *Proc. Natl. Acad. Sci. U.S.A.*, 64, 311, 1969.
15. **Nelson, P., Ruffner, W., and Nirenberg, M.,** Neuronal tumor cells with excitable membranes grown in vitro, *Proc. Natl. Acad. Sci. U.S.A.*, 64, 1004, 1969.
16. **Clark, R. B. and Perkins, J. P.,** Regulation of adenosine 3':5'-cyclic monophosphate concentration in cultured human astrocytoma cells by catecholamines and histamine, *Proc. Natl. Acad. Sci. U.S.A.*, 68, 2757, 1971.
17. **Gilman, A. G. and Nirenberg, M.,** Effect of catecholamines on the adenosine 3':5'-cyclic monophosphate concentrations of clonal satellite cells of neurons, *Proc. Natl. Acad. Sci. U.S.A.*, 68, 2165, 1971.

18. **Schultz, J., Hamprecht, B., and Daly, J.,** Accumulation of adenosine 3':5'-cyclic monophosphate in clonal glial cells: labeling of intracellular adenine nucleotides with radioactive adenine, *Proc. Natl. Acad. Sci. U.S.A.,* 69, 1266, 1972.

19. **Catterall, W. A. and Nirenberg, M.,** Sodium uptake associated with activation of action potential ionophores of cultured neuroblastoma and muscle cells, *Proc. Natl. Acad. Sci. U.S.A.,* 70, 3759, 1973.

20. **Schultz, J. and Hamprecht, B.,** Adenosine 3',5'-monophosphate in cultured neuroblastoma cells: effect of adenosine, phosphodiesterase-inhibitors and benzazepines, *Naunyn Schmiedebergs Arch. Pharmacol.,* 278, 215, 1973.

21. **Klee, W. A. and Nirenberg, M.,** A neuroblastoma × glioma hybrid cell line with morphine receptors, *Proc. Natl. Acad. Sci. U.S.A.,* 71, 3474, 1974.

22. **Traber, J., Fischer, K., and Hamprecht, B.,** Morphine antagonizes the action of prostaglandin in neuroblastoma cells but not of prostaglandin and noradrenaline in glioma and glioma × fibroblast hybrid cells, *FEBS Lett.,* 49, 260, 1974.

23. **Sato, G.,** Ed., *Tissue Culture of the Nervous System,* Plenum Press, New York, 1973.

24. **Fedoroff, S. and Hertz, L.,** Eds., *Cell, Tissue, and Organ Culture in Neurobiology,* Academic Press, New York, 1977.

25. **Hamprecht, B.,** Structural, electrophysiological, biochemical, and pharmacological properties of neuroblastoma-glioma cell hybrids in cell culture, *Int. Rev. Cytol.,* 49, 99, 1977.

26. **Nelson, P. G. and Lieberman, M.,** Eds., *Excitable Cells in Tissue Culture,* Plenum Press, New York, 1981.

27. **Hamprecht, B.,** Cell culture as models for studying neural functions, *Prog. Neuro-Psychopharmacol. Biol. Psychiatr.,* 8, 481, 1984.

28. **Hamprecht, B., Glaser, T., Reiser, G., Bayer, E., and Propst, F.,** Culture and characteristics of hormone-responsive neuroblastoma × glioma hybrid cells, *Methods Enzymol.,* 109, 316, 1985.

29. **Seeds, N. W.,** Biochemical differentiation in reaggregating brain cell culture, *Proc. Natl. Acad. Sci. U.S.A.,* 68, 1858, 1971.

30. **Booher, J. and Sensenbrenner, M.,** Growth and cultivation of dissociated neurons and glial cells from embryonic chick, rat and human brain in flask cultures, *Neurobiology,* 2, 97, 1972.

31. **Schrier, B. K.,** Surface culture of fetal mammalian brain cells: effect of subculture on morphology and choline acetyltransferase activity, *J. Neurobiol.,* 4, 1117, 1973.

32. **Minna, J. D., Yavelow, J., and Coon, H. G.,** Expression of phenotypes in hybrid somatic cells derived from nervous system, *Genetics,* 79, 372, 1975.

33. **Greene, L. A. and Tischler, A. S.,** Establishment of a noradrenergic clonal line of rat adrenal pheochromocytoma cells which respond to nerve growth factor, *Proc. Natl. Acad. Sci. U.S.A.,* 73, 2424, 1976.

34. **Pfeiffer, S. E.,** Ed., *Cell Culture Contributions to Current Frontiers of Neurobiology,* CRC Press, Boca Raton, FL, 1982.

35. **Pfeiffer, S. E.,** Ed., *Neuroscience Approached through Cell Culture,* CRC Press, Boca Raton, FL, 1983.

36. **Weibel, M., Pettmann, B., Daune, G., Labourdette, G., and Sensenbrenner, M.,** Chemically defined medium for rat astroglial cells in primary culture, *Int. J. Dev. Neurosci.,* 2, 355, 1984.

37. **Hamprecht, B.,** Cell cultures as model systems for studying the biochemistry of differentiated functions of nerve cells, in *Biochemistry of Sensory Functions, Mosbacher Colloquium,* 25, Jaenicke, L., Ed., Springer-Verlag, Berlin, 1974, 391.

38. **Reiser, G., Heumann, R., Kemper, W., Lautenschlager, E., and Hamprecht, B.,** Influence of cations on the electrical activity of neuroblastoma × glioma hybrid cells, *Brain Res.,* 130, 495, 1977.

39. **Amano, T., Hamprecht, B., and Kemper, W.,** High activity of choline acetyltransferase induced in neuroblastoma × glia hybrid cells, *Exp. Cell Res.,* 85, 399, 1974.

40. **Heumann, R., Reiser, G., van Calker, D., and Hamprecht, B.,** Polyploid rat glioma cells. Production, oscillations of membrane potential and response to neurohormones, *Exp. Cell Res.,* 139, 117, 1982.

41. **van Calker, D., Müller, M., and Hamprecht, B.,** Adrenergic alpha- and beta-receptors expressed by the same cell type in primary culture of perinatal mouse brain, *J. Neurochem.,* 30, 713, 1978.

42. **Hallermayer, K., Harmening, C., and Hamprecht, B.,** Cellular localization and regulation of glutamine synthetase in primary cultures of brain cells from newborn mice, *J. Neurochem.,* 37, 43, 1981.

43. **Löffler, F., Lohmann, S. M., Walckhoff, B., Walter, U., and Hamprecht, B.,** Immunocytochemical characterization of neuron-rich primary cultures of embryonic rat brain cells by established neuronal and glial markers and by nonspecific antisera against cyclic nucleotide-dependent protein kinases and the synaptic vesicle protein synapsin I, *Brain Res.,* 363, 205, 1986.

44. **McCarthy, K. D. and de Vellis, J.,** Preparation of separate astroglial and oligodendroglial cell cultures from rat cerebral tissue, *J. Cell Biol.,* 85, 890, 1980.

45. **Pettmann, B., Delaunoy, J. P., Courageot, J., Devilliers, G., and Sensenbrenner, M.,** Rat brain glial cells in culture. Effects of brain extracts on the development of oligodendroglia-like cells, *Dev. Biol.,* 75, 278, 1980.

46. **Hallermayer, K. and Hamprecht, B.,** Cellular heterogeneity in primary cultures of brain cells revealed by immunocytochemical localization of glutamine synthetase, *Brain Res.,* 295, 1, 1984.

47. **Weibel, M., Pettmann, B., Artault, J.-C., Sensenbrenner, M., and Labourdette, G.,** Primary culture of rat ependymal cells in serum-free defined medium, *Dev. Brain Res.,* 25, 199, 1985.

48. **Löffler, F.,** Biochemische und immuncytochemische Untersuchungen an glialen und neuronalen Zellkulturen des Gehirns, *Ph.D. thesis,* University of Munich, Federal Republic of Germany, 1983.

49. **Löffler, F., Walckhoff, B., and Hamprecht, B.,** Prostaglandins elevate the level of cyclic AMP in phagocytic cells isolated from primary astroglia-rich mouse brain cell cultures, in preparation.

50. **Hansson, E., Rönnbäck, L., Lowenthal, A., Noppe, M., Alling, C., Karlsson, B., and Sellström, A.,** Brain primary culture — a characterization (part II), *Brain Res.,* 231, 173, 1982.

51. **Hamprecht, B.,** Astroglia cells in culture: receptors and cyclic nucleotides, in *Astrocytes,* Fedoroff, S. and Vernadakis, A., Eds., Academic Press, New York, 1986, 77.

52. **Van Calker, D., Müller, M., and Hamprecht, B.,** Regulation by secretin, vasoactive intestinal peptide, and somatostatin of cyclic AMP accumulation in cultured brain cells, *Proc. Natl. Acad. Sci. U.S.A.,* 77, 6907, 1980.

53. **Reiser, G., Walter, U., and Hamprecht, B.,** Bradykinin regulates the level of guanosine $3',5'$-cyclic monophosphate (cyclic GMP) in neural cell lines, *Brain Res.,* 290, 367, 1984.

54. **Friedl, A.,** Untersuchungen an neuralen Zellkulturen zur Wirkungsweise vasoaktiver Peptidhormone, *Ph.D. thesis,* University of Frankfurt am Main, Federal Republic of Germany, 1986.

55. **Friedl, A., Harmening, C., Schuricht, B., and Hamprecht, B.,** Rat atrial natriuretic peptide elevates the level of cyclic GMP in astroglia-rich brain cell cultures, *Eur. J. Pharmacol.,* 111, 141, 1985.

56. **Friedl, A., Harmening, C., and Hamprecht, B.,** Atrial natriuretic hormones raise the level of cyclic GMP in neural cell lines, *J. Neurochem.,* 46, 1522, 1986.

57. **Friedl, A., Harmening, C., Schmalz, F., Schuricht, B., and Hamprecht, B.,** Elevation by atrial natriuretic hormones of cyclic GMP levels in astroglia-rich cultures from murine brain, J. Neurochem., 589, 1989.

58. **Clyman, R. I., Blacksin, A. S., Manganiello, V. C., and Vaughan, M.,** Oxygen and cyclic nucleotides in human umbilical artery, *Proc. Natl. Acad. Sci. U.S.A.,* 72, 3883, 1975.

59. **Kuno, T., Andresen, J. W., Kanisaki, Y., Waldman, S. A., Chang, L. Y., Saheki, S., Leitman, D. C., Nakane, M., and Murad, F.,** Co-purification of an atrial natriuretic factor receptor and particulate guanylate cyclase from rat lung, *J. Biol. Chem.,* 261, 5817, 1986.

60. **McKinney, M. and Richelson, E.,** Blockade of N1E-115 murine neuroblastoma muscarinic receptor function by agents that affect the metabolism of arachidonic acid, *Biochem. Pharmacol.,* 35, 2389, 1986.

61. **Reiser, G. and Hamprecht, B.,** The influence of bradykinin on intracellular Ca^{++}-activity in cultured neural cells, *Regul. Peptides,* Suppl. 4, 46, 1985.

62. **Reiser, G. and Hamprecht, B.,** Bradykinin causes a transient rise of intracellular Ca^{2+}-activity in cultured neural cells, *Pflügers Arch.,* 405, 260, 1985.

63. **Donié, F.,** Der Einfluß zweier vasoaktiver Peptidhormone auf den Ca^{2+}-Stoffwechsel neuraler Zellen in Kultur, *Diploma thesis,* University of Tübingen, Federal Republic of Germany, 1988.

64. **Reiser, G., Höpp, H.-P., and Hamprecht, B.,** The effect of atriopeptin III on membrane potential and intracellular Ca^{2+}-activity in rat glioma cells, *Regul. Peptides,* Suppl. 4, 101, 1985.

65. **Reiser, G., Höpp, H.-P., and Hamprecht, B.,** Atrial natriuretic polypeptide hormones induce membrane potential responses in cultured rat glioma cells, *Brain Res.,* 402, 164, 1987.

66. **Reiser, G. and Hamprecht, B.,** Bradykinin induces hyperpolarizations in rat glioma cells and in neuroblastoma × glioma hybrid cells, *Brain Res.,* 239, 191, 1982.

67. **Yano, K., Higashida, H., Inoue, R., and Nozawa, Y.,** Bradykinin-induced rapid breakdown of phosphatidylinositol 4,5-biphosphate in neuroblastoma × glioma hybrid NG108-15 cells, *J. Biol. Chem.,* 259, 10201, 1984.

68. **Reiser, G., Binmöller, F.-J., and Hamprecht, B.,** Characterization of the ion conductance regulated by bradykinin in rat glioma cells, *Pflügers Arch.,* 406, R54, 1986.

69. **Higashida, H., Streaty, R. A., Klee, W., and Nirenberg, M.,** Bradykinin activated transmembrane signals are coupled via N_o or N_i to production of inositol 1,4,5-trisphosphate, a second messenger in NG108-15 neuroblastoma × glioma hybrid cells, *Proc. Natl. Acad. Sci. U.S.A.,* 83, 942, 1986.

70. **Reiser, G., Binmöller, F.-J., and Hamprecht, B.,** The regulatory influence of bradykinin and inositol-1,4,5-trisphosphate on the membrane potential in neural cell lines, *Biomed. Biochim. Acta,* 46, S682, 1987.

71. **Höpp, H.-P., Reuter, G., Reiser, G., and Hamprecht, B.,** Angiotensin evokes in polyploid rat glioma cells hyperpolarization-depolarization responses and cross-desensitization with bradykinin, *Brain Res.,* 412, 175, 1987.

72. **Gerzer, R., Hofmann, F., Böhme, E., Ivanova, K., Spies, C., and Schultz, G.,** Purification of soluble guanylate cyclase without loss of stimulation by sodium nitroprusside, *Adv. Cyclic Nucleotide Res.,* 14, 255, 1981.

73. **Rapoport, R. M., Draznin, M. B., and Murad, F.,** Sodium nitroprusside-induced protein phosphorylation in intact rat aorta is mimicked by 8-bromo cyclic GMP, *Proc. Natl. Acad. Sci. U.S.A.,* 79, 6470, 1982.

74. **Propst, F., van Calker, D., Moroder, L., Wünsch, E., and Hamprecht, B.,** The influence of gastrointestinal hormones on the level of cyclic AMP in neuroblastoma × glioma hybrid cells and in cells of primary culture of perinatal mouse brain, in *Hormone Receptors in Digestion and Nutrition,* Rosselin, G., Fromageot, P., and Bonfils, S., Eds., Elsevier/North-Holland, Amsterdam, 1979, 475.

75. **van Calker, D., Müller, M., and Hamprecht, B.,** Regulation by secretin, vasoactive intestinal peptide, and somatostatin of cyclic AMP accumulation in cultured brain cells, *Proc. Natl. Acad. Sci. U.S.A.,* 77, 6907, 1980.

76. **O'Donohue, T. L., Charlton, C. G., Miller, R. L., Boden, G., and Jacobowitz, D.,** Identification, characterization, and distribution of secretin immunoreactivity in rat and guinea pig brain, *Proc. Natl. Acad. Sci. U.S.A.,* 78, 5221, 1981.

77. **Morii, N., Nakao, K., Suguwara, A., Sakamoto, M., Suda, M., Shimokura, M., Kiso, Y., Kihara, M., Yamori, Y., and Imura, H.,** Occurrence of atrial natriuretic polypeptide in brain, *Biochem. Biophys. Res. Commun.,* 127, 415, 1985.

78. **Tanaka, I., Misono, K. S., and Inagami, T.,** Atrial natriuretic factor in rat hypothalamus, atria and plasma: determination by specific radioimmunoassay, *Biochem. Biophys. Res. Commun.,* 124, 663, 1984.

79. **Glembotski, C. C., Wildey, G. M., and Gibson, T. R.,** Molecular forms of immunoactive atrial natriuretic peptide in the rat hypothalamus and atrium, *Biochem. Biophys. Res. Commun.,* 129, 671, 1985.

80. **Jacobowitz, D. M., Skofitsch, G., Keiser, H. R., Eskay, R. L., and Zamir, N.,** Evidence for the existence of atrial natriuretic factor-containing neurons in the rat brain, *Neuroendocrinology,* 40, 92, 1985.

81. **Kawata, M., Nakao, K., Morii, N., Kiso, Y., Yamashita, H., and Sano, Y.,** Atrial natriuretic polypeptide: topographical distribution in the rat brain by radioimmunoassay and immunohistochemistry, *Neuroscience,* 16, 521, 1985.

82. **Samson, W. K.,** Dehydration-induced alteration in rat brain vasopressin and atrial natriuretic factor immunoreactivity, *Endocrinology,* 117, 1279, 1986.

83. **Saper, C. B., Standaert, D. G., Currie, M. G., Schwartz, D., Geller, D. M., and Needleman, P.,** Atriopeptin-immunoreactive neurons in the brain: presence in cardiovascular regulatory areas, *Science,* 227, 92, 1985.

84. **Skofitsch, G., Jacobowitz, D. M., Eskay, R. L., and Zamir, N.,** Distribution of atrial natriuretic factor-like immunoreactive neurons in the rat brain, *Neuroscience,* 16, 917, 1985.

85. **Quirion, R., Dalpe, M., and Dam, T. V.,** Characterization and distribution of receptors for the atrial natriuretic peptides in mammalian brain, *Proc. Natl. Acad. Sci. U.S.A.,* 83, 174, 1986.

86. **Quirion, R., Dalpe, M., De Leon, A., Gutkowska, J., Cantin, M., and Genest, J.,** Atrial natriuretic factor (ANF) binding sites in brain and related structures, *Peptides,* 5, 1167, 1984.

87. **Haskins, J. T., Zingaro, G. J., and Lappe, R. W.,** Rat atriopeptin III alters hypothalamic neuronal activity, *Neurosci. Lett.,* 67, 279, 1986.

88. **Wong, M., Samson, W. K., Dudley, C. A., and Moss, R. L.,** Direct, neuronal action of atrial natriuretic factor in the rat brain, *Neuroendocrinology,* 44, 49, 1986.

89. **Standaert, D. G., Cechetto, D. F., Needleman, P., and Saper, C. B.,** Inhibition of the firing of vasopressin in neurons by atriopeptin, *Nature (London),* 329, 151, 1987.

90. **Poole, C. J. M., Carter, D., and Lightman, S. L.,** Intracerebroventricular atriopeptin III inhibits vasopressin and oxytoxin secretion following haemorrhage in conscious rats, *Neuroendocrinol. Lett.,* 9, 249, 1987.

91. **Samson, W. K., Aguila, M. C., Martinovic, J., Antunes-Rodriguez, J., and Norris, M.,** Hypothalamic action of atrial natriuretic factor to inhibit vasopressin secretion, *Peptides,* 8, 449, 1987.

92. **Binmöller, F.-J., Reiser, G., and Hamprecht, B.,** unpublished observations.

Chapter 15

ATRIAL NATRIURETIC PEPTIDE
AND
THE AUTONOMIC NERVOUS SYSTEM

Juan M. Saavedra, Eero Castren, Jorge S. Gutkind, Masaki Kurihara, Adil J. Nazarali, and Jorge E. B. Pinto

TABLE OF CONTENTS

I. INTRODUCTION

The atrial natriuretic peptide (ANP) is a hormone synthesized in the mammalian cardiac atrium. It is released from the heart into the general circulation in response to atrial stretch as a consequence of increased venous return. ANP is involved in the coordinated control of fluid volume and cardiovascular function.[1,2]

ANP opposes the actions of the water-conservatory peptides vasopressin and angiotensin II by stimulating specific receptors in the kidneys, adrenal zona glomerulosa, and vasculature. The peptide has direct diuretic and natriuretic actions and contributes to the elimination of excess fluid by suppressing renin, aldosterone, and vasopressin release.[3,4]

Since it modulates short- and long-term control of water, electrolyte balance, and blood pressure and is a physiological antagonist of angiotensin II, ANP has been implicated in the pathophysiology of certain forms of hypertension.

The ANP system, however, is probably more widely distributed, and its regulation more complex, than originally thought. It has recently become apparent that ANP and/or closely ANP-related peptides can be produced and released outside of the atria, where they could play the role of local hormones. The most notable example is the presence, formation, release, and activity of ANP in the central nervous system.[5-14] In addition, both ANP[15-18] and ANP receptors[19,20] are located in the sympathetic ganglia and in the adrenal medulla.

It was also apparent that factors other than volume expansion, notably the nervous system and the pituitary gland activation, modulated ANP release from the heart atria into the general circulation.[21] In turn, it was clear that ANP exerted, both directly and indirectly, an inhibitory modulation of peripheral sympathetic outflow.[22]

Since both the sympathetic activity and ANP regulate cardiovascular function and sodium balance, and two systems must be interrelated. It is quite possible that, in addition to its known natriuretic and diuretic effects, and its renin-angiotensin-, aldosterone-, and vaso-pressin-suppressing actions, the inhibition of peripheral sympathetic activity by ANP contributes to the antihypertensive effects of the peptide.

We have studied ANP receptors in the peripheral sympathetic ganglia of spontaneously (genetic) hypertensive rats (SHR). SHR have increased peripheral sympathetic activity,[23] decreased brain ANP receptors,[24] and alterations in peripheral ANP metabolism, including increased plasma ANP levels.[25-27] In SHR, ANP administration decreases high blood pressure.[28]

II. MATERIALS AND METHODS

Groups of eight young (4-week-old) and adult (14-week-old) male SHR and Wistar-Kyoto (WKY) control normotensive rats were obtained from Taconic Farms, Germantown, NY. Blood pressures were measured 1 d before sacrifice with an electrosphygmomanometer (Narco Bio-Systems, Inc., Houston, TX) and photoelectric sensors (IITC, Inc., Landing, NJ). Blood pressures were 94 ± 5 and 89 ± 8 mmHg in young SHR and WKY rats, respectively ($p > 0.10$), and 170 ± 10 and 99 ± 5 mmHg in adult SHR and WKY rats, respectively ($p < 0.05$).

Rats were killed by decapitation. For studies of ANP binding sites, the superior cervical and stellate ganglia were removed immediately, frozen in isopentane at $-30°C$, and 16-μm-thick tissue sections were cut in a cryostat and stored overnight under vacuum at 4°C. ANP binding sites were labeled *in vitro* by incubation with 40 to 500 pM 3-[^{125}I]-iodotyrosyl[28] rat ANP (specific activity 2050 Ci/mmol, Amersham Corp., Arlington Heights, IL). Non-specific binding was determined by incubating adjacent sections with 1 μM unlabeled ANP (rat atrial peptide, 28 amino acids, Peninsula Laboratories, Inc., Belmont, CA). After autoradiography with exposure of the labeled sections to Ultrafilm, binding sites were quantified by comparison with ^{125}I-standards and employing a computerized microdensito-meter.[29,30] Scatchard plots of individual ganglia were produced with the computer program LIGAND.[31] Adjacent tissue sections were stained with Hematoxylin and Eosin.

Emulsion autoradiography was performed as described earlier.[32] Briefly, emulsion-coated coverslips (Kodak NTB 3 emulsion from Eastman Kodak, Rochester, NY) were attached in the dark to previously incubated slides and stored desiccated for varying amounts of time. The emulsion-coated coverslips were developed, as described, while still attached to the slides and the slides were stained with Hematoxylin-Eosin before examination under a microscope.

Unilateral left superior cervical ganglia decentralization was performed by sectioning the preganglionic trunk, 1 cm above the ganglia, under halothane-N_2O-O_2 anesthesia. The animals were sacrificed by cervical dislocation 3 days after the operation and completeness of the left preganglionic denervation was confirmed by visual inspection. Both the decen-tralized and the right control superior cervical ganglia were immediately removed and pro-cessed for autoradiography as described above. Determination of ANP binding site concentrations was performed in individual ganglia after incubation with a single 300-pM concentration of [125I]-ANP.

The ANP-stimulated cyclic GMP accumulation was studied in stellate ganglia from adult SHR and WKY rats. After decapitation, the stellate ganglia were removed immediately and desheathed under microscope. During the procedure, ganglia were bathed with Locke's solution, pH 7.2, containing 136 mM NaCl, 5.6 mM KCl, 20 mM Na_2HCO_3, 1.2 mM NaH_2PO_4, 2.2 mM $CaCl_2$, 1.2 mM $MgCl_2$, and 5.5 mM glucose, and were bubbled with 95% O_2-5% CO_2 at room temperature. Ganglia were preincubated for 30 min in the same fresh buffer with 0.5 mM isobutylmethylxantine and 0.1% bacitracin, followed by incubation at 37°C for 20 min with or without increasing concentrations of unlabeled ANP. The reaction was stopped by boiling the mixture for 5 min. Tissue was then homogenized by Polytron for 1 min. After centrifugation at 12,000 g for 5 min at 4°C, the supernatants were lyophilized, the samples were reconstituted in 50 mM sodium acetate buffer, pH 6.2, and the cyclic GMP content was assayed by radioimmunoassay (New England Nuclear, Boston, MA). Cyclic GMP content was assayed in groups of four to six ganglia for each ANP concentration. Each ganglion was assayed in duplicate. Results are expressed as means ± S.E.M. Single comparisons were done by the Student t-test; $p < 0.05$ was considered significant.

III. RESULTS

Autoradiographic images of both the superior cervical and the stellate ganglia of WKY rats showed a relatively diffuse distribution of ANP binding sites (Figure 1B). In sections from WKY rat ganglia, nonspecific binding was less than 5% of total binding (Figure 1D). The distribution of ANP binding sites corresponded to the diffuse distribution of principal ganglion cells in adjacent stained sections (Figure 1A). Binding to preganglionic and post-ganglionic nerve fibers, and to surrounding connective tissue, was undetectable. Emulsion autoradiography revealed the association of a large percentage of silver grains with the cell bodies of the principal ganglion cells (Figure 2b).

Binding kinetic analysis in sections from both superior cervical and stellate ganglia from young and adult WKY rats indicated the presence of a single class of saturable, high-affinity ANP binding sites (Figure 3 and Table 1). The maximum binding capacity in superior cervical ganglia and stellate ganglia of adult WKY rats was higher than that of young WKY rats, while there were no significant differences in the binding affinities (Table 1).

The number of specific ANP binding sites in both the superior cervical and stellate ganglia of young and adult SHR was very low (less than 15 fmol/mg protein) and could not be quantified reliably under our experimental conditions (Figure 1C).

Superior Cervical Ganglia   Stellate Ganglia

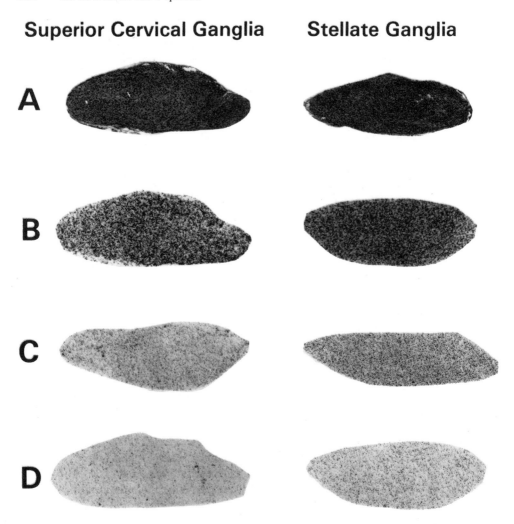

FIGURE 1.   Autoradiography images of [125]-ANP binding to the superior cervical and stellate ganglia from 4-week-old SHR and WKY rats. ANT binding sites were labeled with 0.5 nM [125]-ANP with (nonspecific binding) or without (total binding) 1 μM unlabeled ANP. Sections were exposed to ^{3}H-Ultrofilm for 3 d. (A) Sections from superior cervical and stellate ganglia stained with Hematoxylin and Eosin; (B) total binding in WKY rat; (C) total binding in SHR; (D) section adjacent to B showing nonspecific binding. (Magnification × 5.8.)

There was no difference in the concentration of ANP binding sites after decentralization in superior cervical ganglia from adult WKY rats (right ganglia, control, 119 ± 15 fmol/mg protein; left ganglia, decentralized, 125 ± 38 fmol/mg protein, for groups of 7 and 10 animals, assayed individually).

The basal cyclic GMP content was similar in the stellate ganglia from adult SHR and WKY rats (0.68 ± 0.10 and 0.75 ± 0.06 pmoles cyclic GMP per ganglion in SHR and WKY rats, respectively). In the stellate ganglia of adult SHR and WKY rats, the addition of ANP stimulated cyclic GMP formation in a concentration-dependent manner, and there was no significant difference in the magnitude of response between SHR and WKY rats at any concentration of ANP (Figure 4).

IV. DISCUSSION

Our results of the presence of specific ANP binding sites, and of the ability of ANP to increase cyclic GMP content, indicate the existence of physiologically active ANP receptors

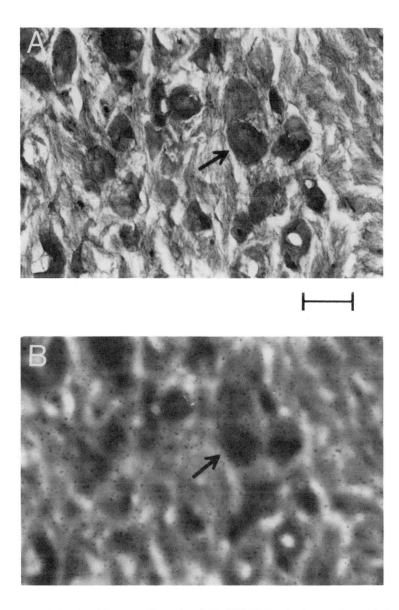

FIGURE 2. Emulsion autoradiography of ^{125}I-ANP binding in the superior cervical ganglia. Sections from a superior cervical ganglia from a 4-week-old WKY rat were incubated with 0.5 n*M* ^{125}I-ANP. Emulsion-coated coverslips were glued to the slides and exposed for 1 week. After development, the slides were stained with Hematoxylin-Eosin and examined under a microscope. Photographs are from the same section with focus on the tissue section (A) or the exposed coverslip (B) Arrows point to a cell body from a principal ganglion cell. Bar represents 10 μm.

in peripheral sympathetic ganglia. At least part of these receptors are associated with principal ganglion cells, as demonstrated by emulsion autoradiography. The lack of changes in the ANP receptor concentration after decentralization suggests that the ganglia ANP receptors probably originate in this tissue and that they are probably not presynaptic receptors located in nerve fibers of central origin. The recent demonstration[20] of ANP binding sites in the adrenal medulla of the tree shrew indicates that ANP receptors may be located in all peripheral tissues of sympathetic origin, including chromaffin cells, which have been reported to contain ANP.[17] However, no significant ANP binding has been detected in the rat adrenal medulla[20]

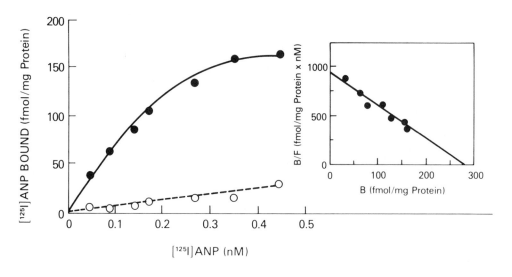

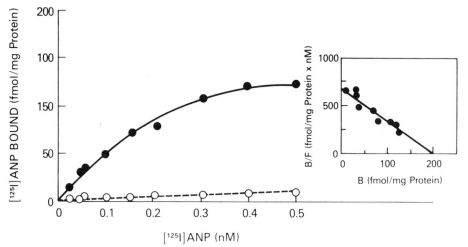

FIGURE 3. ^{125}I-ANP binding in sympathetic ganglia of WKY rats. Saturation curves and Scatchard plots of ^{125}I-ANP binding to the superior cervical ganglia (upper panel) and the stellate ganglia (lower panel) of a 4-week-old WKY rat. Solid lines, specific binding; broken lines, nonspecific binding. Each point represents binding from adjacent sections obtained form a single sympathetic ganglia.

TABLE 1
^{125}I-ANP Binding Sites in the Sympathetic Ganglia of Wistar Kyoto Rats

Age	Ganglia	Binding capacity B_{max} (fmol/mg protein)	Dissociation constant K_d (nM)
4 weeks	Superior		
	Cervical	388 ± 30	0.33 ± 0.03
	Stellate	152 ± 14	0.32 ± 0.04
14 weeks	Superior		
	Cervical	507 ± 43	0.38 ± 0.03
	Stellate	604 ± 38	0.41 ± 0.04

Note: Data represent mean ± S.E.M. from 5 WKY rats, assayed individually by duplicates.

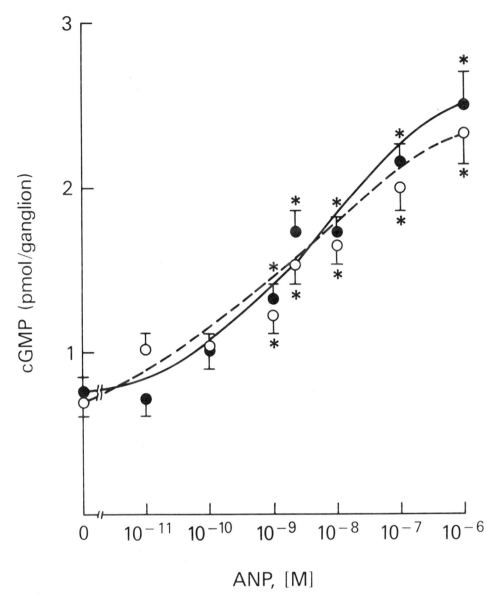

FIGURE 4.   Effect of ANP on the cyclic GMP content in stellate ganglia of adult SHR (open symbols) and WKY rats (closed symbols). Each point represents mean ± S.E.M. of 4 to 6 individual ganglia measured in duplicate. * = p <0.05 vs. basal levels.

and there may be species differences in the distribution of ANP receptors in the peripheral autonomic system.

Our data are consistent with reports of the presence of ANP in sympathetic and para-sympathetic ganglia.[15,16,18,33,34] In the sympathetic ganglia, ANP immunoreactivity is present in small, intensely fluorescent cells, but not in principal ganglion cells.[17,18] In the superior cervical ganglia, at least some ANP may be contained within the cholinergic nerve fibers.[18-35] In addition, no ANP mRNA could be found in the superior cervical ganglia, suggesting that ganglionic cell bodies are not capable of producing ANP and that they are not the source of the peptide.[35] Thus, it is possible that ganglial ANP is of central nervous system origin and reaches the ganglia by axonal transport. This situation is reversed from that of the ANP receptors reported here, which do not change in number after decentralization, are mainly associated with the principal ganglion cells, and are probably postsynaptic.

ANP is also localized in the parasympathetic ganglia,[15] where it could be present in neurons of the afferent vagal pathway, and may have a function in the activation of reflexes that originated in the cardiac baroreceptors.[36]

The presence of ANP receptors is in agreement with the hypothesis of a function of this peptide in the modulation of peripheral sympathetic activity. ANP inhibits the carbachol-stimulated synthesis of catecholamines in sympathetic ganglia,[37] the stimulated norepinephrine release from postganglionic nerve fibers,[38] the synthesis of catecholamines in pheochromocytoma cells,[39] and norepinephrine excretion in rats with experimentally induced high sympathetic tone.[40,41] In addition, ANP administration blunts the increase in sympathetic outflow in response to ANP-induced hypotension[42] and, in SHR, continuous infusion of ANP does not provoke reflex tachycardia, despite an often profound decrease in blood pressure.[43] Peripheral ANP could suppress sympathetic activity through several mechanisms: directly on the sympathetic nerves or sympathetic ganglionic cells through a short feedback loop, indirectly via its vagal action on baroreceptors, or by stimulation of central ANP receptors present in the circumventricular organs and accessible to circulating peptide.

On the other hand, the role of sympathetic nerves in the cardiosuppressive action of ANP, and the depressive effect of sympathetic hyperactivity on ANP release are independent of changes in atrial pressure.[44] Sympathetic denervation abolishes the ANP secretion induced by volume expansion,[45] alpha-adrenergic stimulation increases plasma ANP,[46] and both neuronal and pituitary influences are important in the volume-induced ANP release.[21] In addition, acute stress increases ANP release to the same extent as volume loading.[47,48] Thus, there is growing evidence that ANP is an inhibitory modulator of sympathetic activity, which in turn contributes to the regulation of ANP release.

The alterations in ANP receptors in SHR reported here agree with the proposed regulatory role for the peptide in the peripheral sympathetic system. SHR have increased peripheral sympathetic activity[23] and the marked decrease in ANP binding site concentration in sympathetic ganglia of SHR may represent the loss of an inhibitory influence, with the consequent stimulation of ganglionar catecholamine synthesis leading to increased peripheral sympathetic function in genetic hypertension.

Alterations in ANP receptors of the sympathetic ganglia, however, are not isolated in SHR. Genetically hypertensive rats show increased numbers of angiotensin II receptors in sympathetic ganglia.[49] Angiotensin II is a stimulatory peptide with respect to catecholamine release and ganglionic transmission.[50,51] A similar peptide receptor imbalance, that is, a marked decrease in receptors for an antihypertensive peptide, ANP, together with a marked increase in receptors for the pro-hypertensive peptide angiotensin II, has recently been reported in the circumventricular organs of SHR.[24] A combined central and peripheral imbalance in peptide receptors could be partially responsible for the stimulated peripheral sympathetic activity in genetic hypertension and is in agreement with the postulated physiological antagonism between the renin-angiotensin and ANP systems, both in the periphery[3] and in the central nervous system.[24]

With regard to the alterations in ANP binding-site concentrations reported here, however, some problems of interpretation remain. The ANP receptors in sympathetic ganglia could not only be stimulated by endogenous, ganglionic ANP of central origin, but also by circulating peptides. Adult SHR have higher levels of circulating ANP, an indication of increased atrial peptide release to the general circulation.[25-27] The observed decrease in ANP binding sites, therefore, could be interpreted as a down-regulation mechanism in response to increased peptide stimulation. However, our data from young SHR indicate that low ANP receptor binding in ganglia is already present before the full development of the hypertension and the changes observed could be of genetic origin.

Surprisingly, the ANP-stimulated cyclic GMP formation in stellate ganglia of SHR did not differ from that obtained in age-matched WKY rats. This indicates a discrepancy between the number of ANP binding sites and the ANP-mediated biochemical response in SHR. Recently, the existence of multiple ANP receptors has been demonstrated in many organs,[52-54] and the presence of multiple sites cannot be detected in binding isotherms since the different types of ANP receptors described have identical affinity for the radiolabeled ligand. Only a small percentage of the ANP receptors, however, have been linked to the activation of guanylate cyclase[53] and the nature of the second messenger for most of the ANP binding sites, if any, remains unknown. It could, then, be postulated that the decreased number of ANP binding sites in SHR reflects a specific alteration of those receptors that are uncoupled to the activation of guanylate cyclase.

Our data, and those from others, suggest that the role of ANP in the regulation of cardiovascular and fluid control is more widespread and complex than originally visualized. This role may involve the participation of atrial, or circulating, peptides, acting peripherally and centrally, together with ANP of central origin and ANP acting locally in peripheral organs such as the sympathetic and parasympathetic ganglia. Multiple connections and feedback mechanisms may exist between the ANP and renin-angiotensin system, vasopressin, and the central and peripheral sympathetic systems.

Complex as these interactions may appear, they are certainly not all the mechanisms involved in the regulation of sympathetic ganglionic function. The consideration of peptide mechanisms alone, for example, suggests a role for at least somatostatin, vasoactive intestinal peptide, enkephalin, neuropeptide Y, substance P, and vasopressin since all these peptides, or their receptors, have been located in mammalian sympathetic ganglia.[18,56-61] The elucidation of the mechanisms for peripheral autonomic control is in its infancy and will provide exciting developments for many investigators in the years to come.

REFERENCES

1. **de Bold, A. J., Borenstein, H. B., Veress, A. T., and Sonnenberg, H. A.,** Rapid and potent natriuretic response to intravenous injection of atrial myocardial extract in rats, *Life Sci.,* 28, 89, 1981.
2. **de Bold, A. J.,** Atrial natriuretic factor: a hormone produced by the heart, *Science,* 230, 767, 1985.
3. **Cantin, M. and Genest, J.,** The heart and the atrial natriuretic factor, *Endocrine Rev.,* 6, 107, 1985.
4. **Needleman, P.,** The expanding physiological roles of atrial natriuretic factor, *Nature (London),* 321, 199, 1986.
5. **Saavedra, J. M.,** Regulation of atrial natriuretic peptide receptors in the rat brain, *Cell. Mol. Neurobiol.,* 7, 151, 1987.
6. **Saavedra, J. M., Castren, E., Gutkind, J. S., and Nazarali, A. J.,** Regulation of brain atrial natriuretic peptide and angiotensin receptors: quantitative autoradiographic studies, *Int. Rev. Neurobiol.,* in press.
7. **Quirion, R., Dalpe, M., Lean, A. D., Gutkowska, J., Cantin, M., and Genest, J.,** Atrial natriuretic factor (ANF) binding sites in brain and related structures, *Peptides,* 5, 1167, 1984.
8. **Quirion, R., Dalpe, M., and Dam, T. V.,** Characterization and distribution of receptors for atrial natriuretic peptides in mammalian brain, *Proc. Natl. Acad. Sci. U.S.A.,* 83, 174, 1986.
9. **Glembotski, C. C., Wildey, G. M., and Gibson, T. R.,** Molecular forms of immunoreactive atrial natriuretic peptide in the rat hypothalamus and atrium, *Biochem. Biophys. Res. Commun.,* 129, 671, 1985.
10. **Haskins, J. T., Zingara, G. J., and Lappe, R. W.,** Rat atriopeptin III alters hypothalamic neuronal activity, *Neurosci. Lett.,* 67, 279, 1986.
11. **Kawata, M., Nakao, K., Morii, N., Kiso, Y., Yamashita, H., Imura, H., and Sano, Y.,** Atrial natriuretic polypeptide: topographical distribution in the rat by radioimmunoassay and immunohistochemistry, *Neuroscience,* 16, 521, 1985.
12. **Kurihara, M., Saavedra, J. M., and Shigematsu, K.,** Localization and characterization of atrial natriuretic peptide binding sites in discrete areas of rat brain and pituitary gland by quantitative autoradiography, *Brain Res.,* 408, 31, 1987.

13. **Shibasaki, T., Naruse, M., Naruse, K., Masuda, A., Kim, Y. S., Imaki, T., Yamauchi, N., Demura, H., Inagami, T., and Shizume, K.,** Atrial natriuretic factor is released from rat hypothalamus in vitro, *Biochem. Biophys. Res. Commun.*, 136, 590, 1986.

14. **Tanaka, I. and Inagami, T.,** Release of immunoreactive atrial natriuretic factor from rat hypothalamus in vitro, *Eur. J. Pharmacol.*, 122, 353, 1986.

15. **Debinski, W., Gutkowska, J., Kuchel, O., Racz, K., Buu, N. T., Cantin, M., and Genest, J.,** ANF-like peptide(s) in the peripheral autonomic nervous system, *Biochem. Biophys. Res. Commun.*, 134, 279, 1986.

16. **Debinski, W., Gutkowska, J., Kuchel, O., Racz, K., Buu, N. T., Cantin, M., and Genest, J.,** Presence of an atrial natriuretic factor-like peptide in the rat superior cervical ganglia, *Neuroendocrinology*, 46, 236, 1987.

17. **Inagaki, S., Kubota, Y., Kitto, S., Kangawa, K., and Matsuo, H.,** Immunoreactive atrial natriuretic polypeptides in the adrenal medulla and sympathetic ganglia, *Regul. Peptides*, 15, 249, 1986.

18. **Papka, R. E., Trauring, H. H., and Wekstein, M.,** Localization of peptides in nerve terminals in the paracervical ganglion of the rat by light and electron microscopic immunohistochemistry: encephalin and atrial natriuretic factor, *Neurosci. Lett.*, 61, 285, 1985.

19. **Gutkind, J. C., Kurihara, M., Castren, E., and Saavedra, J. M.,** Atrial natriuretic peptide receptors in sympathetic ganglia: biochemical response and alterations in genetically hypertensive rats, *Biochem. Biophys. Res. Commun.*, 149, 65, 1987.

20. **Fuchs, E., Flugge, G., Shigematsu, K., and Saavedra, J. M.,** Binding sites for atrial natriuretic peptide in Tree Shrew and primate adrenal glands in *Am. Soc. Hypertension Symp. Ser., Vol I, Biologically Active Atrial Peptides,* Brenner, B. M. and Laragh, J. H., Eds., Raven Press, New York, 1987, 232.

21. **Eskay, R., Zukowska-Grojec, Z., Haass, M., Dave, J. R., and Zamir, N.,** Characterization of circulating atrial natriuretic peptide in conscious rats: regulation of release by multiple factors, *Science*, 232, 636, 1986.

22. **Kuchel, O., Debinski, W., Racz, K., Buu, N. T., Garcia, R., Cusson, J., Larochelle, P., Cantin, M., and Genest, J.,** Minireview: an emerging relationship between peripheral sympathetic nervous activity and atrial natriuretic factor, *Life Sci.*, 16, 1545, 1987.

23. **Grobecker, H., Roizen, M. F., Weise, V., Saavedra, J. M., and Kopin, I. J.,** Sympatho-adrenal medullary activity in young, spontaneously hypertensive rats, *Nature (London)*, 258, 267, 1975.

24. **Saavedra, J. M., Correa, F. M. A., Plunkett, L. M., Israel, A., Kurihara, M., and Shigematsu, K.,** Binding of angiotensin and atrial natriuretic peptide in brain of hypertensive rats, *Nature (London)*, 230, 758, 1986.

25. **Imada, T., Takayanagi, R., and Inagami, T.,** Changes in the content of atrial natriuretic factor with the progression of hypertension in spontaneously hypertensive rats, *Biochem. Biophys. Res. Commun.*, 133, 759, 1985.

26. **Morii, N., Nakao, K., Kihara, M., Sugawara, A., Sakamoto, M., Yamori, Y., and Imura, H.,** Decreased content in left atrium and increased plasma concentration of atrial natriuretic polypeptide in spontaneously hypertensive rats (SR) and SHR stroke-prone, *Biochem. Biophys. Res. Commun.*, 135, 74, 1986.

27. **Gutkowska, J., Horky, K., Lachance, C., Racz, K., Garcia, R., Thibault, G., Kuchel, O., Genest, J., and Cantin, M.,** Atrial natriuretic factor in spontaneously hypertensive rats, *Hypertension*, 8 (Suppl. 1), 137, 1986.

28. **Garcia, R., Thibault, G., Gutkowska, J., Horky, K., Hamet, P., Cantin, M., and Genest, J.,** Chronic infusion of low doses of atrial natriuretic factor (ANF Arg 101-Tyr 126) reduces blood pressure in conscious SHR without apparent changes in sodium excretion, *Proc. Soc. Exp. Biol. Med.*, 179, 396, 1985.

29. **Israel, A., Niwa, M., Plunkett, L. M., and Saavedra, J. M.,** High-affinity angiotensin receptors in rat adrenal medulla, *Regul. Peptides*, 11, 237, 1985.

30. **Israel, A., Plunkett, L., and Saavedra, J. M.,** Quantitative autoradiographic characterization of receptors for angiotensin II and other neuropeptides in individual brain nuclei and peripheral tissues from single rats, *Cell. Mol. Neurobiol.*, 5, 211, 1985.

31. **Munson, P. J.,** Ligand: a computerized analysis of ligand binding data in *Methods in Enzymology*, Vol. 92, *Immunochemical Techniques, Part E,* Langone, J. J. and van Vunakis, H., Academic Press, New York, 1983, 543.

32. **Scott Young, W., III, and Kuhar, M. J.,** A new method for receptor autoradiography: [^{3}H]opioid receptors in rat brain, *Brain Res.*, 179, 255, 1979.

33. **Morii, N., Nakao, K., Itoh, H., Shiono, S., Yamada, T., Sugawara, A., Saito, Y., Mukoyama, M., Arai, H., Sakamoto, M., and Imura, H.,** Atrial natriuretic polypeptide in spinal cord and autonomic ganglia, *Biochem. Biophys. Res. Commun.*, 145, 196, 1987.

34. **Nehls, M., Reinecke, M., Lang, R. E., Forssmann, W. G.,** Biochemical and immunological evidence for a cardiodilantin-like substance in the snail neurocardiac axis, *Proc. Natl. Acad. Sci. U.S.A.*, 82, 7762, 1985.

35. **Debinski, W., Kuchel, O., Buu, N. T., Nemer, M., Cantin, M., and Genest, J.,** Atrial natriuretic factor in peripheral sympathetic ganglia originates in preganglionic nerve fibers, *Clin. Res.,* 35, 273A, 1987.

36. **Mark, A. L., Thoren, P., O'Neill, T. P., Morgan, D., Needleman, P., and Brody, M. J.,** Atriopeptins stimulate cardiac sensory receptors with vagal afferents in rats, *Clin. Res.,* 33, 596A, 1985.

37. **Debinski, W., Kuchel, O., Buu, N. T., Cantin, M., and Genest, J.,** Atrial natriuretic factor partially inhibits the stimulated catecholamine synthesis in superior cervical ganglia of the rat, *Neurosci. Lett.,* 77, 92, 1987.

38. **Nakamaru, M. and Inagami, T.,** Atrial natriuretic factor inhibits norepinephrine release evoked by sympathetic nerve stimulation in isolated perfused rat mesenteric arteries, *Eur. J. Pharmacol.,* 123, 459, 1986.

39. **Racz, K., Kuchel, O., Buu, N. T., Debinski, W., Cantin, M., and Genest, J.,** Atrial natriuretic factor, catecholamines and natriuresis. *N. Engl. J. Med.,* 314, 321, 1986.

40. **Debinski, W., Kuchel, O., Garcia, R., Buu, N. T., Racz, K., Cantin, M., and Genest, J.,** Atrial natriuretic factor inhibits the sympathetic nervous activity in one-kidney, one-clip hypertensin in the rat, *Proc. Soc. Exp. Biol. Med.,* 181, 173, 1986.

41. **Debinski, W., Kuchel, O., Buu, N. T., Garcia, R., Cantin, M., and Genest, J.,** Involvement of the adrenal glands in the action of the atrial natriuretic factor, *Proc. Soc. Exp. Biol. Med.,* 181, 318, 1986.

42. **Zukowska-Grojec, Z., Haass, M., and Zamir, N.,** Atriopeptin III (AP III) infusion antagonizes reflexive increases in plasma norepinephrine (NE) in conscious rats, *J. Cardiovasc. Pharmacol.,* 8, 1312, 1986.

43. **Lappe, R. W., Smits, J. F. M., Todt, J. A., and Wendt, R. L.,** Failure of atriopeptin II to cause arterial vasodilation in the conscious rat, *Circ. Res.,* 56, 606, 1985.

44. **Sasaki, A., Kida, O., Kangawa, K., Matsuo, H., and Tanaka, K.,** Involvement of sympathetic nerves in cardiosuppressive effects of α-human atrial natriuretic polypeptide (α-hANP) in anesthetized rats. *Eur. J. Pharmacol.,* 120, 345, 1986.

45. **Pettersson, A., Ricksten, S. E., Towle, A. C., Hedner, J., and Hedner, T.,** Effect of blood volume expansion and sympathetic denervation on plasma levels of atrial natriuretic factor (ANF) in the rat, *Acta Physiol. Scand.,* 124, 309, 1985.

46. **Sanfield, J. A., Shenker, Y., Grekin, R. J., and Rosen, S. G.,** Epinephrine increases plasma immunoreactive atrial natriuretic hormone levels in humans, *Am. J. Physiol.,* 252, E740, 1987.

47. **Horky, K., Gutkowska, J., Garcia, R., Thibault, G., Genest, J., and Cantin, M.,** Effect of different anesthetics on immunoreactive atrial natriuretic factor concentrations in rat plasma, *Biochem. Biophys. Res. Commun.,* 129, 651, 1985.

48. **Blizard, D. A. and Morris, M.,** Acute stress increases plasma concentrations of atrial natriuretic peptides, *Proc. Soc. Exp. Biol. Med.,* 184, 123, 1987.

49. **Pinto, J. E. B., Nazarali, A. J., and Saavedra, J. M.,** Angiotensin II binding sites in the superior cervical ganglia of spontaneously hypertensive and Wistar-Kyoto rats after preganglionic denervation, *Brain Res.,* 475, 146, 1988.

50. **Haefely, W. E.,** Non-nicotinic chemical stimulation of autonomic ganglia, in *Handbook of Experimental Pharmacology,* Vol. 53 *Pharmacology of Ganglionic Transmission,* Kharkevich, D. A., Ed., Springer, New York, 1980, 341.

51. **Peach, M. J. and Ackerly, J. A.,** Angiotensin antagonists and the adrenal cortex and medulla, *Fed. Proc.,* 35, 2502, 1976.

52. **Wildey, G. M. and Glembotski, C. C.,** Cross-linking of atrial natriuretic peptide to binding sites in rat olfactory bulb membranes, *J. Neurosci.,* 6, 3767, 1986.

53. **Leitman, D. C., Andresen, J. W., Catalano, R. M., Waldman, S. A., Tuan, J. J., and Murad, F.,** Atrial natriuretic peptide binding, cross-linking, and stimulation of cyclic GMP accumulation and particulate guanylate cyclase activity in cultured cells, *J. Biol. Chem.,* 263, 3720, 1988.

54. **Schenk, D. B., Johnson, L. K., Schwartz, K., Sista, H., Scarborough, R. M., and Lewicki, J. A.,** Distinct atrial natriuretic factor receptor sites on cultured bovine aortic smooth muscle and endothelial cells, *Biochem. Biophys. Res. Commun.,* 127, 433, 1985.

55. **Takayanagi, R., Snajdar, R. M., Imada, T., Tamura, M., Pandey, K. N., Misono, K. S., and Inagami, T.,** Purification and characterization of two types of atrial natriuretic factor receptors from bovine adrenal cortex: guanylate cyclase-linked and cyclase-free receptors, *Biochem. Biophys. Res. Commun.,* 144, 244, 1987.

56. **Hökfelt, T., Johansson, O., Ljungdahl, A., Lundberg, J. M., and Schultzberg, M.,** Peptidergic neurones, *Nature (London),* 515, 1980.

57. **Lundberg, J. M. and Hokfelt, T.,** Coexistence of peptides and classical neurotransmitters, *TINS,* 6, 325, 1983.

58. **Hökfelt, T., Elfvin, L. G., Elde, R., Schultzberg, M., Goldstein, M., and Luft, R.,** Occurrence of somatostatin-like immunoreactivity in some peripheral sympathetic noradrenergic neurons, *Proc. Natl. Acad. Sci. U.S.A.,* 74, 3587, 1977.

59. **Lindh, B., Hökfelt, T., Elfvin, L.-G., Terenius, L., Fahrenkrug, J., Elde, R., and Goldstein, M.,** Topography of NPY-, somatostatin-, and VIP-immunoreactive, neuronal subpopulations in the guinea pig celiac-superior mesenteric ganglion and their projection to the pylorus., *J. Neurosci.,* 6, 2371, 1986.

60. **Niwa, M., Shigematsu, K., Plunkett, L., and Saavedra, J. M.,** High-affinity substance P binding sites in rat sympathetic ganglia, *Am. J. Physiol.,* 249, H694, 1985.

61. **Kiraly, M., Audigier, S., Tribolet, E., Barberis, C., Dolivo, M., and Dreifuss, J. J.,** Biochemical and electrophysiological evidence of functional vasopressin receptors in the rat superior cervical ganglion, *Proc. Natl. Acad. Sci. U.S.A.,* 83, 5335, 1986.

Chapter 16

CENTRAL NERVOUS SYSTEM ACTIONS OF ATRIAL NATRIURETIC PEPTIDE

Hiroo Imura and Kazuwa Nakao

TABLE OF CONTENTS

I. INTRODUCTION

Soon after the discovery of atrial natriuretic peptide (ANP) from human and rat atria, the existence of ANP-like immunoreactivity (ANP-LI) in the central nervous system (CNS) had been demonstrated by radioimmunoassay (RIA)[1-3] and immunohistochemistry.[4-7] RIA studies showed that the concentration of ANP-LI is highest in the hypothalamus and septum in rats.[1] Immunohistochemical studies[4-7] have obtained strikingly similar results, demonstrating that ANP-LI-containing nerve cells and fibers are abundantly distributed in brain areas which are considered to be involved in the regulation of fluid volume and blood pressure. These areas are also known to have ANP receptors, as demonstrated by the binding of ^{125}I-α-ANP.[8,9] These observations suggest that brain ANP plays an important role in regulating blood pressure and water homeostasis.[10-12]

In this chapter, we will first discuss molecular forms of brain ANP and then possible physiological actions of ANP in the CNS based on studies performed mainly in rats.

II. MOLECULAR FORMS OF ANP IN THE BRAIN

Multiple forms of ANP with high or low molecular weight have been isolated from mammalian atria.[13-16] The cloning of the ANP precursor has shown its primary structure to be composed of 126 amino acids, which is called γ-ANP (ANP 1-126).[17] γ-ANP is now known to be the major storage form in the atrium in man and rats.[18,19] On the other hand, accumulating evidence suggests that the major circulating form is a low molecular weight form consisting of 28 amino acids in both man and rats, which is called α-ANP.[19,20] Molecular forms of ANP in the coronary sinus blood (immediately after secretion from the atrium) in man and in the perfusate from isolated beating rat heart are also known to be predominantly α-ANP.[19] These results suggest that the conversion from γ-ANP (the precursor) to α-ANP occurs just before and/or during the process of secretion from cardiocytes or transport into the blood.

In contrast to the storage form of ANP in the atrium, the gel filtration studies of brain ANP in rats have demonstrated that the predominant molecular form in the brain is a low molecular weight form, eluting at the position of α-ANP.[1,21] Further studies with reverse-phase high performance liquid chromatography (RP-HPLC) have demonstrated two major small molecular forms comigrating with α-ANP(4—28) (ANP[102—126]) and α-ANP(5—28) (ANP[103—126]), as shown in Figure 1. Molecular forms of ANP in other species have been studied more recently. Both α-ANP(4—28) and α-ANP(5—28) have been isolated and identified from pig brain.[22] Human and monkey brains also contain predominantly low molecular weight forms, when studied by gel filtration,[10] which are detected by RIA directed toward the ring portion of α-ANP, but not detected by RIA directed toward the N-terminal end of α-ANP. All these results indicate that the processing of the precursor in the brain differs from that in the atrium and that the major molecular forms in the brain are not α-ANP, but α-ANP(4—28) and (5—28). A single arginine residue preceding α-ANP in the precursor (position 98 of γ-ANP) becomes a processing site in the heart. On the other hand, two basic amino acid residues, Arg-Arg, at positions 3 and 4 of α-ANP (positions 101 and 102 of γ-ANP) become processing sites in the brain, thus giving rise to α-ANP(4—28) and α-ANP(5—28). It is of interest to point out that α-ANP(3—28) (ANP[101—126]) is more active than α-ANP in binding brain ANP receptors.[8]

Figure 2 illustrates the processing and secretion of ANP in the heart and brain. In the heart, γ-ANP is converted to α-ANP during the process of secretion. On the other hand, γ-ANP in the brain is converted to a large extent to α-ANP(4—28) and α-ANP(5—28) in secretory granules and these peptides as well as a small amount of γ-ANP are cosecreted from nerve terminals by membrane depolarization.

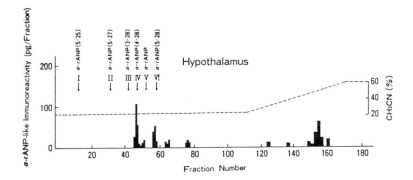

FIGURE 1. Reverse phase HPLC profile of rat hypothalamic extract on a TSK-GEL ODS 120 T column. Major small molecular weight forms co-migrated with α-ANP(4—28) and α-ANP(5—28).

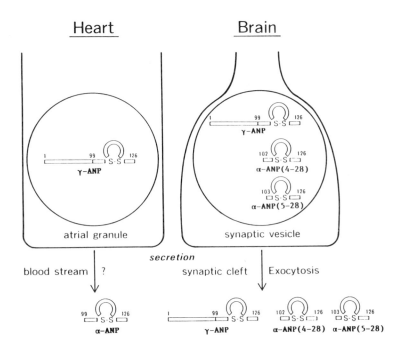

FIGURE 2. Schematic representation of molecular forms of ANP in the heart and brain.

III. POSSIBLE INVOLVEMENT OF ANP IN THE CENTRAL CONTROL OF BLOOD PRESSURE AND FLUID BALANCE

Since ANP-LI-containing neurons are densely distributed in the AV3V region which is responsible for the central cardiovascular control in rats, our group and others have studied the effect of ANP on fluid balance and blood pressure.

A. ANTIDIPSOGENIC ACTION

We first observed that the intracerebroventricular (icv) injection of α-ANP dose-dependently inhibited water intake induced by the icv injection of angiotensin II (ANG II) in rats.[23] The icv injection of ANP also dose-dependently inhibited water intake induced by 24-h water deprivation, whereas it had no significant effect on carbachol-induced drinking.[23]

The icv injection of α-ANP alone did not alter water intake in normal rats given water *ad libitum*. It had no significant effect on food intake and locomotor activity, suggesting the specificity of the antidipsogenic action of ANP. Similar results were obtained by Antunes-Rodrigues et al.[24] in rats.

In order to elucidate whether the antidipsogenic action of ANP is of physiological significance, we studied the effect of icv injection of anti-α-ANP antiserum on water intake in rats. The icv injection of the antiserum (1:2 and 1:5 dilution) significantly potentiated water intake induced by ANG II and water deprivation.[25] This suggests the physiological significance of endogenous ANP in regulating water intake in rats.

B. INHIBITION OF SALT APPETITE

Several lines of evidence suggest the interrelationship between the enhanced brain renin-angiotensin system and exaggerated salt appetite in spontaneously hypertensive rats (SHR). Since the AV3V region is considered to be a critical region in regulating salt appetite, we studied the effect of icv infusion of α-ANP on salt intake in SHR and normotensive Wistar Kyoto rats (WKY).[26] α-ANP was infused into the lateral ventricle at the rate of 100 to 500 ng/h by Alzet osmotic minipump during a 5-d period. Rats were allowed to preferentially drink 0.3 mol/l NaCl solution or tap water. The infusion of α-ANP decreased the intake of hypertonic saline solution in SHR. No significant effect was observed in WKY, which have a lower salt appetite than SHR. Antunes-Rodrigues et al.[27] and Fitts et al.[28] performed short-term experiments and observed that the infusion of ANP into the third ventricle significantly attenuated saline intake in salt-deprived rats. These results suggest that brain ANP is involved in the regulation of salt intake.

C. CENTRAL DEPRESSOR ACTION

ANG II is a well-known pressor substance when given into the ventricle. Since ANP is antagonistic to the dipsogenic action of ANG II, we next studied whether ANP antagonizes the pressor action of ANG II.[29] The icv injection of ANG II caused a prompt rise in blood pressure in conscious, unrestrained rats. This pressor effect of ANG II was dose-dependently inhibited by the icv injection of α-ANP (Figure 3). Since plasma ANP did not change by the icv injection of α-ANP, it is unlikely that centrally administered α-ANP leaked into the peripheral circulation and attenuated the ANG II-induced blood pressure increase. Casto et al.[30] reported that the icv injection of α-ANP abolished the pressor action of ANG II in chloralose-urethane anesthetized WKY and SHR, whereas it failed to affect the pressor response in conscious SHR. These results suggest that ANP antagonizes the pressor action of ANG II, at least in normal rats.

D. INHIBITION OF VASOPRESSIN SECRETION

It is known that the icv injection of ANG II enhances vasopressin release and that the increased vasopressin release is partly responsible for the pressor effect of ANG II. Since ANP-LI-containing nerve cells are abundant in the paraventricular nucleus, we studied the effect of icv injection of α-ANP on vasopressin release in conscious, unrestrained rats. The icv injection of 5 ng α-ANP significantly blunted the plasma vasopressin increase induced by 100 ng of ANG II.[31] There was a dose-response relationship in the inhibitory action of ANP. Similar findings were reported by other groups.[32]

The site of action of ANP in inhibiting vasopressin release has been controversial. Samson[33] first reported that the intravenous injection of ANP inhibited vasopressin secretion induced by dehydration and hemorrhage. This suggested that ANP might act at the level of neurohypophysis, However, his later study[34] and others[35] showed that ANP given by a systemic route inhibits vasopressin release only at large doses and provided evidence suggesting that the major site of action of ANP is at the hypothalamic level. Our observations are consistent with the hypothalamic site of action.

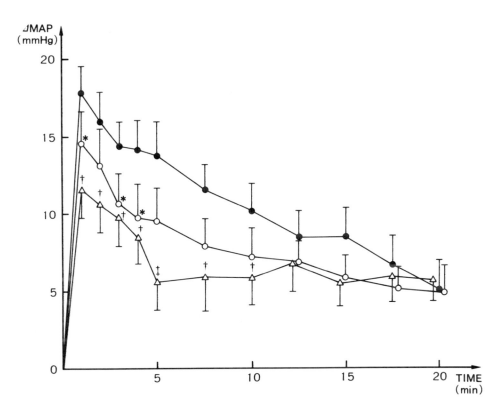

FIGURE 3.   Effect of the icv injection of 100 ng of ANG II with or without ANP on the mean arterial pressure. Control rats (closed circle) received ANG II alone. Experimental groups first received ANG II alone. After complete recovery, they were injected icv with either 200 ng of α-human ANP (open circle) or 1 μg of α-human ANP (open triangle) 5 min prior to the second ANG II injection. Means ± S.E.M. are shown. *$p < 0.05$, $p < 0.01$, and $p < 0.001$, compared with the first experiment. (Redrawn from Itoh, H., Nakao, K., Morii, N., Yamada, T., Shiono, S., Sakamato, M., Sugawara, A., Saito Y., Katsuura, G., Shiomi, T., Eigyo, M., Matsushita, M., and Imura, N., *Brain Res. Bull.*, 16, 45, 1986. With permission.)

E. INHIBITION OF ANG II-INDUCED ACTH SECRETION

Immunohistochemical studies have shown that ANP-LI immunoreactive cell bodies are present in parvocellular components of the paraventricular nucleus and that ANP-LI nerve fibers extend to the external layer of the median eminence.[4,5] These observations suggest possible involvements of brain ANP in the neuroendocrine control of anterior pituitary hormone secretion. We observed in rats that the icv injection of ANG II caused an increase in plasma corticosterone and that α-ANP given icv dose-dependently inhibited the ANG II-induced corticosterone increase.[36] Although the physiological significance of ANG II-induced ACTH secretion is not known, ACTH affects blood pressure and body fluid balance through the actions of corticosterone and aldosterone.

F. DIURETIC, NATRIURETIC, AND KALIURETIC ACTION

The icv injection of α-ANP is known to cause diuresis, which is partly explained by the decrease of vasopressin secretion. Shoji et al.[37] however, reported that increased diuresis, natriuresis, and kaliuresis induced by the icv infusion of α-ANP in dogs could not be explained by a slight decrease in plasma vasopressin observed during the experiment. The exact mechanism by which centrally administered ANP enhances diuresis, natriuresis, and kaliuresis is unknown, but the possibility that ANP affects efferent renal sympathetic nerve activity is considered. More direct study on the renal sympathetic nerve activity is required to draw such a conclusion.

G. INTERACTION OF BRAIN ANP AND ANG II IN REGULATING CARDIAC ANP SECRETION

In order to elucidate the interrelationship between the brain and the cardiac ANP system, we studied the effect of icv injection of ANG II on plasma ANP levels.[38,39] The icv injection of 10 ng to 10 μg of ANG II in conscious, unrestrained rats had no significant effect on plasma ANP levels. However, the icv injection of ANG II significantly enhanced plasma ANP responses to volume expansion induced by saline injection. This potentiating effect of ANG II on cardiac ANP secretion was markedly blunted by the intravenous injection of V_1-receptor antagonist.[38] We also observed that the intravenous injection of less than 10 ng of arginine vasopressin did not affect basal plasma ANP levels, but significantly augmented the plasma ANP response to volume expansion.[40] These results suggest that vasopressin is an important mediator in the potentiating action of centrally administered ANG II on cardiac ANP secretion. We also observed that the icv injection of α-rat ANP(4—28) significantly blunted this potentiating effect.[39] It is of interest that ANG II and ANP are antagonistic in this respect too.

H. STRUCTURE-ACTIVITY RELATIONSHIP IN THE CENTRAL ACTION OF ANP

As mentioned above, ANP in the brain is not α-ANP, but α-ANP(4—28) and α-ANP(5—28). We therefore studied the structure-activity relationship using analogs of α-ANP.[41] The antidipsogenic actions of α-rat ANP, α-rat ANP(4—28), α-rat ANP(5—28), and α-human ANP were almost equipotent in rats stimulated with ANG II (Table 1). Thus, endogenous ANPs, α-ANP(4—28) and α-ANP(5—28), are as active as α-ANP in the antidipsogenic activity, and central actions obtained with α-ANP can be extrapolated to the actions of endogenous ANPs, α-ANP(4—28) and α-ANP(5—28).

I. SUMMARY

It is known that the renin-angiotensin system exists in the brain and that ANG II possesses several central actions, such as enhancement of drinking, salt intake and vasopressin release, and a rise of blood pressure. Thus, the central renin-angiotensin system plays a role in increasing blood volume and raising blood pressure. On the other hand, the brain has the ANP system and centrally administered ANP inhibits drinking, salt intake and vasopressin release, and lowers blood pressure. ANG II and ANP are antagonists in peripheral tissues, such as blood vessels and the adrenal cortex. The antagonistic relationship also exists in the central control of body fluid and blood pressure, as shown in Figure 4.

IV. MECHANISM OF ACTION OF ANP IN THE BRAIN

The presence of ANP-LI in nerve terminals and the presence of ANP receptors in the same brain areas suggest that ANP released from the axon terminals plays a role as either a neurotransmitter or a neuromodulator. Wong et al.[42] recorded single neuron electrical activity *in vivo* and observed that the microiontophoretical application of α-ANP inhibited spontaneous firing rates in the majority of neurons in the AV3V region. Using brain slices, Okuya and Yamashita[43] also recorded single neuron activity *in vitro*. The application of α-ANP also inhibited spontaneous electrical activity in most of the cells in the AV3V region, and magnocellular portion of the paraventricular nucleus. These results suggest that ANP acts on the postsynaptic membrane of neurons in these areas, acting as either a neuromodulator or a neurotransmitter.

TABLE 1
Comparative Inhibitory Potency of icv Administration of ANPs on Water Intake Induced by icv Injection of Angiotensin II (AII)

Treatment		Water intake (ml/30 min)
AII (0.1 nmol)		13.4 ± 0.4
AII (0.1 nmol)		
plus α-rANP	0.3 nmol	12.1 ± 0.8
α-rANP	1.5 nmol	10.9 ± 0.7*
α-hANP	1.5 nmol	11.3 ± 0.5**
α-rANP(4—28)	1.5 nmol	10.3 ± 0.9**
α-rANP(5—28)	1.5 nmol	10.6 ± 0.8**
α-rANP(7—23-amide)	1.5 nmol	13.1 ± 1.9

Note: Values are means ± S.E.M. Significantly different from AII (0.1 nmol) alone: *$p <0.05$, **$p <0.01$ (Duncan's test for multiple comparisons).

From Itoh, H., Nakao, K., Katsuura, G., Morii, N., Yamada, T., Shiono, S., Sakamoto, N., Sugawara, A., Saito, Y., Eigyo, M., Matsushita, A., and Imura, H., *Neurosci. Lett.*, 9, 254, 1986. With permission.

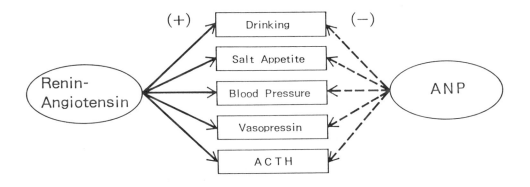

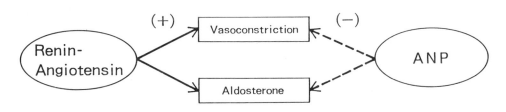

FIGURE 4. Schematic representation of antagonistic actions of the renin-angiotensin and ANP systems in the central and peripheral control of blood pressure and body fluid homeostasis. (Redrawn from Nakao, K., Morii, N., Itoh, H., Yamada, T., Shiono, S., Sugawara, A., Saito, Y., Mukoyama, M., Arai, H., Sakamoto, M., and Imura, H., *J. Hypertens.*, 4 (Suppl. 6), S492, 1986. With permission.)

The transmembrane signaling mechanism in ANP-responsive neurons is not understood yet. ANP is known, after binding its receptor, to stimulate particulate guanylate cyclase in blood vessels and other peripheral tissues. Fiscus et al.[44] observed that ANP enhances the accumulation of cyclic GMP in several discrete regions of rat brain. Using cultured rat glioma cells (C6-2B) and rat pheochromocytoma cells (PC12), they further found that ANP stimulated the accumulation and efflux of cyclic GMP. Although the function of cyclic GMP in the brain remains unclear at present, these observations suggest that the molecular mechanism of action of ANP in the nervous system is at least partly identical to that in peripheral tissues.

The post-receptor signal transduction system causes responses in postsynaptic neurons. To further study the cellular response, we investigated the effect of icv injection of ANP and ANG II on concentrations of dopamine (DA), norepinephrine (NE), and serotonin and their metabolites in the rat brain.[45] The icv injection of ANG II increased DA and its metabolite levels in the septum and hypothalamus, whereas α-ANP decreased them. The simultaneous icv injection of ANP and ANG II significantly reduced the ANG II effect on DA and its metabolite. On the other hand, NE and serotonin contents did not change significantly. In this study, however, we did not study the contents of monoamines in each nucleus. In addition, the icv injection of α-ANP tended to lower, though not significantly, the NE content in the septum. Since the central effect of ANG II is reported to be partly mediated by NE, further studies are required to elucidate the role of NE in mediating ANP action. In summary, both ANP and ANG II seem to act through monoaminergic systems, especially DA neurons, by binding their respective receptors in the same neurons, thus exhibiting opposite effects.

V. CONCLUSION

The distribution of ANP-LI neurons and ANP receptors in the brain suggests roles of ANP in the central control of blood pressure and body fluid homeostasis. The icv injection of ANP inhibits drinking, salt appetite, blood pressure rise, and vasopressin and ACTH releases induced by ANG II. This suggests that the brain renin-angiotensin and ANP systems regulate fluid balance in an opposite way. There is an interaction between the central renin-angiotensin and central ANP systems and the cardiac ANP system. In conclusion, the renin-angiotensin and ANP systems are important modulators of the cardiovascular functions acting in concert in the CNS and in peripheral tissues.

REFERENCES

1. **Morii, N., Nakao, K., Sugawara, A., Sakamoto, M., Suda, M., Shimokura, M., Kiso, Y., Kihara, M., Yamori, Y., and Imura, H.,** Occurrence of atrial natriuretic polypeptide in brain, *Biochem. Biophys. Res. Commun.,* 127, 413, 1985.
2. **Morii, N., Nakao, K., Itoh, H., Shiono, S., Yamada, T., Sugawara, A., Saito, Y., Mukoyama, M., Arai, H., Sakamoto, M., and Imura, H.,** Atrial natriuretic polypeptide in spinal cord and autonomic ganglia, *Biochem. Biophys. Res. Commun.,* 145, 196, 1987.
3. **Tanaka, I., Misono, K. S., and Inagami, T.,** Atrial natriuretic factor in rat hypothalamus, atria, and plasma: determination by specific radioimmunoassay, *Biochem. Biophys. Res. Commun.,* 124, 663, 1984.
4. **Kawata, M., Ueda, S., Nakao, K., Morii, N., Kiso, Y., Imura, H., and Sano, Y.,** Immunohistochemical demonstration of α-atrial natriuretic polypeptide-containing neurons in rat brain, *Histochemistry,* 83, 1, 1985.
5. **Kawata, M., Nakao, K., Morii, N., Kiso, Y., Yamashita, H., Imura, H., and Sano, Y.,** Atrial natriuretic polypeptide: topographical distribution in the rat brain by radioimmunoassay and immunohistochemistry, *Neuroscience,* 16, 521, 1985.

6. **Saper, C. B., Standaert, D. G., Currie, M. G., Schwartz, D., Geller, D. M., and Needleman, P.,** Atriopeptin-immunoreactive neurons in the brain: presence in cardiovascular regulatory areas, *Science,* 227, 1047, 1985.

7. **Jacobowitz, D. M., Skofitsch, G., Keiser, H. R., Eskay, R. L., and Zamir, N.,** Evidence for the existence of atrial natriuretic factor-containing neurons in the rat brain, *Neuroendocrinology,* 40, 92, 1985.

8. **Quirion, R., Dalpe, M., and Dam, T. V.,** Characterization and distribution of receptors for the atrial natriuretic peptides in mammalian brain, *Proc. Natl. Acad. Sci. U.S.A.,* 83, 174, 1986.

9. **Saavedra, J. M., Israel, A., Kurihara, M., and Fuchs, E.,** Decreased number and affinity of rat atrial natriuretic peptide (6—33) binding sites in the subfornical organ of spontaneously hypertensive rats, *Circ. Res.,* 58, 389, 1986.

10. **Nakao, K., Morii, N., Itoh, H., Yamada, T., Shiono, S., Sugawara, A., Saito, Y., Mukoyama, M., Arai, H., Sakamoto, M., and Imura, H.,** Atrial natriuretic polypeptide in brain — implication of central cardiovascular control, *J. Hypertens.,* 4 (Suppl. 6), S492, 1986.

11. **Itoh, H., Nakao, K., Morii, N., Sugawara, A., Yamada, T., Shiono, S., Saito, Y., Mukoyama, M., Arai, H., Sakamoto, M., and Imura, H.,** Central actions of atrial natriuretic polypeptide in spontaneously hypertensive and normotensive rats, *Jpn. Circ. J.,* 51, 1208, 1987.

12. **Standaert, D. G., Saper, C. B., and Needleman, P.,** Atriopeptin: potent hormone and potential neuromediator, *TINS,* 8, 509, 1985.

13. **Kangawa, K. and Matsuo, H.,** Purification and complete amino acid sequence of α-human atrial natriuretic polypeptide, *Biochem. Biophys. Res. Commun.,* 118, 131, 1984.

14. **Kangawa, K., Fukuda, A., and Matsuo, H.,** Structural identification of beta- and gamma-human atrial natriuretic polypeptide, *Nature (London),* 313, 397, 1985.

15. **de Bold, A G.,** Atrial natriuretic factor: a hormone produced by heart, Science 203, 767, 1985.

16. **Needleman, P., Adams, S. P., Cole, E. R., Currie, M. G., Geller, D. M., Michener, M. L., Saper, C. B., Schwartz, D., and Standaert, D. G.,** Atriopeptins as cardiac hormones, *Hypertension,* 4, 469, 1985.

17. **Kangawa, K., Tawaragi, Y., Oikawa, S., Mizuno, A., Sakuragawa, Y., Nakazato, H., Fukuda, A., Minamino, N., and Matsuo, H.,** Identification of rat atrial natriuretic polypeptide and characterization of cDNA encoding its precursor, *Nature (London),* 313, 152, 1984.

18. **Nakao, K., Sugawara, A.,Morii, N., Sakamoto, M., Suda, M., Soneda, J., Ban, T., Kihara, M., Yamori, Y., Shimokura, M., Kiso, Y., and Imura, H.,** Radioimmunoassay for α-human and rat atrial natriuretic polypeptide, *Biochem. Biophys. Res. Commun.,* 124, 815, 1984.

19. **Nakao, K., Sugawara, A., Shiono, S., Saito, Y., Morii, N., Yamada, T., Itoh, H., Mukoyama, M., Arai, H., Sakamoto, M., and Imura, H.,** Secretory form of atrial natriuretic polypeptide as cardiac hormone in humans and rats, *Can. J. Physiol. Pharmacol.,* 65, 1756, 1987.

20. **Sugawara, A., Nakao, K., Morii, N., Sakamoto, M., Suda, M., Shimokura, M., Kiso, Y., Kihara, M., Yamori, Y., Nishimura, K., Soneda, J., Ban, T., and Imura, H.,** α-Human atrial natriuretic polypeptide is released from the heart and circulates in the body, *Biochem. Biophys. Res. Commun.,* 129, 439, 1985.

21. **Shiono, S., Nakao, K., Morii, N., Yamada, T., Itoh, H., Sakamoto, M., Sugawara, A., Saito, Y., Katsuura, G., and Imura, H.,** Nature of atrial natriuretic polypeptide in rat brain, *Biochem. Biophys. Res. Commun.,* 135, 728, 1986.

22. **Sudoh, T., Kangawa, K., Minamino, N., and Matsuo, H.,** Identification in porcine brain of a novel natriuretic peptide distinct from atrial natriuretic peptide, *Nature (London),* 332, 78, 1988.

23. **Nakamura, M., Katsuura, G., Nakao, K., and Imura, H.,** Antidipsogenic action of α-human atrial natriuretic polypeptide administered intracerebroventricularly in rats, *Neurosci. Lett.,* 58, 1, 1985.

24. **Antunes-Rodrigues, J., McCann, S. M., Rogers, L. C., and Samson, W. K.,** Atrial natriuretic factor inhibits dehydration and angiotensin II-induced water intake in the conscious, unrestrained rat, *Proc. Natl. Acad. Sci. U.S.A.,* 82, 8720, 1985.

25. **Katsuura, G., Nakamura, M., Inouye, J., Kono, M., Nakao, K., and Imura, H.,** Regulatory role of atrial natriuretic polypeptide in water drinking in rats, *Eur. J. Pharmacol.,* 121, 285, 1986.

26. **Itoh, H., Nakao, K., Katsuura, G., Morii, N., Shiono, S., Sakamoto, M., Sugawara, A., Yamada, T., Saito, Y., Matsushita, A., and Imura, H.,** Centrally infused atrial natriuretic polypeptdie attenuates exaggerated salt appetite in spontaneously hypertensive rats, *Circ. Res.,* 59, 342, 1986.

27. **Antunes-Rodrigues, J., McCann, S. M., and Samson, W. K.,** Central administration of atrial natriuretic factor inhibits saline preference in the rat, *Endocrinology,* 118, 1726, 1986.

28. **Fitts, D. A., Thunhorst, R. L., and Simpson, J. B.,** Diuresis and reduction of salt appetite by lateral ventricular infusions of atriopeptin II, *Brain Res. Bull.,* 348, 118, 1985.

29. **Itoh, H., Nakao, K., Morii, N., Yamada, T., Shiono, S., Sakamoto, M., Sugawara, A., Saito, Y., Katsuura, G., Shiomi, T., Eigyo, M., Matsushita, A., and Imura, H.,** Central action of atrial natriuretic polypeptide on blood pressure in conscious rats, *Brain Res. Bull.,* 16, 745, 1986.

30. **Casto, R., Hilbig, J., Schroeder, G., and Stock, G.,** Atrial natriuretic factor inhibits central angiotensin II pressor responses, *Hypertension,* 9, 473, 1987.

31. **Yamada, T., Nakao, K., Morii, N., Itoh, H., Shiono, S., Sakamoto, M., Sugawara, A., Saito, Y., Ohno, H., Kanai, A., Katsuura, G., Eigyo, M., Matsushita, A., and Imura, H.,** Central effect of atrial natriuretic polypeptide on angiotensin II-stimulated vasopressin secretion in conscious rats, *Eur. J. Pharmacol.,* 125, 453, 1986.

32. **Iitake, K., Share, L., Crofton, J. T., Brooks, D. P., Ouchi, Y., and Blaine, E. H.,** Central atrial natriuretic factor reduces vasopressin secretion in the rat, *Endocrinology,* 119, 438, 1986.

33. **Samson, W. K.,** Atrial natriuretic factor inhibits dehydration and hemorrhage-induced vasopressin release, *Neuroendocrinology,* 40, 277, 1985.

34. **Samson, W. K., Aguila, M. C., Martinovic, J., Antunes-Rodrigues, J., and Norris, M.,** Hypothalamic action of atrial natriuretic factor to inhibit vasopressin secretion, *Peptides,* 8, 449, 1987.

35. **Janus Zewicz, P., Larose, P., Ong, H., Gutkowska, J., Genest, J., and Cantin, M.,** Effect of atrial natriuretic factor on plasma vasopressin in conscious rats, *Peptides,* 7, 989, 1986.

36. **Itoh, H., Nakao, K., Katsuura, G., Morii, N., Yamada, T., Shiono, S., Sakamoto, M., Sugawara, A., Saito, Y., Eigyo, M., Matsushita, A., and Imura, H.,** Possible involvement of central atrial natriuretic polypeptide in regulation of hypothalamo-pituitary-adrenal axis in conscious rats, *Neurosci. Lett.,* 69, 254, 1986.

37. **Shoji, M., Kimura, T., Matsui, K., Ota, K., Iitaka, K., Inoue, M., Yasujima, M., Abe, K., and Yoshinaga, K.,** Effects of centrally administered atrial natriuretic peptide on renal functions, *Acta Endocrinol.,* 115, 433, 1987.

38. **Itoh, H., Nakao, K., Yamada, T., Morii, N., Shiono, S., Sugawara, A., Saito, Y., Mukoyama, M., Arai, H., and Imura, H.,** Brain renin-angiotensin — central control of atrial natriuretic polypeptide secretion from heart, *Hypertension,* 11 (Suppl. I), I-57, 1988.

39. **Itoh, H., Nakao, K., Yamada, T., Morii, N., Shiono, S., Sugawara, A., Saito, Y., Mukoyama, M., Arai, H., and Imura, H.,** Central interaction of brain atrial natriuretic polypeptide (ANP) system and brain renin-angiotensin system in ANP secretion from heart — evidence for possible brain-heart axis, *Can. J. Physiol. Pharmacol.,* 66, 255, 1988.

40. **Itoh, H., Nakao, K., Yamada, T., Morii, N., Shiono, S., Sugawara, A., Saito, Y., Mukoyama, M., Arai, H., Katsuura, G., Eigyo, M., Matsushita, A., and Imura, H.,** Modulatory role of vasopressin in secretion of atrial natriuretic polypeptide in conscious rats, *Endocrinology,* 120, 2186, 1987.

41. **Itoh, H., Nakao, K., Katsuura, G., Morii, N., Shiono, S., Yamada, T., Sugawara, A., Saito, Y., Watanabe, K., Igano, K., Inoue, K., and Imura, H.,** Atrial natriuretic polypeptides: structure-activity relationship in the central action — a comparison of their anti-dipsogenic actions, *Neurosci. Lett.,* 74, 102, 1987.

42. **Wong, M., Samson, W. K., Dudley, C. A., and Mass, R. L.,** Direct neuronal action of atrial natriuretic factor in the rat brain, *Neuroendocrinology,* 44, 49, 1986.

43. **Okuya, S. and Yamashita, H.,** Effects of atrial natriuretic polypeptide on rat hypothalamic neurones in vitro, *J. Physiol.,* 389, 717, 1987.

44. **Fiscus, R. R., Robles, B. T., Waldman, S. A., and Murad, F.,** Atrial natriuretic factors stimulate accumulation and efflux of cyclic GMP in C6-2B rat glioma and PC12 rat pheochromocytoma cell cultures, *J. Neurochem.,* 48, 522, 1987.

45. **Nakao, K., Katsuura, G., Morii, N., Itoh, H., Shiono, S., Yamada, T., Sugawara, A., Sakamoto, M., Saito, Y., Eigyo, M., Matsushita, A., and Imura, H.,** Inhibitory effect of centrally administered atrial natriuretic polypeptide on brain dopaminergic system in rats, *Eur. J. Pharmacol.,* 131, 171, 1986.

Chapter 17

NEUROENDOCRINE ACTIONS OF THE ATRIAL NATRIURETIC PEPTIDES

Willis K. Samson

TABLE OF CONTENTS

I. INTRODUCTION

As discussed in previous chapters, the hypothalamic distribution of ANP-like immu-noreactivity (Chapter 12) and ANP binding sites (Chapter 13) predicted central nervous system actions of the peptides related to their peripheral actions to control hydromineral balance. Indeed, our group[1] and that of Imura and co-workers (Chapter 16) have discussed several brain actions of ANP which complement those peripheral effects, including hypo-thalamic actions to inhibit vasopressin (AVP) secretion,[2,3] water intake,[4,5] and salt appetite.[6] These actions of ANP all can be demonstrated to involve a potentially significant antagonism by ANP of the central actions of angiotensin II (A II). This is most clearly illustrated by Imura and Nakao in Chapter 16 (Figure 4).

We and the Imura group were impressed, however, by the presence of ANP containing axonal projections in hypothalamic and rostral diencephalic sites not related to fluid and electrolyte homeostasis, but instead to regions of the CNS known to be important in the control of anterior pituitary function.[7-9] In particular, the presence of ANP immunoreactivity and ANP binding sites[10,11] in the preoptic and anterior hypothalamic areas and in the external layer of the median eminence suggested possible neuroendocrine effects of the peptides unrelated to their actions on AVP secretion and fluid intake. This chapter details findings which indicate significant hypothalamic actions of ANP suggesting potent neuromodulatory effects of the peptides, and further details evidence for the interaction of brain-derived ANP with established neurotransmitter and neuropeptide systems within the brain.

II. ANP AND THE HYPOTHALAMO-PITUITARY-GONADAL AXIS

A. INHIBITION OF GONADOTROPIN SECRETION

Several lines of evidence pointed to a potential effect of ANP on luteinizing hormone (LH) secretion. ANP fibers innervate preoptic hypothalamic structures known to be important in the generation of phasic LH secretion and the presence of ANP in the external layer of the median eminence suggested that it either gained access to the hypothalamo-hypophyseal portal vessels for delivery to the anterior pituitary gland, where receptors had been identi-fied,[10] or that it might interact with neurotransmitter- and neuropeptide-containing elements within the tissue to modify the release of LH-releasing hormone (LHRH) into the portal circulation. The initial description by Standaert et al.[12] that intravenous infusion of ANP could lower plasma LH levels in the rat agreed with results that we had obtained simulta-neously.[13] Infusions of ANP (rat atriopeptin III or rat ANF-28, 0.1 μg ANP/kg/min, 30 min, i.v.), which resulted in a two- to threefold elevation in circulating ANP levels, sig-nificantly inhibited LH secretion in both the castrated male and ovariectomized (OVX) female rat (Figure 1). In females, the effect was dose-related and relatively long lasting. These results confirmed our hypothesis that ANP might exert actions on LH secretion, but they did not identify the site of action of ANP. Since neither the median eminence nor the anterior pituitary gland are located behind the blood brain barrier, and since ANP receptors are present in both those sites, we examined these tissues *in vitro* for clues to the site of action of peripherally administered ANP to alter LH release.

In agreement with the findings of several other groups,[14-16] we were unable to detect any significant effect of ANP in doses ranging from 10—12 to 10—6 *M* on basal or LHRH-stimulated LH release from dispersed anterior pituitary cells cultured *in vitro* (Figure 2). Nor were we and others[14-16] able to demonstrate significant and reproducible effects of ANP on the basal or stimulated release of thyrotropin (TSH), adrenocorticotropin (ACTH), pro-lactin (PRL), or growth hormone (GH). Thus, although ANP exposure stimulates guanylate cyclase activity in pituitary cell preparations, these effects do not seem to be functionally

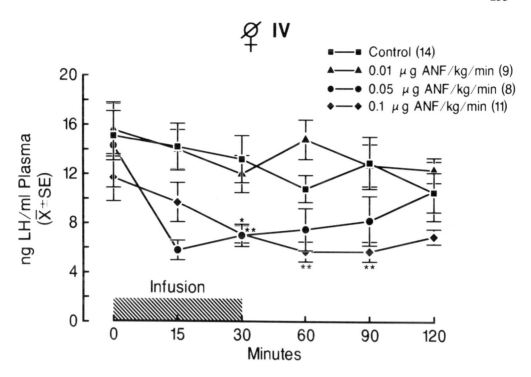

FIGURE 1. Plasma luteinizing hormone (LH) levels in conscious, unrestrained, ovariectomized female rats prior to (0 min), during (15 min), and after a 30 min, intravenous infusion of 1 ml saline alone (control) or 1 ml saline containing atrial natriuretic factor (ANF) at the indicated dose rates. Numbers in parenthesis indicate group size. *p <0.05, **p<0.025. (From Samson, W. K., Aguila, M. C., and Bianchi, R. *Endocrinology*, in press. With permission.)

correlated with hormone secretion[14] and the role of the ANP receptors detected in the anterior pituitary gland remains unknown.

If one assumes that ANP in circulating plasma is excluded form the CNS by the blood brain barrier, then the only other site at which it can act to inhibit LH secretion would be the median eminence. Similarly, ANP infused behind the blood brain barrier, into the third cerebroventricle (3V), would gain access to this site and the inhibition of LH secretion should also be seen. This was indeed the case (Figure 3). These studies suggested that ANP of either central or peripheral origin could play a role in the hypothalamic control of LH secretion. Two experimental procedures further established this possibility.

Exposure of median eminence fragments *in vitro* to the catecholamines, norepinephrine and dopamine, results in dose-related stimulation of LHRH release[17] and, while ANP alone had no effect of the release of LHRH, it significantly reduced and even reversed the stimulatory action of the catecholamines in this tissue.[13] Therefore, ANP of peripheral origin or ANP containing axonal endings within the median eminence can potentially exert significant effects on LH secretion via presynaptic actions in the median eminence.

The ability of centrally administered ANP to inhibit LH secretion in the conscious rat, together with our previous demonstration[18] of the ability of iontophoresed or micropressure-ejected ANP (in doses of less than 10 to 18 g) to inhibit neuronal activity in the preoptic-septal areas and the presence of ANP containing nerve terminals in this region, suggest that the peptide might also act within the rostral diencephalon to inhibit LH release. These regions are known to be important in the generation of cyclic LH secretion and, furthermore, it is well established[19] that the endogenous opioid peptides play crucial, inhibitory roles in the regulation of this phasic form of hormone release. We reasoned that if ANP were acting

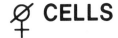

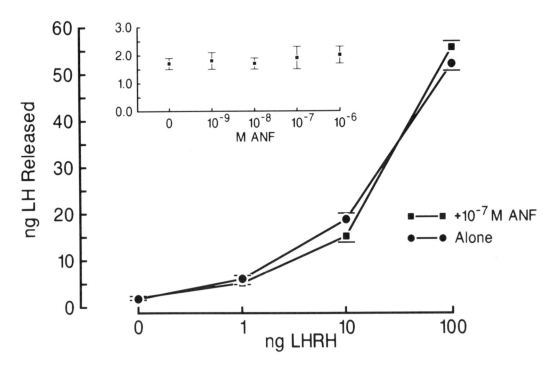

FIGURE 2. Effect of atrial natriuretic factor (ANF) on basal (inset) or luteinizing hormone-releasing hormone (LHRH)-stimulated LH release from cultured anterior pituitary cells of ovariectomized female rats. Cells were incubated in the presence of control medium by itself or medium containing ANF or LHRH alone and in combination with 10 to 7 *M* ANF (n = 7 all groups). (From Samson, W. K., Aguila, M. C. and Bianchi, R., *Endocrinology*, in press. With permission.)

within the preopticseptal regions to modulate the neural control of LH secretion, any interaction with brain opiate systems in the expression of this action might be uncovered by pretreatment of the animals with the opiate antagonist, naloxone. Indeed, naloxone pretreatment completely abolished the ability of ANP to inhibit LH secretion, establishing these rostral CNS sites as potential sites of action of ANP and providing further evidence for the interaction of ANP with endogenous, neuropeptide systems.

In summary, ANP can interact with brain catecholamine systems as well as other neuropeptide-containing neurons to exert significant inhibitory effects on gonadotropin secretion. These effects appear, from a variety of approaches, to be exerted predominantly at the level of the hypothalamus. Whether circulating ANP of cardiac origin can play any significant role in the tonic or phasic regulation of LH secretion remains to be established. Similarly, to prove the physiological significance of the LH-inhibiting action of centrally derived ANP, one would have to remove or neutralize the neural product from these regions. Lesion studies would not answer this question since extensive damage would preclude accurate interpretation of the results. To date, no technique for creating mutants which lack neural ANP exists. We have attempted, however, to sequester centrally released ANP by passive immunoneutralization with microinjections of anti-ANP serum. Initial experiments have revealed a potentially significant role for endogenous ANP in the control of basal LH secretion since injection of 2 μl anti-ANP (rabbit, anti-rat ANP, Peninsula Laboratories) into the third cerebroventricle resulted in a significant ($p < 0.05$, paired t-test), albeit transient, increase

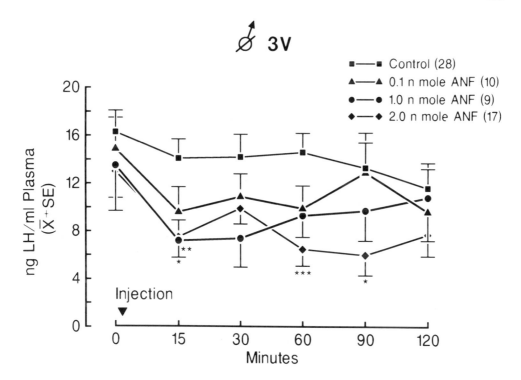

FIGURE 3. Plasma luteinizing hormone (LH) levels in conscious, unrestrained, orchidectomized male rats prior to (0 min) and after third cerebroventricular (3V) injection of 2 μl saline alone (control) or 2 μl saline containing atrial natriuretic factor (ANF) at the doses indicated. Numbers in parenthesis indicate group size. *p <0.05, **p <0.025, ***p <0.005. (From Samson, W. K., Aguila, M. C., and Bianchi, R., *Endocrinology*, in press. With permission.)

in LH secretion (plasma ANF levels, ng/ml; before antiserum injection, 10.6 ± 3.3; 30 min later, 19.5 ± 3.6; 60 min later, 12.1 ± 3.5; 120 min later, 11.5 ± 2.5; n = 6).

B. DOPAMINE-MEDIATED PROLACTIN INHIBITION

Reports of the ability of centrally administered ANP to alter brain levels of dopamine[20] (see Chapter 16) and to inhibit dopamine-beta-hydroxylase activity in tumor cell lines,[21] suggested that central ANP might be involved in the hypothalamic control of prolactin (PRL) secretion since the major expression of that control is via dopamine, the predominate hypothalamic PRL-release inhibiting factor (PIF). While in the case of PRL, i.v. infusions of ANP failed to alter PRL levels in plasma, third cerebroventricular infusions of the peptide resulted in significant, long-lasting, dose-related inhibitions of PRL secretion in the conscious, unrestrained rat (Figure 4[22]). Since no significant action of ANP to alter basal, stimulated (by oxytocin, thyrotropin-releasing hormone, angiotensin II, or vasoactive intestinal peptide) or inhibited (by dopamine) PRL release from dispersed anterior pituitary cells was observed *in vitro*[22] we hypothesized a hypothalamic action of the peptide.

This hypothalamic effect could be exerted either by some inhibition of the release into the hypophyseal portal circulation of a putative PRL releasing factor (PRF) or by stimulation of the release of PIF. While we knew that ANP did not alter the release of at least one of the putative peptidergic PRFs, oxytocin,[2,23] we were unable to determine if the releases of one of the other PRFs examined in our *in vitro* studies[22] could be altered by ANP administration because of the already low levels of these peptides in plasma. Instead, we reasoned that if the predominant effect of ANP to inhibit PRL secretion were due to its action to stimulate the release of the major PIF, dopamine, then pretreatment of the animals with

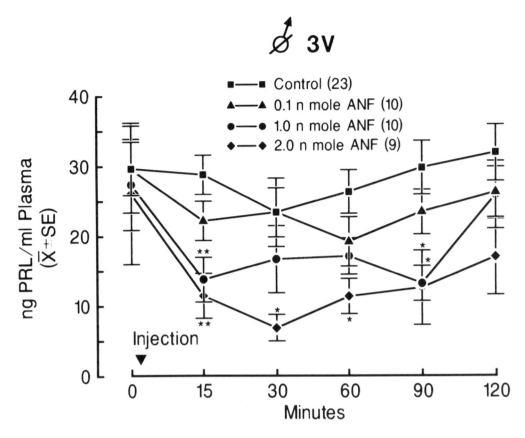

FIGURE 4.   Plasma prolactin (PRL) before and after third cerebroventricular injection of control saline (2 µl) or saline containing the doses of atrial natriuretic factor (ANF) indicated. Numbers in parenthesis indicate groups size. *$p < 0.025$, **$p < 0.005$. (From Samson, W. K. and Bianchi, R., *Can. J. Physiol. Pharmacol.*, 66, 554, 1988. With permission.)

either a dopamine receptor blocker or with the dopamine depletor, alpha-methyl-para-tyrosine (ampt), would prevent the action of centrally administered ANP.[24]

Administration of the D2-dopamine receptor blocker, domperidone, prior to central administration of ANP completely prevented its PRL inhibitory action and when given after the inhibitory effect of ANP had been established, the blocker reversed the ANP effect (Figure 5). Prior depletion of tubero-infundibular dopamine stores with ampt also prevented the central PRL-inhibitory action of ANP (Figure 6). Thus, it is unnecessary to invoke the participation of any inhibitory actions of ANP on the release of putative PRFs since dopaminergic blockade and depletion studies revealed the significant interaction of ANP with dopamine systems regulating PRL secretion.[24] Whether this interaction is expressed in the median eminence or at the level of the dopamine-producing perikarya in the arcuate nucleus is unclear; however, the fact that the lengthy intravenous infusions of ANP can prevent the steroid-induced PRL surge seen in OVX female rats suggests a median eminence site of action (Figure 7).

III. HYPOTHALAMIC ACTIONS UNRELATED TO REPRODUCTION

A. INHIBITION OF ADRENOCORTICOTROPIN SECRETION

As discussed in Chapter 16 Imura and co-workers[25] demonstrated the ability of ANP to interrupt the hypothalamic signals controlling adrenocorticotropin (ACTH) release. These

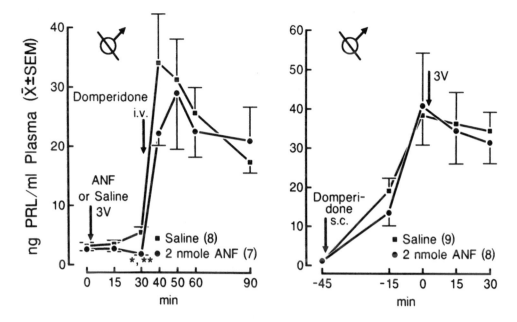

FIGURE 5. Plasma prolactin (PRL) levels in orchidectomized male rats before and after third cerebroventricular injection of 2 μl saline or saline containing 2 nmole atrial natriuretic factor (ANF). The D2-dopamine receptor blocker was given either before or after injection of ANF. *p = 0.005 versus saline infused controls, **p = 0.03 versus preinfusion levels. (From Samson, W. K., Bianchi, R., and Mogg, R., *Neuroendocrinology*, 47, 268, 1988. With permission.)

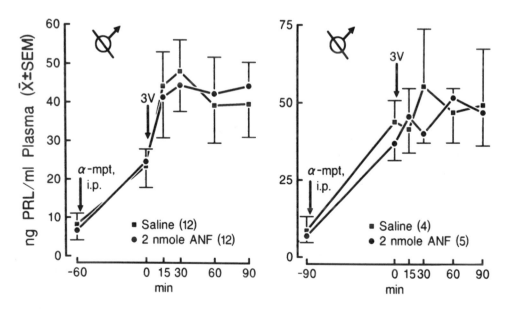

FIGURE 6. Prior treatment of orchidectomized male rats with the tyrosine hydroxylase inhibitor, alpha methyl-para-thyrosine (ampt), prevents the ability of centrally administered atrial natriuretic factor (ANF, 2 nmol) to inhibit prolactin (PRL) secretion. (From Samson, W. K., Bianchi, R., and Mogg, R., *Neuroendocrinology*, 47, 268, 1988. With permission.)

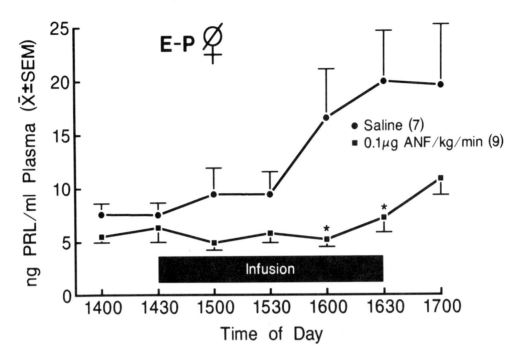

FIGURE 7.   Lengthy intravenous infusion of atrial natriuretic factor (ANF) prevents the prolactin surge seen in control rats. Ovariectomized rats were treated with estrogen and progesterone to induce the PRL surge. *$p < 0.05$.

effects not only might play significant physiological roles in the actions of ACTH on fluid and mineral homeostasis, but also might serve as a mechanism for the integration of stress-related ACTH secretion. Certainly the innervation of the parvocellular paraventricular nucleus by ANP neurons originating in the AVPV (see Chapter 12) suggests a neuromodulatory action of ANP on neurons projecting to the median eminence that contain corticotropin releasing factor. Single neurons in this region of the hypothalamus do respond to the application of ANP.[26,27] Whether these results with central administration of ANP in rats can explain, at least in part, the ability of peripherally administered ANP to inhibit corticosteroid secretion remains to be established.

B. STIMULATION OF GROWTH HORMONE SECRETION

In our hands, third cerebroventricular administration of ANP failed to significantly alter growth hormone (GH) secretion in conscious rats (Figure 8). However, our experiments were conducted at midday when levels of GH in individual rats are quite variable. Imura's group instead examined the effect of central administration of ANP during the early morning when the lowest levels of the hormone are present in plasma.[28] In their studies,[29] intracerebroventricular administration of ANP resulted in a significant elevation of plasma GH levels in both anesthetized and conscious rats. Similar central administration of ANP potentiated the GH response to subsequent i.v. GH-releasing hormone (GRF) infusion; however, the GH releasing effect of central ANP infusion was not affected by pretreatment with anti-GRF serum. These results led the authors to speculate that the GH-elevating effect of ANP was due to an inhibition of somatostatin release into the hypophyseal portal circulation. Indeed, high doses of ANP inhibited somatostatin release from hypothalamic fragments in their studies. Our failure to observe any effect of ANP on GH release *in vivo* was probably related to the time of day the experiments were conducted and our inability to demonstrate an inhibition of somatostatin release from our median eminence explants[13] might have been due to the differing tissue incubated or to the low levels present in the medium to begin

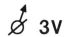

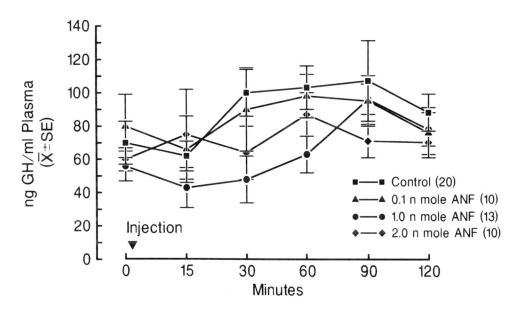

FIGURE 8. Plasma growth hormone (GH) levels in orchidectomized male rats prior to and after third cerebrov-entricular injection of 2 μl saline (control) alone or containing the indicated doses of atrial natriuretic factor (ANF).

with. In any event, the data of Murakami and co-workers[29] strongly suggests potential actions of ANP on the hypothalamic control of GH secretion.

C. FAILURE TO MODIFY THYROTROPIN RELEASE

As mentioned above, exposure of cultured anterior pituitary cells to ANP failed to alter either basal or stimulated thyrotropin (TSH) release *in vitro*. Similarly, neither peripheral nor central administration of the peptide significantly altered TSH secretion *in vivo*. While peripheral circulating concentrations of ANP can be altered in hypo- or hyperthyroid states,[30] we have been unable to demonstrate a significant effect of ANP on the central mechanisms controlling the secretion of thyrotropic factors from the anterior pituitary gland.

IV. A PROPOSED NEUROMODULATORY ROLE FOR ANP IN THE HYPOTHALAMIC CONTROL OF ANTERIOR PITUITARY FUNCTION

While considerable, unresolvable argument exists over the exact definition of a neu-romodulatory agent vis-a-vis a neurotransmitter, we can now say that many of the proposed, necessary criteria for either status have been demonstrated for ANP. First, it is produced in neurons[31] in a prohormone form and processed prior to secretion.[32] Release from neural explants has been demonstrated[33] and direct membrane effects on other neurons documented,[18,26,27,34] most notably hyperpolarization of the receptive element. Distinct neuronal fiber systems containing ANP[7-9] and discreet populations of ANP receptor binding[10,11] within the brain suggest organized systems of ANP elements. Finally, the ability of ANP to influence the release of AVP, LHRH, somatostatin, dopamine, and perhaps even corticotropin-re-leasing factor, together with its ability to antagonize the neural actions of angiotensin II and to interact with brain opioid and catecholamine systems, strongly suggest that not only does the peptide function to "modulate" neural activity within the brain, but also that we will read much more in the future about its actions within the central nervous system.

ACKNOWLEDGMENTS

Support for our studies on the neuroendocrine actions of ANP was provided by the American Heart Association (Texas Affiliate) and the NIH (HD09988, Project II). I thank Judy Scott for her excellent secretarial assistance and wish Renee Bianchi, my research associate who conducted most of the experiments, good luck in her planned graduate studies.

REFERENCES

1. **Samson, W. K.,** Atrial natriuretic factor and the central nervous system, *Clin. Endocrinol. Metab.,* 16, 146, 1987.
2. **Samson, W. K., Aguila, M. C., Martinovic, J., Antunes-Rodrigues, J., and Norris, M.,** Hypothalamic action of atrial natriuretic factor to inhibit vasopressin secretion, *Peptides,* 8, 449, 1987.
3. **Yamada. T., Nakao, K., Morii, N., Itoh, H., Shiono, S., Sakamoto, M., Sugawara, A., Saito, Y., Ohno, H., Kancir, A., Katsuura, G., Eigyo, M., Matsushita, A., and Imura, H.,** Central effect of atrial natriuretic polypeptide on angiotensin II-stimulated vasopressin secretion in conscious rats, *Eur. J. Pharmacol.,* 125, 453, 1986.
4. **Antunes-Rodrigues, J., McCann, S. M., Rogers, L. C., and Samson, W. K.,** Atrial natriuretic factor inhibits water intake in conscious rats, *Proc. Natl. Acad. Sci. U.S.A.,* 82, 8720, 1985.
5. **Katsuura, G., Nakamura, M., Inouye, K., Kono, M., Nakao, K., and Imura, H.,** Regulatory role of atrial natriuretic polypeptide in rats, *Eur. J. Pharmacol.,* 121, 285, 1986.
6. **Antunes-Rodrigues, J., McCann, S. M., and Samson, W. K.,** Central administration of atrial natriuretic factor inhibits salt intake in the rat, *Endocrinology,* 118, 1726, 1986.
7. **Kawata, M., Nakao, K., Morii, N., Kiso, Y., Yamashita, H., Imura, H., and Sano, Y.,** Atrial natriuretic polypeptide: topographical distribution in the rat brain by radioimmunoassay and immunohistochemistry, *Neuroscience,* 16, 521, 1985.
8. **Skoftisch, G., Jacobowitz, D. M., Eskay, R. L., and Zamir, N.,** Distribution of atrial natriuretic factor-like immunoreactive neurons in the rat brain, *Neuroscience,* 16, 917, 1985.
9. **Standaert, D. G., Needleman, P., and Saper, C. B.,** Organization of atriopeptin-like immunoreactive neurons in the central nervous system of the rat, *J. Comp. Neurol.,* 253, 315, 1986.
10. **Quirion, R., Dalpe, M., DeLean, A., Gutkowska, J., Cantin, M., and Genest, J.,** Atrial natriuretic factor (ANF) binding sites in brain and related sites, *Peptides,* 5, 1167, 1984.
11. **Bianchi, C., Gutkowska, J., Ballak, M., Thibault, G., Garcia, R., Genest, J., and Cantin, M.,** Radioautographic localization of I-125 atrial natriuretic factor binding sites in the brain, *Neuroendocrinology,* 44, 365, 1986.
12. **Standaert, D. G., Cicero, T., and Needleman, P.,** Atriopeptin inhibits the release of luteinizing hormone, *Fed. Proc.,* 45, 174, 1986.
13. **Samson, W. K., Aguila, M. C., and Bianchi, R.,** Atrial natriuretic factor inhibits luteinizing hormone secretion in the rat: evidence for a hypothalamic site of action, *Endocrinology,* in press.
14. **Simard, J., Hubert, F. F., Labrie, F., Assayag, E., and Heisler, S.,** Atrial natriuretic factor-induced cGMP accumulation in rat anterior pituitary cells in culture is not coupled to hormonal secretion, *Regul. Peptides,* 15, 269, 1986.
15. **Heisler, S., Simard, J., Assayag, E., Mehri, Y., and Labrie, F.,** Atrial natriuretic factor does not affect basal-, forskolin-, and CRF-stimulated adenylate cyclase activity, cAMP formation of ACTH secretion, but does stimulate cGMP synthesis in anterior pituitary, *Mol. Cell. Endocrinol.,* 44, 125, 1986.
16. **Abou-Samra, A., Catt, K. J., and Aguillera, G.,** Synthetic atrial natriuretic factors (ANFs) stimulate guanylate $3',5'$-monophosphate production but not hormone release in rat pituitary cells: peptide contamination with a gonadotropin-releasing activity of certain ANFs, *Endocrinology,* 120, 18, 1987.
17. **Negro-Vilar, A., Ojeda, S. R., and McCann, S. M.,** Catecholamine modulation of luteinizing hormone-releasing hormone release by median eminence terminals *in vitro, Endocrinology,* 104, 1749, 1979.
18. **Wong, M., Samson, W. K., Dudley, C. A., and Moss, R. L.,** Direct, a neuronal action of atrial natriuretic factor in the rat brain, *Neuroendocrinology,* 44, 1986.

19. **Kalra, P. S. and Kalra, S. P.,** control of gonadotropin secretion, in *The Pituitary Gland,* Imura, H., Ed., Raven Press, New York, 1985, 189.

20. **Nakao, K., Katsuura, G., Morii, N., Itoh, H., Shiono, S., Yamada, T., Sugawara, A., Sakamota, M., Saito, Y., Eigyo, M., Matsushita, A., and Imura, H.,** Inhibitory effect of centrally administered atrial natriuretic polypeptide on brain dopaminergic system in rats, *Eur. J. Pharmacol.,* 131, 171, 1986.

21. **Racz, K., Kuchel, O., Buu, N. T., Debinski, W., Cantin, M., and Genest, J.,** Atrial natriuretic factor, catecholamines, and natriuresis, *N. Engl. J. Med.,* 314, 1986.

22. **Samson, W. K. and Bianchi, R.,** Further evidence for hypothalamic site of action of atrial natriuretic factor: inhibition of prolactin secretion in the conscious rat, *Can. J. Physiol. Pharmacol.,* 66, 554, 1988.

23. **Samson, W. K., Lumpkin, M. D., and McCann, S. M.,** Evidence for a physiological role for oxytocin in the control of prolactin secretion, *Endocrinology,* 119, 554, 1986.

24. **Samson, W. K., Bianchi, R., and Mogg, R.,** Evidence for dopaminergic mechanism for the prolactin inhibitory effect of atrial natriuretic factor, *Neuroendocrinology,* 47, 268, 1988.

25. **Itoh, H., Nakao, K., Katsuura, N., Morii, N., Yamada, T., Shiono, S., Sakamoto, M., Sugawara, A., Saito, Y., Eigyo, M., Matsushita, A., and Imura, H.,** Possible involvement of central atrial natriuretic polypeptide in regulation of hypothalamo-pituitary-adrenal axis in conscious rats, *Neurosci. Lett.,* 69, 254, 1986.

26. **Haskins, J. T., Zingarro, C. J., and Lappe, R.,** Rat atriopeptin III alters hypothalamic neuronal activity, *Neurosci. Lett.,* 67, 279, 1986.

27. **Standaert, D. G., Cechetto, D. F., Neddleman, P., and Saper, C. B.,** Inhibition of firing of vasopressin neurons by atriopeptin, *Nature (London),* 151, 1987.

28. **Murakami, Y., Kato, Y., Kabayama, Y., Tojo, K., Inoue, T., and Imura, H.,** Involvement of growth hormone (GH)-releasing factor in GH secretion induced by serotonergic mechanisms in conscious rats, *Endocrinology,* 119, 1089, 1986.

29. **Murakami, Y., Kato, Y., Inoue, T., Koshiyama, H., Ishikawa, Y., Hattori, N., and Imura, H.,** Stimulation of central atrial natriuretic polypeptide of growth hormone secretion in rats, Abstr. 535, Endocrine Society Meeting, Indianapolis, 1987.

30. **Kohno, M., Takaori, K., Matsuura, T., Murakawa, K., Kanayama, Y., and Takeda, T.,** Atrial natriuretic peptide in atria and plasma in experimental hyperthyroidism and hypothyroidism, *Biochem. Biophys. Res. Commun.,* 134, 178, 1986.

31. **Gardner, D. C., Deschepper, C. F., Ganong, W. F., Hane, S., Fiddes, J., Baxter, J. D., and Lewicki, J.,** Extra-atrial expression of the gene for atrial natriuretic factor, *Proc. Natl. Acad. Sci. U.S.A.,* 83, 6697, 1986.

32. **Shiono, S., Nakao, K., Morii, N., Yamada, T., Itoh, H., Sakamoto, M., Sugawara, A., Saito, Y., Katsuura, G., and Imura, H.,** Nature of atrial natriuretic polypeptide in rat brain, *Biochem. Biophys. Res. Commun.,* 135, 728, 1986.

33. **Shibasaki, T., Naruse, M., Naruse, K., Masuda, A., Kim, Y. S., Imaki, T., Yamauchi, N., Demura, H., Inagami, T., and Shijume, K.,** Atrial natriuretic factor is released from rat hypothalamus *in vitro, Biochem. Biophys. Res. Commun.,* 136, 590, 1986.

34. **Okuya, S. and Yamashita, H.,** Effects of atrial natriuretic polypeptide on rat hypothalamic neurons *in vitro, J. Physiol. (London),* 389, 717, 1987.

Chapter 18

EFFECT OF ATRIAL NATRIURETIC PEPTIDE IN NORMAL AND HYPERTENSIVE HUMANS

Eric A. Espiner and A. Mark Richards

TABLE OF CONTENTS

I. INTRODUCTION

Since the discovery of atrial peptides in human atrial tissue extracts,[1] leading to their synthesis and general availability for experimental studies, there have been numerous studies documenting the effects of atrial natriuretic peptide (ANP) in humans. Most of these studies show clear-cut effects of the peptide on urinary sodium and urine volume, with variable effects on arterial pressure and hormone secretion. Much of this variation in the published literature can be attributed to the wide range of doses employed and differences in study conditions in which sodium intake, posture, and the extent of placebo-controlled observations have varied greatly. Before considering the effects of ANP in detail, it is important to review briefly what is currently known concerning the regulation and metabolism of the hormone in normal humans.

ANP is synthesized and stored in atrial cardiocytes as the precursor ANP(1—126),[2] which is converted to the biologically active ANP(99—126) during secretion.[3] Amino acid sequence analysis of human coronary sinus plasma extracts confirm that this peptide makes the major contribution to ANP immunoreactivity,[4] which is consistent with other chromatographic studies showing that ANP(99—126) is the main circulating form in human plasma.[5,6] Recent studies also indicate that the propeptide (ANP[1—98] or deleted forms) is cosecreted along with ANP(99—126) and circulates in plasma.[7] However, studies of the effects of atrial peptides are virtually confined to the 28-amino-acid C-terminal peptide, and the actions of the propeptide, if any, remain unknown. As discussed elsewhere, the secretion of ANP(99—126) appears to be determined largely by stretch receptors within the atrial myocyte. In keeping with this, a wide range of clinical disorders characterized by central hypervolemia are associated with elevated levels of plasma ANP.[8] Similarly, physiological circumstances producing central blood volume expansion — including high sodium intake, supine posture, and exercise — are associated with small increments in peripheral venous ANP concentrations.[8] In the authors' laboratory, levels of endogenous resting venous plasma immunoreactive ANP (IR-ANP) range from 5 to 24 pmol/1 in normal subjects.[6] Values as high as 400 to 600 pmol/1 may be observed in patients with severe congestive heart failure and/or tachyarrhythmia. Such a wide pathophysiological range — approximately 100-fold — is similar to that observed in plasma renin activity (PRA) and provides a basis for the interpretation of the effects of administered hormone in normal humans. It should be noted that the arterial plasma ANP concentration is approximately double the venous level,[9] reflecting the rapid uptake and clearance of the hormone within the microcirculation.[10] Erect posture reduces the metabolic clearance of ANP in normal subjects.[11] These findings, together with the rapid half-life (approximately 3 min),[10] need to be borne in mind when interpreting the effect of exogenous ANP. Despite the rapid metabolism, there is no evidence to suggest that venous plasma hormone levels fluctuate greatly or rapidly in normal subjects, nor in those with severe heart failure, and any diurnal rhythm appears to be insignificant.[12]

In reviewing the effects of ANP administration in humans, knowledge of the plasma level attained, as well as the factor(s) determining end organ and receptor sensitivity, must be considered. For example, it is already clear that the preexisting renal tubular avidity for sodium reabsorption greatly diminishes the natriuretic effect of ANP, whereas increases in renal perfusion pressure appear to increase the response. For reasons of convenience, the renal, hemodynamic, and endocrine effects of ANP in normal humans will be reviewed separately, followed by a brief review of the responses found in subjects with hypertension.

II. NORMAL SUBJECTS

A. RENAL FUNCTION AND URINARY ELECTROLYTE EXCRETION

Initial studies using large bolus injections of human ANP confirmed the potent natriuretic and diuretic effect of the peptide in normal subjects.[13] Compared with placebo injections,

Richards et al. found that urinary sodium excretion increased fourfold after 100 μg ANP and urinary volume calcium, magnesium, and phosphorus excretion doubled within 30 min of the injection. Potassium and creatinine excretion rates were not affected. Similar effects on urine volume, sodium, chloride, and potassium excretion were obtained by Kuribayashi[14] using bolus injections of 25 and 50 μg hANP. Endogenous creatinine clearance was reported to increase threefold after the larger dose. In a further study,[15] the injection of 50 μg hANP was associated with a brief increase in urine volume and urine sodium excretion, and the urine sodium excretion rate almost doubled within 30 min of the injection. Associated with these events was a 2.8-fold increase in urinary cyclic GMP excretion. These early studies showed that large doses of human ANP caused a rapid, but brief, natriuresis and diuresis without consistently increasing potassium excretion. Because of the rapid metabolism of ANP, more revealing information of the renal action of the hormone is provided by studies using constant infusions where the action of ANP can be related to steady-state levels achieved in venous plasma. As listed in Table 1, numerous studies* have documented the effect of atrial peptides infused into normal subjects at doses ranging from 2.25 to 200 ng/kg/min. In only a few of these studies were placebo (time-controlled) infusions undertaken and in many cases the peptides were infused without carrier protein to prevent adsorption to syringe and infusion tubes.[16,17] Furthermore, sodium status varied greatly (and was not always controlled) and conditions of posture were not uniform. Despite these and other experimental variations, it is clear that large infusions (70 to 200 ng/kg/min) of either rANP or hANP evoke a substantial diuresis and natriuresis (two- to fivefold above control levels), and usually cause a proportionate increase in chloride, calcium, phosphorus, and magnesium, but not potassium, excretion. These infusion rates also uniformly reduced blood pressure. In detailed studies of renal function, employing bladder catheters and water loading to maximize urine flow, Weidmann et al.[18] showed that large doses of hANP (100 ng/kg/min) increased GFR and more impressively increased the filtration fraction (by as much as 37%), even though arterial pressure fell. Very large doses (200 ng/kg/min) caused a greater fall in blood pressure and did not further increase natriuresis — in fact, natriuresis was less well sustained at the highest infusion rate. Lower infusion rates[21,23-25] (10 to 47 ng/kg/min), achieving plasma ANP levels in the pathophysiological range (50 to 320 pmol/l), did not generally decrease blood pressure, but were associated with variable natriuresis and diuresis (Table 1). In some cases,[23,25,26] responses matched those produced by much larger infusion rates, whereas in others[21,24] there was no significant natriuresis or diuresis. Responses to rat and N-terminal-deleted peptides were not clearly different from those of hANP. Natriuresis was usually associated with increases in calcium, magnesium, and chloride excretion, but phosphaturia was less evident at the lower infusion rate and kaliuresis again did not occur. A remarkably reproducible renal response to ANP (14 ng/kg/min) was reported by Biollaz et al.,[25] who studied a group of six salt-loaded normal subjects on two occasions at an interval of 1 week. The same group,[22] infusing 70 ng/kg/min for 4 h, observed waning natriuresis and diuresis as blood pressure fell 2 to 3 h after commencement of infusion. Similar findings of waning responsiveness to prolonged ANP infusions were reported by Waldhausl.[30] These results, taken together with the effect of very large doses[18] and results from animal studies,[31] strongly suggest that reductions in blood pressure (and therefore in renal perfusion pressure) severely limit a continuing natriuretic response to ANP in man. The natriuretic effect of ANP is also greatly reduced in normal subjects equilibrated on a low-salt diet.[19,23] In subjects ingesting 10 mmol sodium daily, Cuneo et al.[23] found that peak natriuresis was only 10% of that observed in the same subjects ingesting 200 mmol sodium daily — despite identical levels of plasma ANP (320 pmol/1) in the two studies. Interestingly,

---

* Step incremental infusions as employed by some groups[16,36,45] have not been considered because of the difficulty in interpreting renal responses to rapid changes in ANP levels.

TABLE 1
Renal Response to ANP Infusions in Normal Humans

Peptide infused	Infusion rate (ng/kg/min)	Duration (min)	Sodium intake (mmol/d)	Posture	ANP conc. (pmol/l) Basal	ANP conc. (pmol/l) Steady state	Renal response Na	Renal response Volume	Renal response Comments	Blood pressure	Ref.
hANP	200+	45	"Normal"	Supine	19 ± 4	414 ± 65	↑ (273%)	↑ (333%)	GFR ↓ FF ↑	↓	18
hANP	100*	45	"Normal"	Supine	19 ± 4	208 ± 30	↑ (224%)	↑ (495%)	GFR ↑ FF ↑	↓	18
hANP	100*	45	140	Supine	18 ± 4	180 ± 18	↑	↑	K NS	↓ (9.8%)	19
hANP	100*	45	310	Supine	15 ± 3	170 ± 10	↑	↑	K NS	↓ (5.3%)	19
hANP†	100	20	200	Supine	NA	NA	↑ (250%)	↑ (350%)		↓	20
rANP† (102—126)	100	60	Uncontrolled	Seated	19 ± 3	868 ± 54	↑ (450%)	↑ (200%)	K NS, FF ↑	↓	21
rANP† (101—126)	70	240	ca. 240	Supine	31 ± 6	1070 ± 92	↑ (270%)	↑ (250%)	K & P NS, FF ↑	↓ at 2 to 3 h	22,29
hANP	47	60	200	Seated	12.6 ± 2.8	320 ± 40	↑ (300%)	↑ (180%)	K & P NS	NS	23
rANP† (102—126)	30	60	Uncontrolled	Seated	19 ± 3	238 ± 70	NS	NS		NS	21
hANP†	25	40	180	Supine	NA	NA	NS	NS		↓ (6.2%)	24
rANP† (101—126)	14	120	250	Supine	40 ± 7	152 ± 14	↑ (200%)	NS	K & P NS, FF ↑	NS	25,29
rANP† (101—126)	10	60	Uncontrolled	Seated	19 ± 3	49 ± 11	NS	NS		NS	21
rANP† (101—126)	7	240	ca. 300	Supine	36 ± 6	75 ± 7	↑ (24%)	NS	K & P NS, FF ↑	NS	22,29
hANP (101—126)	6	120	200	Seated	3 ± 0.5	26 ± 2	↑ (220%)	↑	K & P NS, FF ↑	NS	26
hANP	3.6	180	ca. 200	Seated	3.8 ± 1.5	20.9 ± 1.9	↑ (60%)	↑ (28%)	K NS	NS	27
hANP	2.25	180	150	Seated	8 ± 2	16 ± 2	↑ (30%)	NS	K & P NS	↓	28

Note: Parentheses are percentage change from control levels. Abbreviations: NA, not available; NS, not significant; FF, filtration fraction; K, potassium; P, phosphorus; ↑, increase; ↓, decrease.

+   Preceded by bolus (100 μg).
*   Preceded by bolus (50 μg).
†   No carrier protein added to infusate.

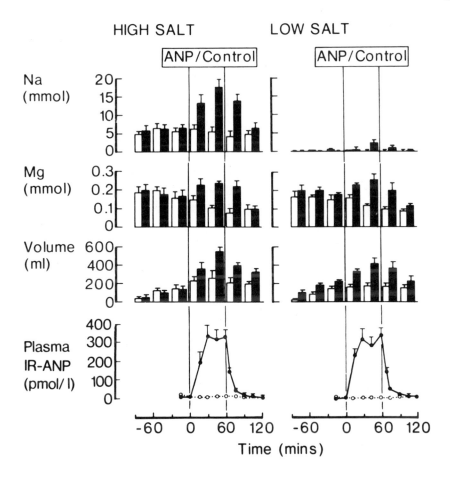

FIGURE 1. Mean (± SEM) urinary sodium, magnesium, and volume excretion during control (□) and hANP (■) infusions (47 ng/kg/min for 60 min) in six normal subjects equilibrated on daily sodium intakes of 200 mmol (left) and 10 mmol (right). Plasma ANP levels (bottom panel) are also shown on infusion (continuous line) and control (interrupted line) days.

responses in urine volume and magnesium excretion were similar on the two different diets (Figure 1). Weidmann et al.[19] also observed a reduced natriuresis during infusions (100 ng/kg/min) given to subjects equilibrated on 17 mmol sodium daily when compared to those subjects receiving 140 mmol sodium daily. In addition, this group noted a much greater diuretic and natriuretic effect in subjects equilibrated on 310 mmol sodium daily when compared to the responses observed in normal subjects ingesting 140 mmol sodium daily. Thus, in addition to the effects of systemic arterial pressure, it appears that low-salt intake attenuates and high-salt intake augments the natriuretic effect of ANP. Whether renin-angiotensin activity, renal hemodynamic response, or other renal tubular response to sodium is responsible for these differences remains to be clarified, but it is obvious that "volume" and sodium status must be carefully considered when interpreting the response of the kidney to ANP.

Speculation concerning the natriuretic effect of ANP infused to achieve plasma levels observed in normal subjects[32] appears to be resolved by several recent studies.[26-28] As shown in Table 1, at least three reports show increased sodium excretion at mean steady-state plasma ANP levels ranging from 16 to 26 pmol/1 for periods of 2 to 3 h. In all of these studies, which were placebo-controlled, infusions contained carrier proteins to reduce adsorption of ANP and standardized conditions of posture and sodium intake were employed.

Richards et al.[26] found that 6 ng/kg/min more than doubled the sodium excretion rate as well as increasing calcium, magnesium, and urine volume. The filtration fraction increased by 14% when compared to the control day. Virtually identical results were obtained using the N-terminally deleted peptide hANP(101 — 126). Using even smaller doses (3.6 ng/kg/min), Anderson[27] reported a 60% increase in sodium excretion and a smaller (28%), but significant, increase in urine volume on the ANP-infusion day. In a recently completed study,[28] our group has found clear-cut natriuretic effects of infused ANP (2.25 ng/kg/min) at venous plasma concentrations entirely within the range for normal resting subjects (see Figure 2). In this study, calcium and magnesium excretion were significantly increased by ANP, but there was no significant change in urine volume or creatinine, potassium, or phosphate excretion, and the filtration fraction did not differ between infusion and control placebo studies. An interesting feature of the reports using very low infusion rates, is the persisting natriuresis after plasma ANP levels have returned to baseline levels, Presumably, this persistence of ANP action relates to the continuing production (or action) of the second messenger "cyclic GMP",[33] which appears to be a marker of ANP hormonal action,[15] even at physiological levels in normal humans.[28]

While the above studies indicate that ANP is likely to have important effects on renal function and sodium homeostasis in normal humans, a number of outstanding questions remain. Not least among these is the importance of small dietary variations in sodium intake and the specific effect of the renin-angiotensin system in determining renal responsiveness to ANP. Finally, much more work is required to clarify the underlying mechanism of the renal action of ANP in humans. From studies already reported, it appears likely that increases in both GFR and, more importantly, filtration fraction serve to promote natriuresis and diuresis, as reported in experimental animals.[31] A direct action of ANP on renal tubular function[34] also has strong experimental support. Unlike diuretics such as furosemide,[35] the natriuretic action of ANP in humans does not appear to be affected by inhibitors of renal prostaglandin formation.[36] Whereas studies in experimental animals and in humans (see below) show that ANP may suppress renin-angiotensin, aldosterone secretion, and possibly AVP, it appears unlikely that inhibition of these hormones — with the possible exception of angiotensin II — contribute significantly to the acute renal effects of ANF in man.[37]

B. HEMODYNAMIC ACTION

Initial studies in normal subjects[13] showed that large bolus injections (100 μg/h hANP) induced an immediate fall in arterial pressure and a significant increase in heart rate, as measured by the Oxford technique of continuous pressure and heart rate recording.[38] Compared with the placebo (control) study, the fall in arterial pressure (mean 5.5 mmHg) was maximal at 2 min, but a small and sustained hypotensive effect and increase in heart rate was recorded for the 3 h of observation after ANP injection. As shown in Table 1, continuous infusions employing doses above 50 ng/kg/min reduced blood pressure and in most cases also increased heart rate. Weidmann et al.[18] reported a 7 and 12% fall in systolic and diastolic pressure, respectively, during ANP infusion (100 ng/kg/min for 45 min) and an increase in heart rate of 10 to 16% above preinfusion levels. These hemodynamic changes remained for the 45-min period of observation after discontinuation of ANP infusion. Surprisingly, the hypotensive and tachycardic effect of these infusions was similar in salt-restricted and salt-loaded normal subjects.[19] Dose-dependent effects of rANP infusions on intraarterial blood pressure were reported by Bussien et al. in normal salt-loaded subjects.[39] Commencing with 14.5 ng/kg/min, the rate was increased at 15-min intervals until a fall of 10 to 20 mmHg in systolic pressure was obtained, after which a constant infusion was maintained for a further 60 min. Diastolic pressure fell and heart rate increased progressively during the incremental infusion period, whereas systolic pressure only fell at very high infusion rates (290 to 580 ng/kg/min). Again, the hypotensive effect persisted for at least 60 min

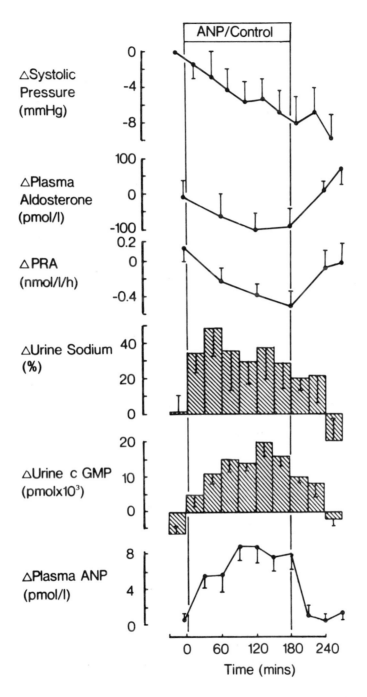

FIGURE 2. Response to intravenous infusions of hANP (2.25 ng/kg/min for 180 min) in six normal subjects equilibrated on a daily Na intake of 150 mmol. Values (mean ± SEM) are plotted as change (Δ) from time-matched levels on the control day for systolic pressure, plasma aldosterone, PRA, and urinary excretion of sodium and cGMP. Change in plasma ANP on the infusion day is also shown (bottom panel).

postinfusion. The same group[22] observed similar hemodynamic changes (in salt-loaded normal subjects) after 2 to 3 h of infusing 50 ng/kg/min. Infusions of less than 50 ng/kg/min have not obviously affected systemic pressure, as measured by cuff sphygmomanometry. However, in a recent study using continuous intraarterial pressure monitoring, we noted a significant fall in both systolic and mean arterial pressure during physiological doses (2.25 ng/kg/min) when compared to time-matched placebo recordings (Figure 2). The absence of a significant fall in blood pressure in many of the above studies does not, of course, necessarily imply a lack of vascular action of ANP since homeostatic mechanisms may well be activated to restore pressure to normal. In fact, rise in heart rate and increase in sympathetic activity (as indicated by significant increases in plasma norepinephrine levels), was observed by Cuneo et al.[23] during ANP infusions of 47 ng/kg/min, which did not significantly affect blood pressure. Presumably, these changes represent arterial baroreceptor-mediated increases in sympathetic outflow to the heart in order to maintain blood pressure in these circumstances.

In attempts to clarify the mechanism by which ANP exerts its vasodepressor actions in humans, a number of studies have examined the effect of the hormone on hemodynamic function and regional blood flow. A dose-dependent effect of ANP to increase skin blood flow of the left forearm was documented by Bussien et al.[39] Skin blood flow increased soon after starting infusions (14 ng/kg/min) and tended to fall with larger doses once hypotension occurred. Direct intraarterial infusion of hANP in normal subjects was shown by Bolli et al.[17] to increase forearm blood flow within 1 min and lowered forearm vascular resistance in a dose-dependent fashion without increasing systemic venous ANP levels. The maximum vasodilator response amounted to 60% of that produced by sodium nitroprusside. Similar results were reported by Fujita et al.,[40] who found the vasodilator action to be closely coupled to both ipsilateral venous plasma ANP and cGMP levels, In this study, vasodilatation by ANP was inhibited by coinfusions of calcium chloride sufficient to raise ipsilateral venous plasma calcium from 9.5 to 11-12 mg%. Extrapolating from changes in ipsilateral venous plasma ANP levels during brachial arterial infusion of ANP, Bolli et al.[17] suggested that ANP increments as low as 15 pmol/l in venous plasma may be associated with a 10% increase in forearm blood flow. On the other hand, Takeshita et al.[41] found that systemic infusions of hANP (30 ng/kg/min), while decreasing systolic blood pressure, did not change forearm vascular resistance. However, the expected increase in forearm vascular resistance accompanying lower body negative pressure (which reduced right atrial pressure) was significantly less during ANP infusions when compared to placebo control studies. Since the forearm vascular response to intraarterial infusion of norepinephrine was not reduced by this dose of ANP, the authors suggested that the ANP infusion attenuated the reflex sympathetic activation mediated by cardiopulmonary baroreceptors. In contrast to most other studies, the same group found no significant increase in heart rate associated with these hypotensive infusions of hANP and attributed this result to the low dose infused, along with the inhibition of baroreflex control mechanisms, as shown by the studies using lower body negative pressure. Evidence that ANP may oppose the pressor effects of circulating hormones, including norepinephrine[42] and angiotensin II,[43] provides another mechanism for the vasorelaxant effect of ANP on the arterial circulation. Such a mechanism, while well established from *in vitro* and animal experiments,[31] has so far only been assessed at relatively high levels of ANP in man (e.g., 45 ng/kg/min,[43] achieving venous levels of 300 pmol/l) and its physiological role is yet to be established.

In addition to its arterial vasorelaxant effect, ANP infusions reduce central venous pressure[24,41] and pulmonary wedge pressure.[21] During 100 ng/kg/min rANP infusion given to supine normal subjects, a 30% fall in pulmonary wedge pressure was the only significant hemodynamic change observed by Cody et al.[21] Cardiac index, arterial pressure, and systemic vascular resistance did not change in these supine subjects. However, in seated (as opposed to supine) normal subjects, in whom blood pressure fell with the same dose of ANP, the fall in cardiac filling pressure would also be expected to reduce cardiac output. These effects of ANP in normals indicate that the hormone reduces venous return to the heart (at least at high infusion rates) and may also explain the changes observed in regional blood flow. For instance, observations[25] that infusions of 7 and 14 ng/kg/min reduced hepatic and renal blood flow, respectively, in normal humans without affecting systemic pressure are consistent with regional autonomic-mediated responses to a fall in cardiac output.

Another potential mechanism by which ANP may modify blood pressure is reduction of plasma volume. Weidmann et al.[18] using high infusion rates of ANP (100 ng/kg/min), observed prompt increases in hematocrit and serum protein concentrations which were in excess of any possible hemoconcentration effect resulting from diuresis. Hematocrit and protein levels fell some 45 min after infusions were terminated. These increases in hematocrit were on average greater in subjects receiving a high-salt intake (12% rise) than in those receiving a normal (9.5% rise) or low-salt (4.5% rise) intake.[19] Similar, though smaller, changes were observed in both seated and supine normal subjects by Cody et al.,[21] infusing 100 ng/kg/min. Presumably, these changes reflect a fluid shift from vascular to extravascular space and are consistent with an ANP-induced increase in capillary filtration.[44] Richards et al.[26] observed a 4 to 6% increase in hematocrit (compared to time-matched samples during placebo infusion) with infusions of 6 ng/kg/min, achieving steady-state plasma levels of 26 pmol/l. Even with infusions achieving plasma ANP levels completely within the normal range, there was a trend for hematocrit to increase, although values did not achieve statistical significance.[28] Thus, it is possible that quite small increments in ANP, well within the range encountered in normal subjects, may diminish plasma volume acutely, with a consequent fall in cardiac filling pressure.

It is clear from the above that the hemodynamic actions of ANP are extremely diverse and difficult to dissect using clinical studies in humans. As noted with renal effects, some of the actions of ANP on the circulation persist long after infusions are terminated and after plasma ANP levels have returned to control levels. In view of the complex interplay of hemodynamic actions and their persistence, it is perhaps not surprising that alarming hypotensive reactions have been reported during and after ANP infusions by several groups. Some,[18,22,39,45] but not all,[46] episodes have occurred with high infusion rates or several hours after infusions had commenced. Typically, the episode of hypotension is unheralded, is often associated with bradycardia, and may occur well after cessation of the ANP infusion.[47] The mechanism remains obscure and clearly indicates the need for close supervision of all subjects receiving ANP infusions, regardless of dose.

C. NEUROENDOCRINE EFFECTS

Inhibition of renin and aldosterone secretion appear to be the main endocrine actions of ANP, but for several reasons many of the studies performed in humans have given inconsistent or contradictory results. First, most studies have examined the effect of ANP in supine subjects receiving a normal or high sodium intake so that the renin-angiotensin axis is already relatively suppressed. Second, the failure to allow for the well-established diurnal rhythm and the effects of posture on renal and adrenal hormones may complicate interpretation — especially when placebo time-controlled studies are omitted. Finally, the apparent endocrine effects of ANP may well be modified by reflex responses to concurrent hemodynamic actions. Thus, the failure to observe any change in the renin-aldosterone axis in the presence of significant sympathetic stimulation, volume contraction, or hypotension may in fact represent an inhibitory effect of the hormone on the renin-aldosterone axis. Early studies using bolus injections[13] or brief infusions of ANP[48] not surprisingly failed to show any significant changes in renin-aldosterone activity. However, high infusion rates (100 ng/kg/min) given after a bolus of 50 μg to supine normal subjects were reported to inhibit plasma aldosterone levels even though PRA increased.[19] Since hypotension and significant increase in plasma norepinephrine (at least two-fold) occurred with these infusions, presumably any suppressive effect by ANP on renin was overridden by sympathetic activation. Lower infusion rates (<100 ng/kg/min) producing less or no sympathetic activation are variously reported to reduce aldosterone, but not renin,[24,49] reduce both renin and aldosterone,[21,23] or affect neither hormone.[22,25,36,45] Cuneo et al.,[23] infusing 47 ng/kg/min, found that all elements of the renin-aldosterone system were suppressed at plasma ANP levels approximating 320 pmol/l. Whereas inhibition was more readily demonstrated in subjects equilibrated on a low-salt diet, the percentage inhibition (approximately 40%) was in fact similar in subjects ingesting 200 mmol sodium daily. Almost identical inhibition was observed by Cody et al., using higher doses (100 ng/kg/min).[21] In some studies, a rebound activation of aldosterone[21] or both renin and aldosterone[22] has occurred upon cessation of ANP infusions — findings which provide further support for an inhibitory effect of ANP, which appears to be of brief duration under these experimental conditions. Lower infusion rates, calculated to mimic physiologically attainable levels, are also inhibitory to both plasma renin[26,27,46] and aldosterone.[26] Richards et al.[26] reported that plasma renin, angiotensin II, and aldosterone fell to half time-matched placebo-controlled values during infusions of 6 ng/kg/min in seated, sodium-loaded subjects. Similar doses (7 ng/kg/min), as well as reducing PRA and plasma aldosterone, markedly reduced the response of both hormones to erect posture in normal subjects[11] receiving a normal salt intake.[50] Finally, as shown in Figure 2, ANP infusions for 3 h — raising venous plasma ANP levels in normal subjects by as little as 8 pmol/l — significantly reduced both PRA and aldosterone to 50 and 64% of control values, respectively.[28] Although it is possible that ANP lowers hormone levels by increasing their clearance rate from plasma, this mechanism appears unlikely in view of the reports that even quite low doses of ANP (7 ng/kg/min) reduce, rather than increase hepatic blood flow.[25] Such an effect would tend to mask, rather than account for, any fall in plasma hormone concentration during ANP infusion. All these studies therefore give strong support to an inhibitory effect of small physiological ANP increments on both renin and aldosterone secretion in normal subjects. It is possible that inhibition is in fact greater at lower levels of ANP infusion, where homeostatic reflexes (including augmented ACTH and sympathetic activation) are less evident or avoided.

Although it is established that even small changes in ANP effect renin and aldosterone, the mechanisms underlying these inhibitory effects remains unclear. From evidence quoted above, it appears that both renin and aldosterone may be equally sensitive to inhibition — provided sudden hypotension and acute sympathetic activation does not occur. The possibility that the inhibitory effect on aldosterone is simply a consequence of renin inhibition appears unlikely in view of the findings that ANP also inhibits angiotensin II-induced aldosterone stimulation.[43,46,51] ANP infusions (45 ng/kg/min) greatly reduced peak aldosterone levels induced by large pressor doses of angiotensin II (10 ng/kg/min).[43] In a more recent study[46] much lower ANP infusion rates (7 ng/kg/min), inducing increments of approximately 30 pmol/l, significantly flattened the angiotensin-aldosterone dose response curve of normal sodium-restricted subjects, but did not affect the aldosterone (or cortisol) response to physiological increments in ACTH. Since the same infusion rate (7 ng/kg/min) also reduced basal renin and angiotensin II levels, it is possible that both renal and adrenal actions occur independently and at concentrations of endogenous ANP attainable in normal subjects. The effect of ANP on potassium-induced changes in aldosterone secretion are as yet unknown. A preliminary report[52] has shown no effect of ANP (100 μg bolus injection) on aldosterone secretion induced by metoclopramide. Whether renin inhibition is due to a direct effect of ANP on juxtaglomerular cells[53] or results from the natriuretic action of ANP to increase distal tubular sodium concentration is still uncertain. However, the similar percent inhibition of renin in subjects ingesting 200 or 10 mmol sodium daily,[23] despite greatly different natriuretic responses to the hormone, argues against a direct *macula densa* effect alone.

A variety of other hormonal effects of ANP, many of them inconsistent, have been reported in humans. In human adrenal cell cultures, ANP is reported to inhibit both basal and ACTH-induced cortisol and DHA release, as well as aldosterone.[54] However, most clinical studies (but not all[19,49]) failed to show any inhibitory effect of ANP on plasma cortisol of ACTH levels. Ohashi et al.[49] reported that plasma cortisol (but not ACTH or DHA) was significantly lower than time-matched placebo-control values some 20 to 40 min after ANP infusions (100 ng/kg/min) were terminated. Weidmann et al.[19] also reported a fall in plasma cortisol during ANP infusions (100 ng/kg/min), but no placebo-control studies were performed. At physiologically attainable levels of ANP, no inhibition of the cortisol response to incremental ACTH infusion was found in normal subjects.[46] Since some groups[21,23] have observed a rebound rise in plasma cortisol after cessation of ANP infusions, the possibility remains that higher doses of ANP are inhibitory to the hypothalamic-pituitary adrenal axis in humans, but further studies are clearly required.

Although data from animal experiments show an inhibitory effect of ANP on AVP secretion,[55] most,[23,25,37,45] but not all,[20] groups have failed to confirm such an effect in normal humans. The difficulty of measuring a fall in plasma AVP reliably in well-hydrated normal subjects, however, needs to be kept in mind. Fujio et al.[20] reported that 100 ng/kg/min hANP, given to six salt-loaded normal subjects for 20 min suppressed plasma AVP levels from detectable (0.3 to 0.5 pg/ml) to undetectable levels at 20 to 30 min. AVP values were unaffected in a control study in which a similar volume of "saline" was substituted for the ANP infusion. Coincident with this fall in plasma AVP was a striking rise in free-water clearance. Interpretation of these results is made difficult by the absence of adequate placebo-control data, in particular the rate of urine excretion and changes in free-water clearance on the control day.

As discussed in the section on hemodynamic effects, high infusion rates of ANP may also increase plasma norepinephrine[19,23] without necessarily affecting systemic blood pressure.[23] Using incremental infusions of hANP (11.5, 23, and 46 ng/kg/min each for 30 min), Cusson et al.[45] found no significant changes in plasma dopamine, norepinephrine, or epinephrine levels in seven normal control subjects. Dopamine beta hydroxylase activity also remained unchanged. Since a brisk fall in blood pressure occurred in three of the seven normal subjects, it could be argued that sympathetic function (as judged by stable plasma norepinephrine levels) was suppressed by ANP in these subjects. Infusion rates producing ANP levels in the physiological attainable range[26,28] caused no significant change in plasma catecholamine levels. It seems likely, therefore, that large doses of ANP may induce a secondary response from the sympathetic system, whereas smaller changes in ANP levels appear to make little difference to plasma catecholamines. However, since plasma norepinephrine is not necessarily a marker of sympathetic activity, it would be wrong to assume that even physiological increments in ANP have no affect on sympathetic function. More work is therefore needed to assess any interaction of administered ANP and the sympathetic system in normal man.

D. SUMMARY

Short-term infusions of ANP in normal man have clear-cut renal, hemodynamic, and endocrine effects — the patterns of which depend upon the dose infused and the subjects' sodium status and blood pressure. Interpretation of the effects of large doses of ANP is complicated by homeostatic reflex changes occurring in response to the protean hemodynamic actions of the hormone. As shown in Figure 2, studies using very low infusion rates, achieving plasma ANP levels in the upper normal range, show significant natriuresis as well as inhibitory effects of the hormone on blood pressure, plasma renin, and aldosterone levels in normal subjects. These results point to multiple actions at physiological ANP levels and emphasize the potential of ANP to affect sodium and fluid homeostasis in normal humans.

However, more studies — especially using longer periods of infusion and eventually using ANP antagonists — are required to assess the importance of the hormone in the day-to-day regulation of sodium homeostasis in normal man.

III. ESSENTIAL HYPERTENSION

The multiple actions of ANP at even physiological plasma concentrations clearly suggest a role for this peptide in the regulation of blood pressure. This raises the possibility that deficiencies in ANP synthesis and release, or in end-organ responses to ANP, may contribute to the pathophysiology of hypertension. Several groups have demonstrated that circulating concentrations of ANP are, if anything, elevated in hypertension — particularly in severe and/or complicated cases.[56,57] Several published studies document the renal, hemodynamic, and endocrine effects of various doses of ANP infused in patients with untreated essential hypertension.[45,58-60] As described in normal subjects, interpretation and comparison of data from ANP infusions in hypertension must be viewed in relation to other factors, including dose and duration of infusions, baseline sodium status, posture, and the extent of true matched-control data. Reviewed here are studies already published, together with some preliminary observations from data in preparation.[61]

A. RENAL FUNCTION AND URINARY ELECTROLYTE EXCRETION
Richards et al., adhering to the same protocol used for their original study of normal subjects,[13] gave bolus intravenous injections of 100 μg α-hANP to six male patients with mild to moderate untreated essential hypertension in a placebo-controlled study.[58] Sodium excretion rose to sixfold time-matched placebo values in the 30 min after the injection of ANP and remained elevated for 2 to 5 h. Smaller, briefer increments in urine volume and calcium, magnesium, and phosphorus excretion were also observed. Urine potassium, osmolality, pH, and creatinine were unchanged. Caution is necessary when comparing these results with those from similarly studied normal volunteers[13] as the two groups were not closely matched for age or weight. However, urine volume and excretion of sodium, calcium, and magnesium were all significantly greater in the hypertensive group. There was a significant positive correlation between baseline blood pressure and the natriuretic responses to ANP. This was true within each group — normotensive or hypertensive — and when all data were combined. The observation is consistent with other experimental evidence suggesting that renal perfusion pressure exerts a major influence on the renal response to ANP.[31,62]

Weidmann et al. measured a comprehensive range of variables in a group of ten patients with severe essential hypertension infused with ANP.[59] Dietary sodium was not rigidly standardized, but the preinfusion sodium excretion rate of 271 ± 38 μmol/min suggests the patients were sodium replete. Since this study (and the group's preceding, similar study conducted in normal subjects) lacks time-matched control data, changes in urinary indices are related to baseline (preinfusion) values. ANP, 50 μg bolus, followed by 100 ng/kg/min for 45 min, resulted in a mean plateau venous plasma ANP value of 407 ± 53 pmol/l and a maximum increase in sodium excretion of 665%. Sharp increases were also observed in urine flow (772%) and the excretion rates of chloride (1524%), phosphate (518%), and magnesium (303%). Increases in uric acid (95%) and potassium (104%) excretion were less marked. GFR and renal blood flow rose acutely within 15 min, but then returned to control values, whereas the marked natriuresis persisted. When data from normal and hypertensive subjects were compared, increases in urine flow and excretion of sodium, chloride, potassium, calcium, phosphate, and magnesium were all found to be more pronounced in the hypertensive group.

Janssen et al.[60] reported some of the effects of prolonged infusions (up to 4 h) of relatively low doses of ANP (7 and 14 ng/kg/min) in three patients with essential hypertension during both high (200 mmol/d) and moderately restricted (50 mmol/d) sodium intake. Urinary indices were not completely documented in this publication, but the authors state that natriuresis was observed with doses in both sodium-replete and -restricted states. Their illustration of hourly urinary sodium excretion during infusions of 14 ng/kg/min in sodium-replete subjects suggests at least a doubling of baseline values. Natriuresis was severely curtailed if marked hypotension occurred during infusions.

Cusson et al. infused hANP at rates of 11.5, 23, and 46 ng/kg/min over three successive 30-min periods in five patients with mild, untreated essential hypertension and in seven normal volunteers.[45] In this placebo-controlled study, patients received a standard dietary sodium intake (150 mmol/d) and studies were conducted with patients supine. Plasma ANP values rose from a basal value of 4 ± 1 pmol/l to 23 ± 3, 60 ± 13, and 77 ± 17 pmol/l during successive steps of the infusion. Similar values were achieved in the normal subjects. With ANP infusions natriuresis increased in a step-wise fashion to 1.4-, 2.4-, and 5.0-fold the time-matched placebo values. Similar effects were observed in the normal control group. However, comparison of hypertensive and normotensive groups is made difficult by differences in posture, basal urine flow, and sodium excretion and by hypotensive reactions in the normotensives. Nevertheless, the absolute values of both urine flow and sodium excretion rate tended to be greater in the hypertensive group at all infusion rates. No clear effect on potassium excretion was observed. An original contribution from this study was measurement of urine cGMP excretion, which rose in a step-wise fashion to a similar extent in both groups.

Tonolo et al.[61] infused ANP at doses of 3 and 6 ng/kg/min for successive 2-h periods in a placebo-controlled study of eight patients with mild to moderate essential hypertension. Mean baseline 24-h urine sodium excretion was approximately 130 mmol/d and patients were studied supine. Significant natriuresis (60%) was observed only during infusions of 6 ng/kg/min when compared to the placebo study. Trends toward increased urine flow and excretion of magnesium and calcium were not statistically significant.

The above studies show that, overall, urine volume and electrolyte responses to ANP are preserved in essential hypertension. Natriuresis had been observed at doses ranging between 7 and 100 ng/kg/min, with infusions varying from 45 min to 4 h in duration, and in patients with mild to severe hypertension ingesting as little as 50 and as much as 200 mmol/d (or more) of sodium. Where comparisons between similarly studied normotensive and hypertensive subjects have been possible, natriuresis appears to be enhanced in hypertension. This observation requires confirmation by further studies incorporating rigidly standardized study conditions and careful matching of subjects for characteristics other than blood pressure. The correlation of baseline blood pressure with natriuresis induced by ANP,[58] the antinatriuresis noted by Janssen et al. during hypotensive reactions,[60] and the apparent overall enhancement of renal responses to ANP in hypertension are all features consistent with a crucial role for renal perfusion pressure in determining the natriuretic response to ANP.

B. HEMODYNAMIC ACTION

Richards et al.[58] reported that bolus injections (100 μg) of hANP in patients with mild to moderate hypertension (mean arterial pressure, MAP, 117 mmHg) caused a transient 10 mmHg fall (9%) in MAP at 3 min after injection. Pressures returned to placebo values in 7 min. Heart rate rose to a maximum of 14 bpm above placebo levels in 4 min and remained elevated for the 3-h period of observation. The heart rate response was identical to that seen in normal subjects.[13] However, in contrast to the sustained effect on MAP observed in normotensives, the blood pressure fall in hypertensives was brief. This difference was of borderline significance ($p = 0.052$). The patients studied by Weidmann et al.[59] had severe hypertension (MAP 146 mmHg). During infusion of ANP (100 ng/kg/min for 45 min), systolic blood pressure fell by 8% and was further reduced in the 45-min follow-up period by 12%. Diastolic pressure fell by 15 and 8% during and following the infusion, respectively. Heart rate rose by 11 to 13% throughout the infusion and recovery phases. Compared with normal subjects the percentage reductions in systolic blood pressure and increases in heart rate were only slightly more pronounced in the hypertensive group. As the authors comment, the effect of agents which lower blood pressure is generally more profound as basal pressure rises. They felt the difference in response between normotensive and hypertensive groups was notably slight, considering the marked disparity in basal MAP (100 vs. 146 mmHg). The heart rate response was also slightly enhanced in the hypertensive group. Cusson et al.[45] noted that blood pressure "remained stable" during stepped infusion of ANP in patients with mild hypertension, but no data beyond baseline pressures ($135 \pm 3/92 \pm 5$ mmHg) are given. These authors did note a rise in heart rate to 15 bpm above placebo values at the highest ANP infusion rate (46 ng/kg/min). The sudden hypotensive/bradycardic episodes reported by Janssen et al.[60] during ANP infusions of 7 and 14 ng/kg/min, respectively, make it clear that aberrant reactions can occur in subjects with hypertension as well as in normotensives, even after infusions have been terminated.[47]

The effect of ANP infusions on right atrial pressure, pulmonary artery wedge pressure, and cardiac output (Swan-Ganz catheter), in addition to systemic arterial pressure (intraarterial cannula) and heart rate, has been studied by Tonolo et al. in hypertensive subjects.[61] The patients had mild to moderate hypertension (MAP 122 mmHg). Significant falls in systolic (but not diastolic), systemic, and pulmonary arterial pressures were observed after 2-h infusion (3 ng/kg/min) and these falls were more pronounced after a further 2 h at 6 ng/kg/min. Cardiac output fell progressively below placebo values with successive doses of ANP and calculated total peripheral resistance tended to rise. Thus, the fall in blood pressure was attributable to the fall in cardiac output. Fall in right atrial and pulmonary wedge pressures failed to attain statistical significance. Heart rate rose slightly above placebo values. Hematocrit rose with ANP in the studies by both Weidmann et al. and Tonolo et al., the change being greater than that attributable to diuresis alone. Again, these findings suggest an extrarenal effect of ANP — promoting fluid shift from the intra- to the extravascular compartment.

Mechanisms underlying the hypotensive effect of ANP remain uncertain, and are probably multiple. It seems likely that the transient, modest effects, occurring within minutes after bolus injections and occasionally associated with facial flushing, are due to an acute (direct) vasodilatation. On the other hand, the longer-term reductions in pressure, selectively affecting systolic pressure and associated with falls in cardiac output, a trend towards increase peripheral resistance, and a rise in hematocrit (Tonolo et al.), suggest that plasma volume reduction plays an important role during prolonged lower-dose infusions. Inhibition of the renin-angiotensin system and modification of central and reflex nervous vasoregulatory activity may contribute.

In summary, ANP lowers blood pressure in hypertension, but this response may be somewhat blunted in hypertensives when compared with normotensives, particularly when bolus injections and/or short, high-dose infusions are employed. Sustained low-dose infusions significantly lower blood pressure in mild to moderate hypertension, possibly by different mechanisms, and comparison of the relative effects of such infusions in normotensive and hypertensive subjects is awaited.

C. NEUROENDOCRINE EFFECTS

Although clear-cut suppression of plasma renin values below time-matched placebo levels has yet to be demonstrated during infusions of ANP in hypertensive patients, the data from Richards et al.[58] Cusson et al.[45] and Tonolo et al.[61] are consistent in showing a lack of rise in renin in the face of significant natriuretic and/or hypotensive effects. This suggests that, as in normal subjects, ANP directly inhibits renin secretion in human hypertension. However, data from Weidmann et al.[59] suggests that if doses of ANP are sufficient to cause a significant, acute hypotensive effect associated with a rise in plasma norepinephrine values, and presumably a reflex increase in sympathetic activity, then plasma renin activity may actually rise. Plasma aldosterone values are frankly suppressed,[58] and show a downward trend[45] or a significant postinfusion "rebound" rise[59] when bolus and/or short infusions of high doses of ANP are given. In the study by Tonolo et al., sustained low doses of ANP for 4 h caused no significant intra- or postinfusion change in plasma aldosterone. Aldosterone values may be suppressed even though renin values rise[59] — confirming the presence of independent mechanisms for the action of ANP on the two hormones. Most,[45,58] though not all, studies of hypertensives show little effect of ANP on plasma cortisol. Weidmann et al.[59] observed a "rebound" rise in cortisol in parallel with plasma aldosterone when infusions were stopped. Hence, as in normal subjects, the possibility of an inhibitory effect on ACTH secretion remains to be clarified.

In studies employing high doses of ANP,[45,58,59] such as bolus injections and/or short infusions, plasma norepinephrine rose. In contrast, epinephrine values were either frankly lowered[58] or unchanged.[45,59] Low, prolonged doses of ANP, as administered by Tonolo et al., caused no significant change in plasma catecholamine values. These findings make it likely that any increase in plasma norepinephrine follows from an acute sympathetic response to the acute hypotensive effect of ANP. On the other hand, the possibility of a direct, specific inhibitory effect on adrenal medullary secretion of epinephrine is yet to be excluded.

Plasma arginine vasopressin levels were documented by Cusson et al. alone in the five studies considered in this review.[45] These were unchanged.

Overall, neuroendocrine responses to ANP appear to be qualitatively similar in both hypertensive patients and normal subjects. ANP suppresses the activity of the renin-angiotensin-aldosterone system. Hypotensive effects of the peptide may elicit a sympathetic response with a rise in plasma norepinephrine and an over-riding of the primary inhibitory action of the peptide on renin secretion. ANP may directly suppress adrenal secretion of epinephrine from the adrenal medulla, in addition to its confirmed inhibitory effect on aldosterone release from the zona glomerulosa.

D. SUMMARY

ANP has qualitatively similar effects on renal function, urinary electrolytes, hemodynamic parameters, and neuroendocrine systems in patients with essential hypertension as in normal subjects. However, urinary electrolyte responses may be enhanced and hypotensive effects may be somewhat blunted in hypertension. The tantalizing possibility remains that an abnormality in end-organ response to ANP is important in the pathogenesis of hypertension and provides an exciting avenue for further research.

ACKNOWLEDGMENTS

Studies undertaken from the Departments of Endocrinology and Cardiology, The Princess Margaret Hospital, and quoted in this review were generously supported by the National Heart Foundation of New Zealand and the New Zealand Medical Research Council. We are indebted to Mrs. Natalie Purdue for assistance in preparing the manuscript.

REFERENCES

1. **Kangawa, K., Fukuda, A., and Matsuo, H.,** Structural identification of β and g human atrial natriuretic polypeptides, *Nature (London).,* 313, 397, 1985.
2. **Miyata, A., Kangawa, K., Toshimori, T., Hatoh, T., and Matsuo, H.,** Molecular forms of atrial natriuretic polypeptides in mammalian tissues and plasma, *Biochem. Biophys. Res. Commun.,* 129, 248, 1985.
3. **Sugawara, A., Nakao, K., Morii, N., Sakamoto, M., Suda, M., Shimokura, M., Kiso, Y., Kihara, M., Yamori, Y., Nishimura, K., Soneda, J., Ban, T., and Imura, H.,** α-Human atrial natriuretic polypeptide is released from the heart and circulates in the body, *Biochem. Biophys. Res. Commun.,* 129, 439, 1985.
4. **Yandle, T., Crozier, I., Nicholls, G., Espiner, E., Carne, A., and Brennan, S.,** Amino acid sequence of atrial natriuretic peptides in human coronary sinus plasma, *Biochem. Biophys. Res. Commun.,* 146, 832, 1987.
5. **Yamaji, T., Ishibashi, M., and Takaku, F.,** Atrial natriuretic factor in human blood, *J. Clin. Invest.,* 76, 1705, 1985.
6. **Yandle, T. G., Espiner, E. A., Nicholls, M. G., and Duff, H.,** Radioimmunoassay and characterization of atrial natriuretic peptide in human plasma, *J. Clin. Endocrinol. Metab.,* 63, 72, 1986.
7. **Camargo, M. J. F., Sala, C., Laragh, J. H., Cody, R. J., and Atlas, S. A.,** Atrial natriuretic factor release by atrial myocytes in vitro and characterization of circulating forms (Abstr.) in 69th Annu. Meet. U.S. Endocrine Society, 1987.
8. **Espiner, E. A. and Nicholls, M. G.,** Human atrial natriuretic peptide, *Clin. Endocrinol.,* 26, 637, 1987.
9. **Crozier, I. G., Nicholls, M. G., Ikram, H., Espiner, E. A., Yandle, T. G., and Jans, S.,** Atrial natriuretic peptide in humans: production and clearance by various tissues, *Hypertension,* 8 (Suppl. 2), 11, 1986.
10. **Yandle, T. G., Richards, A. M., Nicholls, M. G., Cuneo, R., Espiner, E. A. and Livesey, J. H.,** Metabolic clearance rate and plasma half life of alpha-human natriuretic peptdie in man, *Life Sci.,* 38, 1827, 1986.
11. **Gillies, A. H., Crozier, I. G., Nicholls, M. G., Espiner, E. A., and Yandle, T. G.,** Effect of posture on clearance of atrial natriuretic peptide from plasma, *J. Clin. Endocrinol. Metab.,* 65, 1095, 1987.
12. **Richards, A. M., Tonolo, G., Fraser, R., Morton, J. J., Leckie, B. J., Ball, S. G., and Robertson, J. I. S.,** Diurnal change in plasma atrial natriuretic peptide concentrations, *Clin. Sci.,* 73, 489, 1987.
13. **Richards, A. M., Nicholls, M. G., Ikram, H., Webster, M. W. I., Yandle, T. G., and Espiner, E. A.,** Renal, haemodynamic, and hormonal effects of human alpha atrial natriuretic peptide in healthy volunteers, *Lancet,* 1, 545, 1985.
14. **Kuribayashi, T., Nakazato, M., Tanaka, M., Nagamine, M., Kurihara, T., Kangawa, K., and Matsuo, H.,** Renal effects of human α-atrial natriuretic polypeptide, *N. Engl. J. Med.,* 312, 1456, 1985.
15. **Gerzer, R., Witzgall, H., Tremblay, J., Gutkowska, J., and Hamet, P.,** Rapid increase in plasma and urinary cyclic GMP after bolus injection of atrial natriuretic factor in man, *J. Clin. Endocrinol. Metab.,* 61, 1217, 1985.
16. **Anderson, J., Struthers, A., Christofides, N., and Bloom, S.,** Atrial natriuretic peptide: an endogenous factor enhancing sodium excretion in man, *Clin. Sci.,* 70, 327, 1986.
17. **Bolli, P., Muller, F. B., Linder, L., Raine, A. E. G., Resink, T. J., Erne, P., Kiowski, W., Ritz, R., and Buhler, F. R.,** The vasodilator potency of atrial natriuretic peptide in man, *Circulation,* 75, 221, 1987.
18. **Weidmann, P., Hasler, L., Gnadinger, M. P., Lang, R. E., Uehlinger, D. E., Shaw, S., Rascher, W., and Reubi, F. C.,** Blood levels and renal effects of atrial natriuretic peptide in normal man, *J. Clin. Invest.,* 77, 734, 1986.
19. **Weidmann, P., Hellmueller, B., Uehlinger, D. E., Lang, R. E., Gnadinger, M. P., Hasler, L., Shaw, S., and Bachmann, C.,** Plasma levels and cardiovascular, endocrine, and excretory effects of atrial natriuretic peptide during different sodium intakes in man, *J. Clin. Endocrinol. Metab.,* 62, 1027, 1986.
20. **Fujio, N., Ohashi, M., Nawata, H., Kato, K., Ibayashi, H., Kangawa, K., and Matsuo, H.,** α-human atrial natriuretic polypeptide reduces the plasma arginine vasopressin concentration in human subjects, *Clin. Endocrinol.,* 25, 181, 1986.
21. **Cody, R. J., Atlas, S. A., Laragh, J. H., Kubo, S. H., Covit, A. G., Ryman, K. S., Shaknovich, A., Pondolfino, K., Clark, M., Camargo, M. J. F., Scarborough, R. M., and Lewicki, J. A.,** Atrial natriuretic factor in normal subjects and heart failure patients: plasma levels in renal, hormonal, and hemodynamic responses to peptide infusion, *J. Clin. Invest.,* 78, 1362, 1986.
22. **Biollaz, J., Nussberger, J., Porchet, M., Brunner-Feber, F., Otterbein, E. S., Gomez, H., Waeber, B., and Brunner, H. R.,** Four-hour infusions of synthetic atrial natriuretic peptide in normal volunteers, *Hypertension,* 8 (Suppl. 2), 96, 1986.

23. **Cuneo, R. C., Espiner, E. A., Nicholls, M. G., Yandle, T. G., Joyce, S. L., and Gilchrist, N. L.,** Renal, hemodynamic, and hormonal responses to atrial natriuretic peptide infusions in normal man, and effect of sodium intake, *J. Clin. Endocrinol. Metab.*, 63, 946, 1986.

24. **Ishii, M., Sugimoto, T., Matsuoka, H., Hirata, Y., Ishimitsu, T., Fukui, K., Sugimoto, T., Kangawa, K., and Matsuo, H.,** The haemodynamic, renal and endocrine effects of alpha-human atrial natriuretic polypeptide in normotensive people and patients with essential hypertension, *J. Hypertension,* 4 (Suppl. 6), S542, 1986.

25. **Biollaz, J., Waeber, B., Nussberger, J., Porchet, M., Brunner-Ferber, F., Otterbein, E. S., Gomez, H. J., and Brunner, H. R.,** Atrial natriuretic peptides: reproducibility of renal effects and response of liver blood flow, *Eur. J. Pharmacol.,* 31, 1, 1986.

26. **Richards, A. M., Tonolo, G., Montorsi, P., Findlayson, J., Fraser, R., Inglis, G., Towrie, A., and Morton, J. J.,** Low dose infusions of 26 and 28 amino acid human atrial natriuretic peptides in normal man, *J. Clin. Endocrinol. Metab.,* 66, 465, 1988.

27. **Anderson, J. V., Donckier, J., Payne, N. N., Beacham, J., Slater, J. D. H., and Bloom, S. R.,** Atrial natriuretic peptide: evidence of action as a natriuretic hormone at physiological plasma concentrations in man, *Clin. Sci.,* 72, 305, 1987.

28. **Richards, A. M., Nicholls, M. G., Jans, S., McDonald, D., Espiner, E. A., Grant, S., Fitzpatrick, M. A., Ikram, H., and Yandle, T.,** Atrial natriuretic factor has biological effects in man at physiological plasma concentrations, 67, 1134, 1988.

29. **Biollaz, J., Callahan, L. T., Nussberger, J., Waeber, B., Gomez, H. J., Blaine, E. H., and Brunner, H. R.,** Pharmacokinetics of synthetic atrial natriuretic peptides in normal men, *Clin. Pharmacol. Ther.,* 41, 671, 1987.

30. **Waldhausl, W., Vierhapper, H., and Nowotny, P.,** Prolonged administration of human atrial natriuretic peptide in healthy men: evanescent effects on diuresis and natriuresis, *J. Clin. Endocrinol. Metab.,* 62, 956, 1986.

31. **Atlas, S. A. and Mack, T.,** Effects of atrial natriuretic factor on the kidney and the renin-angiotensin-aldosterone system, *Endocrinol. Metab. Clin. N. Am.,* 16, 107, 1987.

32. Atrial natriuretic peptide (editorial), *Lancet,* 2, 371, 1986.

33. **Leitman, D. C. and Murad, F.,** Atrial natriuretic factor receptor heterogeneity and stimulation of particulate guanylate cyclase and cyclic GMP accumulation, *Endocrinol. Metabol. Clin. N. Am.,* 16, 79, 1987.

34. **Ballermann, B. J. and Brenner, B. M.,** Role of atrial peptides in body fluid homeostasis, *Circ. Res.,* 58, 619, 1986.

35. **Kirchner, K. A., Martin, C. J., and Bower, J. D.,** Prostaglandin E$_2$ but not I$_2$ restores furosemide response in indomethacin-treated rats, *Am. J. Physiol.,* 250, F980, 1986.

36. **Miyamori, I., Ikeda, M., Matsubara, T., Okamoto, S., Koshida, H., Yasuhara, S., Morise, T., and Takeda, R.,** The renal, cardiovascular and hormonal actions of human atrial natriuretic peptide in man: effects of indomethacin, *Br. J. Clin. Pharmacol.,* 23, 425, 1987.

37. **Gnadinger, M. P., Weidmann, P., Rascher, W., Lang, R. E., Hellmuller, B., and Uehlinger, D. E.,** Plasma arginine-vasopressin levels during infusion of synthetic atrial natriuretic peptide on different sodium intakes in man, *J. Hypertens.,* 4, 623, 1986.

38. **Millar-Craig, M. W., Hawes, D., and Whittington, J.,** New system for recording ambulatory blood pressure in man, *Med. Biol. Eng. Comput.,* 16, 727, 1978.

39. **Bussien, J. P., Biollaz, J., Waeber, B., Nussberger, J., Turini, G. A., Brunner, H. R., Brunner-Ferber, F., Gomez, H. J., and Otterbein, E. S.,** Dose-dependent effect of atrial natriuretic peptide on blood pressure, heart rate, and skin blood flow of normal volunteers, *J. Cardiovasc. Pharmacol.,* 8, 216, 1986.

40. **Fujita, T., Ito, Y., Noda, H., Sato, Y., Ando, K., Kangawa, K., and Matsuo, H.,** Vasodilatory actions of α-human atrial natriuretic peptide and high Ca^{2+} effects in normal man, *J. Clin. Invest.,* 80, 832, 1987.

41. **Takeshita, A., Imaizumi, T., Nakamura, N., Higashi, H., Sasaki, T., Nakamura, M., Kangawa, K., Matsuo, H.,** Attenuation of reflex forearm vasoconstriction by α-human atrial natriuretic peptide in men, *Circ. Res.,* 61, 555, 1987.

42. **Uehlinger, D. E., Weidmann, P., Gnadinger, M. P., Shaw, S., and Lang, R. E.,** Depressor effects and release of atrial natriuretic peptide during norepinephrine or angiotensin II infusion in man, *J. Clin. Endocrinol. Metab.,* 63, 669, 1986.

43. **Anderson, J. V., Struthers, A. D., Payne, N. N., Slater, J. D. H., and Bloom, S. R.,** Atrial natriuretic peptide inhibits the aldosterone response to angiotensin II in man, *Clin. Sci.,* 70, 507, 1986.

44. **Huxley, V. H., Tucker, V. L., Verburg, K. M., and Freeman, R. H.,** Increased capillary hydraulic conductivity induced by atrial natriuretic peptide, *Circ. Res.,* 60, 304, 1987.

45. **Cusson, J. R., Hamet, P., Gutkowska, J., Kuchel, O., Genest, J., Cantin, M., and Larochelle, P.,** Effects of atrial natriuretic factor on natriuresis and cGMP in patients with essential hypertension, *J. Hypertens.,* 5, 435, 1987.

46. **Cuneo, R. C., Espiner, E. A., Nicholls, M. G., Yandle, T. G., and Livesey, J. H.,** Effect of physiological levels of atrial natriuretic peptide on hormone secretion: inhibition of angiotensin-induced aldosterone secretion and renin release in normal man, *J. Clin. Endocrinol. Metab.,* 65, 765, 1987.

47. **Franco-Suarez, R., Somani, P., and Mulrow, P. J.,** Bradycardia after infusion of atrial natriuretic factor, *Ann. Int. Med.,* 107, 594, 1987.

48. **Tikkanen, I., Fyhrquist, F., Metsarinne, K., and Leidenius, R.,** Plasma atrial natriuretic peptide in cardiac disease and during infusion in healthy volunteers, *Lancet,* 2, 66, 1985.

49. **Ohashi, M., Fujio, N., Kato, K., Nawata, H., Ibayashi, H., and Matsuo, H.,** Effect of human α-atrial natriuretic polypeptide on adrenocortical function in man, *J. Endocrinol.,* 110, 287, 1986.

50. **Gillies, A. H., Crozier, I. G., Nicholls, M. G., Espiner, E. A., and Yandle, T. G.,** unpublished observation.

51. **Vierhapper, H., Nowotny, P., and Waldhausl, W.,** Prolonger administration of human atrial natriuretic peptide in healthy men: reduced aldosteronotropic effect of angiotensin II, *Hypertension,* 8, 1040, 1986.

52. **Jungmann, E., Haak, T., Walter-Schrader, M.-C., Rosak, C., Fassbinder, W., Althoff, P.-H., and Schoffling, K.,** No effect of human atrial natriuretic peptide upon aldosterone stimulation by metoclopramide in normal man, *Acta Endocrinol.,* 114 (Abstr. 118), 99, 1987.

53. **Pinet, F., Mizrahi, J., Laboulandine, I., Menard, J., and Corvol, P.,** Regulation of prorenin secretion in cultured human transfected juxtaglomerular cells, *J. Clin. Invest.,* 80, 724, 1987.

54. **Higuchi, K., Nawata, H., Kato, K.-I., Ibayashi, H., and Matsuo, H.,** α-human atrial natriuretic polypeptide inhibits steroidogenesis in cultured human adrenal cells, *J. Clin. Endocrinol. Metab.,* 62, 941, 1986.

55. **Samson, W. K.,** Atrial natriuretic factor and the central nervous system, *Endocrinol. Metab. Clin. N. Am.,* 16, 145, 1987.

56. **Sagnella, G. A., Markandu, N., Shore, A., and MacGregor, G. A.,** Raised circulating levels of atrial natriuretic peptides in essential hypertension, *Lancet,* 1, 179, 1986.

57. **Montorsi, P., Tonolo, G., Polonia, J., Hepburn, D., and Richards, A. M.,** Correlates of plasma atrial natriuretic factor in health and hypertension, *Hypertension,* 10, 570, 1987.

58. **Richards, A. M., Nicholls, M. G., Espiner, E. A., Ikram, H., Yandle, T. G., Joyce, S. L., and Cullens, M. M.,** Effects of α-human atrial natriuretic peptide in essential hypertension, *Hypertension,* 7, 812, 1985.

59. **Weidmann, P., Gnadinger, M. P., Ziswiler, H. R., Shaw, S., Bachmann, C., Rascher, W., Uehlinger, D. E., Hasler, L., and Reubi, F. C.,** Cardiovascular, endocrine and renal effects of atrial natriuretic peptide in essential hypertension, *J. Hypertens.,* 4 (Suppl. 2), S71.

60. **Janssen, W. M. T., de Jong, P. E., van der Hem, G. K., and de Zeeuw, D.,** Effect of human atrial natriuretic peptide on blood pressure after sodium depletion in essential hypertension, *Br. Med. J.,* 293, 351, 1986.

61. **Tonolo, G., Gloriosa, N., Manunta, P., Lever, A. F., and Richards, A. M.,** Haemodynamic, renal and hormonal effects of low dose ANF in essential hypertension, in preparation.

62. **Sosa, R. E., Volpe, M., Marion, D. N., Atlas, S. A., Laragh, J. H., Vaughan, E. D., and Maack, T.,** Relationship between renal haemodynamic and natriuretic effects of atrial natriuretic factor, *Am. J. Physiol.,* 250, F520, 1986.

Chapter 19

ATRIAL NATRIURETIC FACTOR IN ESSENTIAL HYPERTENSION: EFFECTS, PHARMACOKINETICS, AND PLASMA MEASUREMENTS

P. Larochelle and J. R. Cusson

TABLE OF CONTENTS

I. EFFECTS OF ATRIAL NATRIURETIC FACTOR IN ESSENTIAL HYPERTENSION

Adolfo de Bold demonstrated in his landmark paper[1] that acute administration of ANF could reduce arterial blood pressure, as well as stimulate diuresis and natriuresis. This reduction in arterial blood pressure was quickly attributed to vasorelaxation[2-3] and the effects of ANF were later examined in different models of hypertension. Garcia et al.[4] reported that the chronic intravenous infusion of ANF, at the relatively low dose of 100 ng/h per rat, corresponding to about 2.0 pmol/kg/min normalized blood pressure in spontaneously hypertensive rats. This finding, later confirmed by Kida et al.,[5] stimulated the research efforts on ANF and hypertension.

Studies on the effects of ANF in human hypertension have all been acute or short-term (hours) experiments. Richards et al.[6] were the first to report the effects of ANF in patients with essential hypertension. As they previously did with normotensive volunteers,[7] the authors administered intravenous bolus of 100 μg of human ANF(99 — 126). This was followed by a transient reduction in blood pressure associated with an increase in heart rate. In this study, ANF stimulated diuresis and excretion of sodium and potassium and reduced plasma aldosterone and epinephrine levels, whereas norepinephrine levels increased. Compared to their previous study of ANF in normotensive volunteers, their patients with essential hypertension appeared to have a greater renal response and a greater inhibition of aldosterone, but a smaller blood pressure reduction.

Weidmann et al.[8] later examined the effects of ANF in essential hypertension. ANF was given as an initial bolus of 50 μg, followed by a constant infusion at the rate of 0.1 μg/kg/min (about 32 pmol/kg/min) during 45 min. Plasma ANF levels increased up to about 400 pmol/l. Their subjects had higher blood pressure than the patients studied by Richards et al.[6] and exhibited more sustained hypotensive response to ANF. Four of these patients had nausea and unchanged or slowed heart rate with marked decreases in blood pressure. The authors also found an increased renal response of their patients when compared to normotensive volunteers. They also demonstrated that ANF produced an early increase in effective renal plasma flow (ERPF) and glomerular filtration rate (GFR), but the persistent reduction in blood pressure was followed by normalization of GFR and reduction of ERPF, producing an increase in filtration fraction. Despite the stimulation of renin secretion by the reduced blood pressure and the intravascular plasma volume, it is noteworthy that plasma aldosterone levels decreased during the ANF infusion and sharply increased after its discontinuation, supporting the inhibitory effects of ANF on aldosterone secretion.[9,10] ANF had no effects on the plasma levels of renin activity and aldosterone in their normotensive controls,[11] as in the studies of Richards et al.[7]

In another study, ANF was administered intravenously in a stepped fashion over 90 min.[12] There were three periods of constant infusion rates of 0.8, 1.6, 3.2 μg/min, respectively, over 30-min periods, corresponding to about 4, 8, and 16 pmol/kg/min. In this placebo-controlled study, ANF did not reduce blood pressure in patients with essential hypertension, but dramatic episodes of hypotension and bradycardia occurred in four of the seven control subjects. The hypertensive patients, like those of Richards et al.[6] and Weidmann et al.,[8] exhibited a greater renal response than did healthy volunteers. Furthermore, Cusson et al.[12] showed a greater stimulation of plasma cGMP levels in these patients, in addition to the greater renal response. The plasma concentrations of ANF increased 5-, 14-, and 18-fold following the three periods and the increase in plasma ANF levels, as well as the disappearance rate following this continuation of the infusion, were similar in the hypertensive patients and in the control subjects. The greater increase in plasma cGMP levels in the patients with essential hypertension, also seen in spontaneously hypertensive rats,[13] is consistent with their greater renal response, however, the urinary excretion of cGMP was not significantly higher in the hypertensive patients. In this study, plasma renin activity tended to increase and aldosterone to decrease in hypertensive patients, whereas in normotensive subjects, plasma renin activity significantly decreased and aldosterone remained unaltered.

Ishii et al.[14,15] studied invasively the hemodynamics and renal effects of ANF in patients with essential hypertension. ANF was infused at 0.025 μg/kg/min (about 8 pmol/kg/min) for 40 min. ANF reduced mean arterial pressure by about 6% and increased the heart rate, diuresis, and natriuresis. ANF reduced blood pressure partly through vasodilation since cardiac output remained unchanged and total peripheral resistances decreased. In that study, central venous pressure was also mildly decreased. Plasma ANF levels increased up to about 220 pmol/l. Plasma aldosterone decreased both in normotensive and hypertensive subjects, but this response was greater in normotensives.

Weder et al.[16] recently reported the effects of infusions of ANF at three different infusion rates for 60 min each under two different sodium intakes. Eight patients with mild essential hypertension received ANF at 0.03, 0.20, and 0.45 μg/kg/min, which corresponds to doses of about 10, 70, and 150 pmol/kg/min. Plasma ANF levels increased to about 300, 1500, and 3000 pmol/l, respectively. Four of the eight patients experienced sudden bradycardia and hypotension, as described previously. Otherwise, ANF lowered blood pressure and increased heart rate with the two greater doses. These effects were persistent for at least 2 h following discontinuation of the infusions. The renal responses to ANF were greater on the higher sodium intake, as has been found in animals.[5] Although the lower infusion rate of ANF inhibited the renin-aldosterone axis, the greater depressor effect of the higher doses was associated with its stimulation.

Janssen et al.[17] reported on the hemodynamic effects of human ANF infused during 4 h at rates of 0.125, 0.25, 0.5, and 1.0 μg/min in three patients with essential hypertension, under sodium intake of 50 and 200 mmol/d. The higher dose and the lower sodium intake increased the depressor effect of ANF and hypotensive and bradycardic episodes occurred twice at the 1.0 μg/min dose and once at 0.5 μg/min.

Volpe et al.[18] recently studied the hemodynamic and hormonal effects of ANF in 13 patients with essential hypertension. Following a bolus dose of 0.5 μg/kg, they infused ANF at 0.05 μg/kg/min (about 16 pmol/kg/min) for 20 min, followed by 0.1 μ/kg/min (about 32 pmol/kg/min) for 20 min. The lower dose reduced aortic mean blood pressure by 5% (p = NS) and the higher dose by 10% (p <0.05). There were no changes in the other hemodynamic measurements at the lower dose, but cardiac index and stroke volume index decreased significantly, whereas pulmonary wedge pressure tended to diminish with the higher dose. Total peripheral resistances were not changed. This is in contrast to the findings of Ishii et al.,[15] who demonstrated a reduction in total peripheral resistances with half the lower dose used by Volpe et al.[18] With regard to the plasma concentrations of ANF, the lower dose increased these levels from 27 to 209 pmol/l and with the higher dose, they reached 544 pmol/l. Both doses were without effects on plasma renin activity, aldosterone, and epinephrine levels, but plasma norepinephrine increased significantly with the higher dose. The renal response to ANF was not determined in this study. Finally, one of their patients had a hypotensive and bradycardic episode on the higher dose, which reverted to normal following atropine.

The vasodepressor effects of ANF seen in the studies appeared to be of two types. First boluses of ANF[6] and short-term infusions of ANF at relatively high rates[8,14-16] are associated with reductions in arterial blood pressure and with an increase in heart rate. The increase in heart rate has been interpreted as a baroreceptor-mediated reflex following vasodilation. However, vasodilatation is demonstrable with lower rates of infusion.[15] The arterial vasodilatation by ANF is probably a direct action through specific receptor sites in the endothelial wall and smooth muscle cells.[19-21] Second, continuous infusions of ANF[8,16-18] have been associated with occasional, but dramatic, episodes of hypotension and bradycardia also seen in normotensive volunteers[12,22] which are believed to be caused by the inhibition by ANF of the sympathoadrenal axis or perhaps with enhanced vagal tone.[23-25] Further studies on the chronic effects of ANF in human hypertension with doses that do not cause the adverse hypotensive episodes are needed.

The increase in renal response of patients with essential hypertension to ANF is consistent with animal experiments.[26] Furthermore, some of the data[6-8,11-12] seem to indicate that patients with essential hypertension are more sensitive to the aldosterone inhibitory effect of exogenous ANF than are normotensive subjects. If these greater renal and aldosterone responses are due to an up-regulation phenomenon at the level of receptors, it remained unclear why such up-regulation occurs in the phase of plasma levels of ANF which are reported to be either normal[27-29] or mildly elevated[30-32] in patients with essential hypertension, and although it is not known if the patients studied[6,8,12] had reduced ANF release, their basal levels were not reduced. The circulating form of ANF in patients with essential hypertension appears to be the same as that found in normotensive subjects.[30]

Perhaps ANF interacts with another factor causing the greater renal response of the patients with essential hypertension. Since the effects of ANF seem to be modulated by the status of blood volume or salt balance,[5,33] a higher salt intake or blood volume in patients with essential hypertension would have been associated with greater renal response to ANF. However, blood volume is generally reported to be normal in patients with essential hypertension, although it has been reported that volemia is relatively elevated compared to arterial compliance.[34] Ishii et al.[14,15] found that patients with essential hypertension had higher central venous pressure when compared to their normotensive controls. In this study, the subjects had been put on the same salt intake of about 8 to 10 g/d. Patients and controls in the studies of Cusson et al.[12] Richards et al.,[6,7] and Weidmann et al.[8,11] were on the same sodium intake diets. Thus, the apparent greater renal and adrenal effects of ANF in patients with essential hypertension should be studied further.

In summary, the studies of the administration of ANF in human hypertension have not yet been able to show the sustained antihypertensive effect seen in spontaneously hypertensive rats, but no comparable "chronic" studies have been done. ANF seems to be more natriuretic in patients with essential hypertension, perhaps in relation to a greater sensitivity of these patients to the inhibitory effect of ANF on aldosterone secretion.

II. PHARMACOKINETICS OF ANF

Only a few studies have attempted to specifically characterize the pharmacokinetics of ANF. Most studies have looked at the effects of ANF administration the hemodynamics, renal or hormonal effects of the peptide. In their initial publication on the use of ANF in humans, Richards et al.[6] mentioned that the half-life of ANF was short, although pharmacokinetic parameters were not calculated. Bussien et al.[35] measured the effects of increasing doses of ANF (1 to 40 μg/min) on blood pressure and skin blood flow. They calculated that there was a cumulative dose-dependent effect on skin blood flow and that blood pressure was reduced in a dose-related fashion. The hypotensive effect persisted for 1 h after the infusion. From the same group, Biollaz et al.[22] reported that the infusion of 5.0 μg/min of ANF for 6 h produced a reduction in blood pressure and they commented on the dissociation of the short half-life of ANF and the relatively long duration of its effect.

More precise pharmacokinetic parameters were calculated in a few studies.[12,36-41] Nakao et al.[36] studied the disappearance of ANF after injections of a bolus dose of 100 μg in healthy volunteers. The distribution half-life was 1.7 min and the elimination half-life was 10.1 min. The volume of distribution was 23 l and the metabolic clearance rate was 1.5 l/min.

Yandle et al.[37] studied the metabolic clearance rate of α-hANF in six normal men and six patients with essential hypertension after an injection of 100 μg i.v. over a 60-s period. They reported a half-life of 2.5 min, with a volume of distribution of the central compartment of 10.4 l and a clearance rate of 2.4 l/min. In three subjects, they also evaluated the same parameters after a constant infusion of 3.3 μg/min over a 60-min period. The calculated half-life was 3.1 min, with a clearance rate of 2.7 l/min and a volume of distribution of 10.7 l.

Gnadinger et al.[38] also studied the kinetics of the hormone after an infusion of 0.1 μg/kg/min over 45 min and reported a half-life of 3.2 min. We have also studied the kinetic disposition of ANF after bolus injection (12.5, 25, 50, and 100 μg)[39] and after infusions of 0.8, 1.6, and 3.6 μg/min for 30 min at each dose level.[12] After bolus injections of 50 and 100 μg, the volume of distribution was between 25 and 35 l and elimination half-life between 4 and 14 min. The relationship between plasma concentrations and BP reduction was not linear. The renal effects and the increase in plasma cGMP concentrations persisted for 3 h, despite plasma concentrations returning to baseline levels. Following infusion of ANF, the calculated elimination half-life was 4.2 ± 0.6 min and the metabolic clearance was 11.6 l/min in normal subjects.

Gillies et al.[40] reported recently that posture influenced the plasma clearance of ANF. They infused ANF at a constant rate of 0.5 μg/min for 2 h. Volunteers were supine for 60 min, erect for 30 min, and supine for 30 min. The calculated clearance rate fell from 7.7 to 5.7/l/min when standing and increased again to 7.6 l/min after lying down. Posture seems to influence the rate of clearance of ANF and possibly is related to changes in hepatic and renal blood flow.

Biollaz et al.[41] confirmed their initial results of a short half-life of ANF during infusion of r-ANF or h-ANF at doses of 0.5 to 5 μg/min. The calculated half-life was 4.3 min and there was no difference in the kinetics of either r- or h-ANF.

Finally, Crozier et al.[42] studied the effect of the subcutaneous administration of ANF in normal volunteers. The concentrations obtained were less than 3% of those obtained after i.v. administration.

The pharmacokinetics of ANF indicate a short half-life and a large volume of distribution, which would indicate uptake or metabolism in a wide variety of vascular beds where the hormone has physiological effects. The kinetics of ANF are not altered in hypertension.

III. PLASMA LEVELS OF ANF IN HYPERTENSION

The plasma levels of ANF have been measured in various types of severity of hypertension and have been reported as being unchanged or increased when compared to the levels in a group of normal controls. These studies vary extensively in the number of subjects studied, the characteristics of these subjects, or the level of the blood pressure.

A. INCREASED PLASMA LEVELS

In the initial report by Sugawara et al.,[31] the plasma levels of ANF were reported to be elevated significantly in patients with essential hypertension. In patients with grade I or II hypertension, the level of ANF was 77.8 ± 9.5 pg/ml (n = 10), compared to 37.8 ± 6.0 pg/ml in 14 normotensive controls. Five of these hypertensives were grade I and had levels of 67.7 ± 10 pg/ml. The plasma levels in 14 patients with treated essential hypertension, but of unknown blood pressure, were found to be 104 ± 12 pg/ml and significantly higher than the other two groups.

Arendt et al.[30] measured ANF levels in 13 normotensive controls and 17 hypertensive patients, with no description of the patients or the blood pressure. Plasma levels were significantly higher in the hypertensive patients (62 ± 20 fmol/ml) than in the normotensive controls (9 ± 2 fmol/ml). They reported similar results in 1987[43] in 51 normal controls

(9.6 ± 1 fmol/ml) and 36 patients with hypertension (61.7 ± 13 fmol/ml) of unknown description.

Sagnella et al.[32] reported the first well-controlled comparison study between normal subjects and patients with essential hypertension. The ANF levels were 8.4 ± 3.7 pg/ml in a group of 24 normal volunteers and 17.1 ± 3.7 pg/ml in a group of patients with mild to moderate essential hypertension. They reported a correlation between ANF levels and age, but only in the normal subjects. There was, however, a correlation between ANF and systolic blood pressure or diastolic blood pressure in the hypertensive subjects. In a further study by the same research team, MacGregor et al.[44] reported similar results in a larger group of subjects, although they reported a correlation with age, even in the hypertensive subjects who had a blood pressure of 173/108 mmHg.

Kohno et al.[45] reported in 1987 that the levels of ANF were higher in a group of 42 patients with essential hypertension (48 ± 25 pg/ml) than in 17 normal controls (31.7 ± 11.8 pg/ml). Antihypertensive treatment for 4 weeks in the group of hypertensive patients reduced the blood pressure to levels of borderline hypertension and also reduced ANF to the levels measured in borderline hypertension.

Montorsi et al.[46] recently reported a well-controlled study comparing 22 pairs of matched normal subjects and patients with mild essential hypertension. There was a small, but statistically significant, difference in the ANF levels — 36 ± 3 pg/ml vs. 45 ± 3 pg/ml. Using unmatched subjects, they also showed a significant difference between untreated or treated hypertension and normal subjects. The levels were 27 ± 2 pg/ml in normal subjects, 52 ± 6 pg/ml in untreated hypertensives, and 62 ± 6 pg/ml in treated hypertensives. There was a correlation between the log ANF and age in the normal subjects and between log ANF and mean arterial pressure in the hypertensive subjects. The presence of LVH was associated with a clear increase in the levels of ANF.

Finally, Wambach et al.[47] reported in a small study comparing 12 hypertensive subjects and 9 normal subjects that plasma levels were significantly higher in a group of hypertensive subjects. They also reported that upright posture produced a reduction in the plasma levels in both groups, while high and low sodium diets produced an increase and a decrease, respectively, in the plasma levels.

B. UNCHANGED PLASMA LEVELS

On the other hand, there are now in the literature a number of reports indicating that the plasma levels of ANF could be similar in patients with essential hypertension and normotensive subjects. Muller et al.[48] reported in 1986 that, as measured by a radioreceptor assay, there was no difference in the plasma levels of 26 normotensive volunteers and 24 patients with essential hypertension (37.9 ± 7 vs. 42.7 ± 5.3 pg/ml). In this study, the two groups were not exactly matched for age, the hypertensive patients being 10 years older, and changing from upright to supine postures did not increase significantly the plasma levels in either group. However, after subdividing the hypertensive patients into groups with high, normal, or low peripheral renin activity, the patients with the low renin activity had a higher basal level of ANF and a significant increase in their ANF values upon recumbency.

Larochelle et al.[49] reported in a group of 48 control subjects and 44 hypertensive patients, matched for age and weight, that the plasma level of ANF was identical in both groups. The mean ANF concentrations were 13.2 ± 1.5 pg/ml in the hypertensive patients and 13.0 ± 1.3 pg/ml in the control subjects. These data were later confirmed in a greater number of subjects.[50] There was a significant correlation in these two groups with age and a significant correlation with systolic blood pressure, but only in the group of normal subjects. Eight patients with renovascular hypertension were found to have a higher level of ANF than a group of patients with essential hypertension at similar levels of blood pressure. In a further study,[64] we have also measured the levels of the N-terminal fraction of ANF (Asn_1-Arg_{98}),

TABLE 1
Variations in cGMP, C and N-Terminal ANF

±	Normal	<90		90 to 104		105 to 114		>115		p value[a]
		No Tx	Tx	No Tx	Tx	No Tx	Tx	No Tx	Tx	
N	77	32	16	74	51	16	15	7	10	
Age (years)	49 ± 2	47 ± 3	54 ± 3	46 ± 1	53 ± 1	46 ± 3	54 ± 3	40 ± 3	59 ± 2	0.008
Systolic BP (mmHg)	116 ± 7	139 ± 2	141 ± 5	151 ± 2	160 ± 3	179 ± 7	186 ± 7	192 ± 8	192 ± 7	0.0001
Diastolic BP (mmHg)	71 ± 1	80 ± 1	79 ± 2	96 ± 1	96 ± 1	108 ± 1	109 ± 1	126 ± 3	127 ± 3	0.0001
cGMP (pmol/l)	4.7 ± 0.2	5.9 ± 0.8	4.7 ± 1.9	5.3 ± 0.4	6.5 ± 0.5[b]	4.2 ± 0.4	6.9 ± 1.3[b]	4.1 ± 1.2	7.1 ± 1.1[b]	0.0004
C-ANF (pmol/l)	11.5 ± 0.7	12.4 ± 1.5	10.2 ± 1.0	9.8 ± 0.6	15.3 ± 1.1[c]	12.4 ± 2.0	22.0 ± 3.8[c]	11.4 ± 1.6	25.4 ± 4.5[c]	0.0001
N-ANF (pmol/l)	580 ± 35	444 ± 37	684 ± 86[b]	443 ± 23	774 ± 46[c]	446 ± 52	953 ± 201[c]	481 ± 82	1304 ± 241[c]	0.0003

Essential hypertension

[a] Anova between all groups.
[b] p <0.05. vs. untreated patients (No Tx)
[c] p <0.005. vs. untreated patients (No Tx)

as well as the C-terminal fraction of ANF (Ser_{99}-Tyr_{126}) (Table 1) in normal subjects, patients with untreated essential hypertension, and patients with treated essential hypertension. As can be seen from this table, the levels of both C- and N-terminal ANF are elevated in the patients with treated essential hypertension, but not in the untreated patients at a similar level of blood pressure. The levels of cyclic GMP, which is thought to be a secondary messenger to the action of ANF,[51] would tend to confirm the validity of the levels of ANF.

Zachariah[29] studied 62 patients with essential hypertension and 38 matched healthy normotensive subjects and found lower plasma levels of ANF in the hypertensive patients (27.4 ± 1.8 vs. 35.3 ± 2.4 pg/ml). They could not find a correlation with age or blood pressure in either group.

Nillson et al.[52] studied 328 controls and 389 hypertensive subjects and were unable to show any significant difference in the plasma ANF levels between the two groups. Treatment with beta blockers, diuretics or a combination of both drugs did not influence the plasma levels to a significant degree. However, they did not observe any age-related increase in ANF. Nakaoka[53] also examined the effects of hypertension and its treatment in 61 healthy normal controls, 32 patients with untreated hypertension, and 31 patients undergoing long-term treatment with beta blockers. Plasma ANF levels of untreated patients and control subjects were similar. However, the administration of atenolol 50 mg/d produced a significant rise in ANF levels from 38.8 ± 9.5 to 68.7 ± 20.6 pg/ml in ten previously untreated subjects.

There have also been some other reports in the literature of measurements of plasma ANF in groups of patients with undefined hypertension. Five of these groups reported no significant difference between the levels in both groups,[54-58] while one group reported a significant increase.[59]

Plasma levels of ANF are influenced by several factors in both normotensive and hypertensive subjects. Sodium intake seems to be an important determinant since there is a one- to threefold difference between values measured under a low or high salt intake.[47] Postural changes can cause similar variations in plasma ANF levels.[47] Salt-sensitive hypertensive patients appear to increase their plasma ANF concentrations more than salt-resistant patients when subjected to a high sodium diet.[60] Patients with low-renin hypertension will also have higher increases in plasma ANF levels than will those with normal or high-renin essential hypertension, at least when changing from upright to recumbent postures[48] or when infused with isotonic saline.[61] This might be due to their presumed greater cardiopulmonary blood volume.

Volpe et al.[62] recently made the interesting observation in essential hypertension that upon unloading of the carotid baroreceptors with neck compression, plasma ANF levels decreased, whereas indices of sympathetic activity were activated. However, it is not known whether normotensives react similarly or differently.

The mechanism underlying the relationship between plasma ANF concentration and arterial pressure in hypertension is unclear. It has been reported by various authors[34,63] that the right atrial or pulmonary arterial pressure is increased in patients with mild essential hypertension, although in none of the studies reported here, were these pressures measured. The lack of increase in the plasma levels of ANF could be interpreted as a deficiency in the secretion of ANF in patients with essential hypertension. It also could be speculated that patients with mild essential hypertension and even more moderate essential hypertension have increased pressures in the right and left atria and, therefore, should have increased plasma levels since the main stimulus for secretion of ANF is stretch or pressure in atria. Elevation of ANF levels in patients with essential hypertension could indicate that these patients do, in fact, have an increase in mean atrial pressures and that these values are a marker of the influence of the increased blood pressure on the myocardial function.

The discrepancy between the various reports showing unchanged vs. elevated plasma

ANF levels can probably be ascribed to differences in the age, chronicity of hypertension, prior use of antihypertensive treatment, duration of treatment, and level of blood pressure of the subjects studied.

Most reports have now indicated that there is a correlation between age and plasma levels of ANF, which could indicate either a reduced metabolism or an increased secretion from a reduced myocardial function. In the presence of the combined effect of age and systolic pressure, it could easily be expected that the plasma levels of ANF would be higher than in a group of younger normal subjects. The chronicity of the hypertension could also be a major factor in the levels of ANF in these patients. The more chronic the hypertension, the more likely would be a measurable effect on the myocardial function and, therefore, the more likely an increase in ANF. Therefore, the combination of age, level of blood pressure, and chronicity of hypertension would become the main determinant of the plasma ANF values.

ACKNOWLEDGMENTS

The authors would like to thank Ms. Lucette Gauthier, Colette Vanier, Marie-Ange Boutin, Suzanne Paris, and France Boulianne, nurses, for their technical assistance. We also acknowledge Mr. Francois Bellavance of the Department of Mathematics and Statistics of the Université de Montréal for advice and Mrs. Carole Tremblay for typing this manuscript.

This work was supported by grant #Ma 9304 from the Medical Research Council of Canada and the Hypertension Group of the MRC. Jean R. Cusson is supported by a fellowship from the Medical Research Council of Canada.

REFERENCES

1. **de Bold, A. J., Borenstein, H. B., Veress, A. T., and Sonnenberg,** A rapid and potent natriuretic response to intravenous injection of atrial myocardial extract in rat, *Life Sci.*, 28, 89, 1981.
2. **Garcia, R., Thibault, G., Nutt, R. F., Cantin, M., and Genest, J.,** Comparative vasoactive effects of native and synthetic atrial natriuretic factor (ANF), *Biochem. Biophys. Res. Commun.*, 119, 685, 1984.
3. **Winquist, R. J.,** Minireview. The relaxant effects of atrial natriuretic factor on vascular smooth muscle, *Life Sci.*, 37, 1081, 1985.
4. **Garcia, R., Thibault, G., Gutkowska, J., Horky, K., Hamet, P., Cantin, M., and Genest, J.,** Chronic infusion of low doses of atrial natriuretic factor (ANF Arg 101 — Tyr 126) reduces blood pressure in conscious SHR without apparent changes in sodium excretion, *Proc. Soc. Exp. Biol. Med.*, 179, 396, 1985.
5. **Kida, O., Kondo, K., and Tanaka, K.,** Natriuretic and hypotensive effects of chronically administered α-human atrial natriuretic polypeptide in sodium-deplete or replete conscious spontaneously hypertensive rats, *J. Hypertens.*, 4 (Suppl. 6), S529, 1986.
6. **Richards, A. M., Nicholls, M. G., Espiner, E. A., Ikram, H., Yandle, T. G., Joyce, S. L., and Cullens, M. M.,** Effects of α-human atrial natriuretic peptide in essential hypertension, *Hypertension*, 7, 812, 1985.
7. **Richards, A. M., Ikram, H., Yandle, T. G., Nicholls, M. G., Webster, M. W. I., and Espiner, E. A.,** Renal, haemodynamic, and hormonal effects of human alpha atrial natriuretic peptide in healthy volunteers, *Lancet*, 1, 545, 1985.
8. **Weidmann, P., Gnadinger, M. P., Ziswiler, H. R., Shaw, S., Bachmann, C., Rascher, W., Uehlinger, D. E., Hasler, L., and Reubi, F. C.,** Cardiovascular, endocrine and renal effects of atrial natriuretic peptide in essential hypertension, *J. Hypertens.*, 4 (Suppl. 2), S71, 1986.
9. **Chartier, L., Schiffrin, E., Thibault, G., and Garcia, R.,** Atrial natriuretic factor inhibits the stimulation of aldosterone secretion by angiotensin II, ACTH and potassium in vitro and angiotensin II-induced steroidogenesis in vivo, *Endocrinology*, 115, 2026, 1984.
10. **Atarashi, K., Franco-Saenz, R., Mulrow, P. J., Snajdar, R., and Rapp, J. P.,** Inhibition of aldosterone production by atrial natriuretic factor, *J. Hypertens.*, 2, 293, 1984.

11. **Weidmann, P., Hasler, L., Gnadinger, M. P., Lang, R. E., Uehlinger, D. E., Shaw, S., Rascher, W., and Reubi, F. C.,** Blood levels and renal effects of atrial natriuretic peptide in normal man, *J. Clin. Invest.,* 77, 734, 1986.

12. **Cusson, J. R., Hamet, P., Gutkowska, J., Kuchel, O., Genest, J., Cantin, M., and Larochelle, P.,** Effects of atrial natriuretic factor on natriuresis and cGMP in patients with essential hypertension, *J. Hypertens.,* 5, 435, 1987.

13. **De Mey, J. G., Defreyn, G., Lenaers, A., Calderon, P., and Roba, J.,** Arterial reactivity, blood pressure, and plasma levels of atrial natriuretic peptides in normotensive and hypertensive rats: effects of acute and chronic administration of atriopeptin III, *J. Cardiovasc. Pharmacol.,* 9, 525, 1987.

14. **Ishii, M., Sugimoto, T., Matsuoka, H., Hirata, Y., Ishimistu, T., Fukui, K., Sugimoto, T., Kangawa, K., and Matsuo, H.,** The haemodynamic, renal and endocrine effects of alpha-human atrial natriuretic polypeptide in normotensive people and patients with essential hypertension, *J. Hypertens.,* 4 (Suppl. 6), S542, 1986.

15. **Ishii, M., Sugimoto, T., Matsuoka, H., Hirata, Y., Ishimitsu, T., Fukui, K., Sugimoto, T., Kangawa, K., and Matsuo, H.,** A comparative study on the hemodynamic, renal and endocrine effects of alpha-human atrial natriuretic polypeptide in normotensive persons and patients with essential hypertension, *Jpn. Circ. J.,* 50, 1181, 1986.

16. **Weder, A. B., Sekkarie, M. A., Takiyyuddin, M., Schork, N. J., and Julius, S.,** Antihypertensive effects of atrial natriuretic factor in men, *Hypertension,* 10, 582, 1987.

17. **Janssen, W. M. T., De Jong, P. E., van der Hem, G. K., and De Zeeuw, D.,** Effect of human atrial natriuretic peptide on blood pressure after sodium depletion in essential hypertension, *Br. Med. J.,* 293, 351, 1986.

18. **Volpe, M., Mele, A. F., Indolfi, C., De Luca, N., Lembo, G., Focaccio, A., Condorelli, M., and Trimarco, B.,** Hemodynamic and hormonal effects of atrial natriuretic factor in patients with essential hypertension, *J. Am. Coll. Cardiol.,* 10, 787, 1987.

19. **Winquist, R. J., Faison, E. P., Waldman, S. A., Schwartz, K., and Rapoport, R. M.,** Atrial natriuretic factor elicits an endothelium-independent relaxation and activates particulate guanylate cyclase in vascular smooth muscle, *Proc. Natl. Acad. Sci. U.S.A.,* 81, 7661, 1984.

20. **Napier, M. A., Valdlen, R. L., Albers-Shonberg, G., Nutt, R. F., Brady, S., Lyle, T., Winquist, R., Faison, E. P., Hermel, L. A. and Blaine, E. H.,** Specific membrane receptors for atrial natriuretic factor in renal and vascular tissues, *Proc. Natl. Acad. Sci. U.S.A.,* 81, 5946, 1984.

21. **Schiffrin, E. L., Chartier, L., Thibault, G., St-Louis, J., Cantin, M., and Genest, J.,** Vascular and adrenal receptors for atrial natriuretic factor in the rat, *Circ. Res.,* 56, 801, 1985.

22. **Biollaz, J., Nussberger, J., Porchet, M., Brunner-Ferber, F., Otterbein, E. S., Gomez, H., Waeber, B., and Brunner, H. R.,** Four-hour infusions of synthetic atrial natriuretic peptide in normal volunteers, *Hypertension,* 8 (Suppl. 2), 96, 1986.

23. **Ackermann, U.,** Cardiovascular effects of atrial natriuretic extract in the whole animal, *Fed. Proc.,* 45, 2111, 1986.

24. **Thoren, P., Mark, A. L., Morgan, D. A., O'Neill, T. P., Needleman, P., and Brody, M. J.,** Activation of vagal depressor reflexes by atriopeptins inhibits renal sympathetic nerve activity, *Am. J. Physiol.,* 251, H1252, 1986.

25. **Allen, D. E. and Gellai, M.,** Cardioinhibitory effect of atrial peptide in conscious rats, *Am. J. Physiol.,* 252, R610, 1987.

26. **Pang, S. C., Hoang, M.-C., Tremblay, J., Cantin, M., Garcia, R., Genest, J., and Hamet, P.,** Effect of natural and synthetic atrial natriuretic factor on arterial blood pressure, natriuresis, and cyclic GMP excretion in spontaneously hypertensive rats, *Clin. Sci.,* 69, 721, 1985.

27. **Larochelle, P., Cusson, J. R., Gutkowska, J., Schiffrin, E. L, Hamet, P., Kuchel, O., Genest, J., and Cantin, M.,** Plasma atrial natriuretic factor concentrations in essential and renovascular hypertension, *Br. Med. J.,* 294, 1249, 1987.

28. **Yamaji, T., Ishibashi, M., Sekihara, H., Takaku, F., Nakaoka, H., and Fujii, J.,** Plasma levels of atrial natriuretic peptide in primary aldosteronism and essential hypertension, *J. Clin. Endocrinol. Metab.,* 63, 815, 1986.

29. **Zachariah, P. K., Burnett, J. C., Jr., Ritter, S. G., and Strong, C. G.,** Atrial natriuretic peptide in human essential hypertension, *Mayo Clin. Proc.,* 62, 782, 1987.

30. **Arendt, R. M., Stangl, E., Zahringer, J., Liebisch, D. C., and Hertz, A.,** Demonstration and characterization of human atrial natriuretic factor in human plasma, *FEBS Lett.,* 189, 57, 1985.

31. **Sugawara, A., Nakao, K., Sakamoto, M., et al.,** Plasma concentration of atrial natriuretic polypeptide in essential hypertension, *Lancet,* 2, 1426, 1985.

32. **Sagnella, G. A., Markanda, N. D., Shose, A. C., and MacGregor, G. A.,** Raised circulating levels of atrial natriuretic peptides in essential hypertension, *Lancet,* 2, 179, 1985.

33. **Cuneo, R. C., Espiner, E. A., Nicholls, M. G., Yandle, T. G., Joyce, S. L., and Gilchrist, N. G.,** Renal, hemodynamic, and hormonal responses to atrial natriuretic peptide infusions in normal man, and effect of sodium intake, *J. Clin. Endocrinol. Metab.,* 63, 946, 1986.

34. **Safar, M. E. and London, G. M.,** Arterial and venous compliance in sustained essential hypertension, *Hypertension,* 10, 133, 1987.

35. **Bussien, J. P., Biollaz, J., Waeber, B., Nussberger, J., Turini, G. A., Brunner, H. R., Brunner-Ferber, F., Gomez, H. J., and Otterbein, E. S.,** Dose-dependent effect of atrial natriuretic peptide on blood pressure, heart rate, and skin blood flow of normal volunteers, *J. Cardiovasc. Pharmacol.,* 8, 216, 1986.

36. **Nakao, K., Sugawara, A., Morii, N., Sakamoto, M., Yamada, T., Itoh, H., Shiono, S., Nishimura, K., Bau, T., Kihara, M., Yamuri, Y., Shikomura, M., Kiro, Y., Kangawa, K., Matsuo, H., and Imura, H.,** Pharmacokinetic study on α-human atrial natriuretic polypeptide in man, in *Peptide Chemistry 1985,* Proc. 23rd Symp. Peptide Chemistry, Kiso, Y., Ed. Protein Research Foundation, Osaka, 1986.

37. **Yandle, T. G., Richards, A. M., Nicholls, M. G., Cuneo, R., Espiner, E. A., and Livesey, J. H.,** Metabolic clearance rate and plasma half-life of alpha-human atrial natriuretic peptide in man, *Life Sci.,* 38, 1027, 1986.

38. **Gnadinger, M. I., Lang, R. F., Hasler, L., Vehlenger, D. F., Shaw, S., and Weidmann, P.,** Plasma kinetics of synthetic alpha-human atrial natriuretic peptide in man, *Miner. Electrolyte Metab.,* 12, 371, 1986.

39. **Cusson, J. R., du Souich, P., Hamet, P., Schiffrin, E. L., Kuchel, O., Tremblay, J., Cantin, M., Genest, J., and Larochelle, P.,** Effects and pharmacokinetics of bolus injections of atrial natriuretic factor in normal volunteers, *J. Cardiovasc. Pharmacol.,* in press.

40. **Gillies, A. H., Crozier, I. G., Nicholls, M. G., Espiner, E. A., and Yandle, T. G.,** Effect of posture on clearance of atrial natriuretic peptide from plasma, *J. Clin. Endocrinol. Metab.,* 65, 1095, 1987.

41. **Biollaz, J., Calhahan, L. T., Nussberger, J., Waeber, H., Gomez, H. J., Blaine, E. H., and Brunner, H. R.,** Pharmacokinetics of synthetic atrial natriuretic peptide in normal men, *Clin. Pharmacol. Ther.,* 41, 671, 1987.

42. **Crozier, P. E., Nicholls, M. G., Ikram, H., Espiner, E. A., and Yandle, T. G.,** Plasma immunoreactive atrial natriuretic peptide levels after subcutaneous α-hANP-injections in normal humans, *J. Cardiol. Pharmacol.,* 10, 72, 1987.

43. **Arendt, R. M., Gerbes, A. L., Stangl, E., Glatthor, C., Schimak, M., Ritter, D., Riedel, A., Zahringer, J., Kernkes, B., and Erdmann, E.,** Baseline and stimulated ANF plasma levels: is an impaired stimulus-response coupling diagnostically meaningful?, *Klin. Wochenschr.,* 65 (Suppl. 8), 122, 1987.

44. **MacGregor, G. A., Sagnella, G. A., Markandu, N. D., Shore, A. C., Buckley, M. G., Cappuccio, P., and Singer, D. R. J.,** Raised plasma levels of atrial natriuretic peptide in subjects with untreated essential hypertension, *J. Hypertens.,* 4 (Suppl. 6), 567, 1986.

45. **Kohno, M. J., Yasunari, K., Matsuura, T., Murakawa, K., and Takeda, T.,** Circulating atrial natriuretic polypeptide in essential hypertension, *Am. Heart J.,* 113, 1160, 1987.

46. **Montorsi, P., Tonolo, G., Polonia, J., Hepburn, D., and Richards, A. M.,** Correlates of plasma atrial natriuretic factor in health and hypertension, *Hypertension,* 10, 570, 1987.

47. **Wambach, G., Gotz, S., Bonner, G., Degenhardt, S., Kaufmann, W.,** Modulation of atrial natriuretic peptide, renin and aldosterone by dietary sodium intake in normotension and essential hypertension, *J. Hypertens.,* 4 (Suppl. 6), S564, 1986.

48. **Muller, F. B., Bolli, P., Kiowski, W., Erne, P., Resink, T., Raine, A. E. G., and Buhler, F. R.,** Atrial natriuretic peptide is elevated in low renin essential hypertension, *J. Hypertens.,* 4 (Suppl. 6), S489, 1986.

49. **Larochelle, P., Cusson, J. R., Gutkowska, J., Schiffrin, E. L., Hamet, P., Kuchel, O., Genest, J., and Cantin, M.,** Plasma atrial natriuretic factor concentrations in essential and renovascular hypertension, *Br. Med. J.,* 294, 1249, 1987.

50. **Larochelle, P., Cusson, J. R., Gutkowska, J., Genest, J., and Cantin, M.,** Mesure du facteur natriurétique de l'oreillette chez des patients avec hypertension essentielle et renovasculaire, *Arch. Mal. Coeur. Vaiss.,* 80, 976, 1987.

51. **Hamet, P., Tremblay, J., Pang, S. C., Skuherska, R., Schiffrin, E. L., Garcia, R., Cantin, M., Genest, J., Palmour, R., Irvin, F. R., Martin, S., and Goldwater, R.,** Cyclic GMP as mediator and biological marker of atrial natriuretic factor, *J. Hypertens,* 4 (Suppl. 2), S49, 1986.

52. **Nillsson, P., Lindholm, L., Schersten, B., Horn, R., Melander, A., and Hesch, R. D.,** Atrial natriuretic peptide and blood pressure in a geographically defined population, *Lancet,* 2, 883, 1987.

53. **Nakaoka, H., Kitahara, Y., Amano, M., Imataka, K., Fujii, J., Ishibashi, M., and Yamaji, T.,** Effect of β-adrenergic receptor blockage on atrial natriuretic peptide in essential hypertension, *Hypertension* , 10, 221, 1987.

54. **Naruse, M., Naruse, K., Obana, K., Kurimoto, F.,, Sakurai, H., Honda, T., Higashida, T., Demura, H., Inagami, T., and Shizume, K.,** Immunoreactive α-human atrial natriuretic polypeptide in human plasma, *Peptides,* 7, 141, 1986.

55. **Andersson, O. K., Persson, B., Aurell, M., Granérus, G., Wysocky, M., Hedner, J., and Hedner, T.**, Basal and stimulated levels of immunoreactive atrial natriuretic peptide (α-hANP) in relation to central venous pressure, renal and central hemodynamics, and sodium excretion in normotensive and hypertensive men, *J. Cardiovasc. Pharmacol.*, 8 (Abstr.), 6, 1986.

56. **Yamaji, T., Ishibashi, M., Sekihara, H., Takaku, F., Nakaoka, H., and Fujii, J.**, Plasma levels of atrial natriuretic peptide in primary aldosteronism and essential hypertension, *J. Clin. Endocrinol. Metab.*, 63, 815, 1986.

57. **Nozuki, M., Mouri, T., Itoh, K., Takahashi, K., Totsune, K., Saito, T., and Yoshinaga, K.**, Plasma concentrations of atrial natriuretic peptide in various diseases, *Tohoku J. Exp. Med.*, 148, 439, 1986.

58. **Hedner, T., Hedner, J., Towle, A. C., Hartford, M., Ljungman, S., Wikstrand, J., and Berglund, G.**, Plasma atrial natriuretic peptide (ANP) in patients with mild to moderate essential hypertension, *J. Cardiovasc. Pharmacol.*, 8 (Abstr.), 1299, 1986.

59. **Nishiuchi, T., Saito, H., Yamasaki, Y., and Saito, S.**, Radioimmunoassay for atrial natriuretic peptide: method and results in normal subjects and patients with various diseases, *Clin. Chim. Acta*, 159, 45, 1986.

60. **Kohno, M., Yasunari, K., Murakawa, K., Kanayama, Y., Matsuura, T., and Takeda, T.**, Effects of high-sodium and low-sodium intake on circulating atrial natriuretic peptides in salt-sensitive patients with systemic hypertension, *Am. J. Cardiol.*, 59, 1212, 1987.

61. **Tunny, T. J., Gordon, R. D., Klemm, S. A., and Hamlet, S. M.**, Effects of acute volume expansion on atrial natriuretic peptide levels in normal subjects, primary aldosteronism and low-renin essential hypertension, *J. Hypertens.*, 4 (Suppl. 6), S509, 1986.

62. **Volpe, M., Mele, A., De Luca, N., Golino, P., Bondiolotti, G., Camargo, M. J., Atlas, S. A,, and Trimarco, B.**, Carotid baroreceptor unloading decreases plasma atrial natriuretic factor in hypertensive patients, *J. Hypertens.*, 4 (Suppl. 6), S519, 1986.

63. **Olivari, M. T., Fiorentini, C., Polese, A., and Gerazzi, M. D.**, Pulmonary hemodynamics and right ventricular function in hypertension, *Circulation,* 57, 1185, 1978.

64. **Larochelle, P. and Cusson, J. R.**, unpublished data.

Chapter 20

THE ROLE OF ATRIAL NATRIURETIC FACTOR IN CONGESTIVE HEART FAILURE

John C. Burnett, Jr.,

TABLE OF CONTENTS

I. INTRODUCTION

The preservation of optimal body fluid homeostasis is dependent upon an integration of cardiac and renal function, which responds to surfeits or deficits in sodium intake to maintain a near constancy of extracellular fluid volume. In such a system, cardiac baro- and mechanoreceptors respond to alterations in intravascular volume and/or pressure and signal intrarenal effector mechanisms to regulate urinary sodium excretion. This sensor-effector cardiorenal axis thus serves to regulate sodium excretion to maintain optimal plasma volume and arterial pressure.[1]

Repeated studies have established the importance of cardiac neurogenic mechanisms in the regulation of renal function.[2] Beginning with the important contributions of de Bold and colleagues, a hormonal system of cardiac origin has also emerged which plays a fundamental role in body fluid homeostasis.[3] This peptide hormone, atrial natriuretic factor (ANF), is synthesized in the cardiac atria and released in response to atrial stretch. ANF acts on the kidney to increase sodium excretion and inhibit the reninangiotensin-aldosterone system in both animals and humans.[3-5] ANF also acts on the peripheral circulation to decrease venous return.[6-8]

The emerging picture of the atrial peptide system as it relates to volume homeostasis is that it operates as a physiologic hormone system to defend the central circulation from volume and/or pressure overload. This is consistent with the observations of Salazar and co-workers that circulating ANF is unchanged in response to chronic alterations in sodium intake.[9] In contrast, circulating ANF is increased in response to increases in atrial pressure, which occur in response to acute intravascular volume expansion or chronic cardiac volume overload associated with congestive heart failure.[5,10,11] The goal of this review is to support a role for the atrial peptide system as a hormone which serve to guard the cardiopulmonary circulation from overfilling. Thus, this chapter will attempt to first focus upon the physiology of ANF and then address its role in acute and chronic congestive heart failure.

II. PHYSIOLOGIC ACTIONS OF ANF ON RENAL FUNCTION, THE RENIN-ANGIOTENSIN-ALDOSTERONE SYSTEM, AND CARDIOVASCULAR HEMODYNAMICS

In 1984, studies investigated the renal action of synthetic ANF in the dog.[3,4] These investigations reported the effect of ANF on renal blood flow, glomerular filtration rate, whole kidney tubular reabsorption of sodium, and renin release. Intrarenal administration of ANF resulted in a marked increase in urine volume and sodium excretion. The marked natriuresis and diuresis were associated with increases in glomerular filtration rate and fractional sodium excretion with decreases in proximal tubule reabsorption, as determined by the lithium clearance techniques.[3] Renin secretion and aldosterone were inhibited despite a decrease in arterial pressure.

A unique renal blood flow response to ANF was observed which was characterized by a significant transient increase despite continued infusion of ANF. This transient increase in renal blood flow was followed by a slight, but significant, decrease that persisted. The mechanism mediating this biphasic renal blood-flow response is unclear; however, the mechanism may be secondary to activation of a slower acting intrarenal vasoconstrictor which modulates glomerular filtration by controlling preglomerular arteriolar resistance in response to alterations in the delivery of sodium to the macula densa in the distal nephron. Despite the transient increase in renal blood flow, the increase in glomerular filtration rate persisted throughout the ANF infusion. The observed decrease in renal blood flow and increase in glomerular filtration rate support the conclusion that the increase in GFR was associated with an increase in postglomerular arteriolar resistance as well. In view of these renal hemodynamic effects, ANF may decrease preglomerular resistance and increase postglomerular resistance, thus increasing glomerular hydrostatic pressure. A direct effect of ANF to increase K_f, the ultrafiltration coefficient, is also possible. Recent studies in both the dog and rat support these two alternative mechanisms in mediating changes in the determinants of the filtration process.[12,13] Thus, these studies suggest that the natriuresis observed during intrarenal infusion of ANF may, in part, be mediated by an augmentation of glomerular filtration rate. However, the natriuretic response to ANF remains, although attenuated, when the increase in glomerular filtration rate is prevented.[14] Thus, while ANF has a potent action on GFR, the natriuresis is not solely dependant upon its increase.

Administration of ANF results in an increase in the fractional excretion of sodium, indicating a decrease in the tubular reabsorption of sodium at one or more nephron segments. The nephron segments altered by ANF remains unclear. Studies support multiple nephron segments. An action of ANF on the proximal tubule is supported by micropuncture, as well as studies employing the lithium clearance technique.[3,15] In view of the absence of ANF receptors in the proximal tubule, the mechanism by which ANF decreases proximal tubule reabsorption may be secondary to an intrarenal hemodynamic action which may preferentially decrease proximal tubule reabsorption. Reports by Schwab et al. of an increase in renal interstitial hydrostatic pressure, an intrarenal physical factor linked to alterations in proximal reabsorption, are consistent with an intrarenal hemodynamic mechanism,.[16]

Micropuncture, as well as *in vitro* isolated cell preparations, have documented an action of ANF on the medullary collecting duct segment.[17,18] These studies support a direct action of ANF on receptor-mediated alterations in tubular reabsorption — actions which may be linked to the cGMP second messenger system.

Atrial natriuretic factor decreases urine osmolality. This action supports a role for ANF in increasing medullary blood flow, resulting in a washout of the medullary concentration gradient.[19] Such an action may contribute to the decreases in reabsorption of sodium in juxtamedullary nephrons. Indeed, the increase in renal interstitial hydrostatic pressure may be the result of increases in hydrostatic pressure within the medullary circulation as previously reported in mineralocorticoid escape, a phenomenon associated with increased circulating ANF.[20,21] The importance of increases in renal interstitial hydrostatic pressure in mediating ANF natriuresis is underscored by the report that prevention of the increase in interstitial pressure markedly attenuates the increase in sodium excretion in response to ANF.[22]

In addition to its natriuretic action, ANF decreases renin secretion despite a decrease in arterial pressure.[3,4] The mechanism by which ANF mediates this inhibition of renin release was investigated in a recent study by Opgenorth and colleagues.[23] Recognizing that increasing tubular delivery of sodium chloride to the macula densa may decrease renin release, these authors tested the hypothesis that ANF-induced reduction in renin release by the kidney is dependent on increased solute delivery to the macula densa. In normal dogs, intrarenal infusion of ANF resulted in a decrease in renin secretion despite a sustained decrease in arterial pressure. In contrast, in the nonfiltering kidney without a functional macula densa, ANF did not inhibit renin secretion. Adenosine, however, known to directly inhibit renin release, did decrease renin secretion in the nonfiltering kidney. Thus, these previous studies support the hypothesis that the mechanism of ANF inhibition of renin release is through a macula densa mechanism. Pharmacologic concentrations of ANF may also directly inhibit renin release from isolated juxtaglomerular cells. Others have reported significant inhibition of renin release from cultured juxtaglomerular cells in response to incubation with ANF.[24] In summary, ANF is a potent natriuretic and diuretic hormone. This natriuretic action is associated with an increase in glomerular filtration rate and decrease in proximal tubule reabsorption, as determined by the clearance of lithium. The mechanisms by which ANF may alter tubular reabsorption may be multiple, including both a direct receptor-mediated cGMP mechanism and indirect mechanism mediated by the intrarenal physical factors. In addition to these renal actions, ANF inhibits renin release.

ANF decreases arterial pressure independent of its natriuretic action.[3,4] The mechanism of this decrease remains unclear. This uncertainty may manifest a multifaceted action of ANF on the determinants of arterial blood pressure regulation, species differences, and the effects of anesthesia in modulating the action of exogenously administered ANF.

ANF *in vitro* relaxes vascular smooth muscle and, when directly administered into the forearm, decreases vascular resistance.[25,26] However, when ANF is administered systemically in normal animals and animals made hypertensive with angiotensin II, ANF does not decrease systemic vascular resistance.[27] Indeed, an increase in systemic vascular resistance is observed in response to marked decreases in cardiac filling pressures and cardiac output. Such observations support the interpretation that ANF decreases arterial pressure by decreasing venous return and cardiac output. Recent studies by Trippodo et al. have demonstrated that ANF decreases mean circulating filling pressure and increases resistance to venous return.[28,29] These investigators have interpreted these observations as compatible with the concept of ANF as a venoconstrictor which increases transfer of intravascular volume into the interstitium by increasing hydrostatic pressure within the venous arteriole.

The increase in systemic vascular resistance in response to ANF-mediated hypotension may, however, be blunted, supporting a subtle arterial vasodilator role for ANF and/or an inhibiting action of ANF on arterial baroreflexes. The localization of the ANF gene and mRNA transcripts in aortic arch adventia supports this latter speculation, as well as reports in animals and humans of blunted sympathetic nerve activity in response to exogenous ANF.[30,31]

Studies by Wangler and colleagues in isolated blood perfused heart preparations have reported that ANF is a coronary vasoconstrictor which results in myocardial ischemia and subsequent decreases in myocardial performance and cardiac output.[32] This coronary vasoconstrictor response has not been confirmed.[33] We investigated the action of ANF both *in vivo* in the anesthetized dog and *in vitro* in the isolated Langdendorf rat heart preparation.[8] Both physiologic and pharmacologic doses of ANF were administered to these preparations and coronary flow and cardiac function measured. No coronary vasoconstriction was observed. Indeed, *in vivo*, a transient coronary vasodilatation was noted. No decrease in myocardial contractility was observed. The decrease in arterial pressure in studies in the dog at pharmacologic doses was associated with decreases in cardiac filling pressure and cardiac output. In summary, the mechanism of the decrease in arterial pressure in response to ANF is best explained by a decrease in venous return, resulting in a decrease in cardiac filling pressure and volume with a subsequent decrease in cardiac output. A role for ANF in modulating cardiovascular reflexes is also suggested in recent studies.

These previous studies have focused upon the pharmacologic action of the atrial peptide system. The physiologic role of ANF in cardiovascular-volume regulation continues to emerge. Studies by Salazar et al. investigated whether long-term elevations in sodium intake lead to chronic adjustments in circulating ANF and associated alterations in urinary sodium excretion.[9] In these studies, chronic sodium loading to mimic increases in sodium diet presumably unassociated with increases in atrial pressure did not increase circulating ANF. Despite no increase in plasma ANF, plasma renin and aldosterone were suppressed and sodium excretion was increased during increases in sodium intake. These studies support the concept that the regulation of volume homeostasis in response to physiologic changes in sodium diet may not involve the atrial peptide system.

In contrast, acute intravascular volume loading (i.e., 3 to 10% body weight saline volume expansion) increased atrial pressures with parallel increases in circulating ANF and associated natriuresis.[34] Subsequent studies by the same investigators administered exogenous ANF to mimic circulating concentrations achieved during acute intravascular volume loading (Table 1).[7] The lowest dose of ANF infusion resulted in an increase in circulating ANF of 31 ± 3 pg/ml, resulting in a significant increase in absolute sodium excretion, fractional excretion

TABLE 1A
Effects of ANF Infusion on Cardiac Systemic Hemodynamics

ANF dose (μg/kg/min)	RAP (mmHg)	PCWP (mmHg)	SVR (dyn/s/cm^{-5})	MAP (mmHg)	C.O. (l/min)	HR (bpm)	Hct (%)
Control	−1.3 ± 0.4	2.4 ± 0.5	2296 ± 180	120 ± 4	4.5 ± 0.4	108 ± 5	40 ± 1
.0025	−1.6 ± 0.4	2.1 ± 0.6	2496 ± 233	120 ± 4	4.2 ± 0.4	106 ± 6	40 ± 1
.005	−2.2 ± 0.5[a]	1.9 ± 0.6	2672 ± 227[a]	121 ± 4	3.9 ± 0.4[a]	106 ± 5	39 ± 1
.01	−2.3 ± 0.5[a]	1.6 ± 0.6[a]	2895 ± 248[a]	120 ± 4	3.6 ± 0.3[a]	105 ± 5	40 ± 1
.3	−2.2 ± 0.5[a]	1.2 ± 0.7[a]	3020 ± 261[a]	106 ± 4[a]	3.1 ± 0.3[a]	108 ± 7	42 ± 1[a]
Recovery	−2.5 ± 0.5[a]	1.9 ± 0.5[a]	3633 ± 342[a]	120 ± 4	2.9 ± 0.3[a]	105 ± 5	40 ± 1

Note: ANF, atrial natriuretic factor; RAP, right atrial pressure; PCWP, pulmonary capillary wedge pressure; SVR, systemic vascular resistance; MAP, mean arterial pressure; C.O., cardiac output; HR, heart rate; HCT, hematocrit.

[a] $p < 0.05$, compared to control.

of sodium and lithium, and a significant decrease in urine osmolality. A greater change in circulating ANF (96 ± 12 pg/ml) was required to significantly decrease right atrial pressure, cardiac output, and plasma renin activity, and to increase systemic vascular resistance and total and fractional excretion of potassium. The highest dose to mimic pharmacologic concentrations of ANF was required to decrease arterial pressure and renal vascular resistance. This important study demonstrated that (1) ANF is natriuretic and diuretic at physiologic concentrations, (2) at low concentrations, ANF appears to decrease whole kidney proximal tubular reabsorption of sodium and does not affect glomerular filtration rate, (3) a greater, but physiologic, change in circulating ANF is required to significantly decrease cardiac output, cardiac filling pressure, and plasma renin activity than is required to significantly increase sodium excretion, and (4) a decrease in systemic arterial pressure and vascular resistance does not occur at physiologic concentrations of ANF.

Studies by Schwab et al. extend these previous physiologic studies and support the hypothesis that the increase in sodium excretion in response to acute intravascular fluid volume expansion is, in part, mediated by ANF.[35] These investigators studied rats with and without intact right atrial appendages (i.e., the latter appendectomized to remove ANF-secreting endocrine tissue) before and following acute volume expansion which increased central venous pressure. Increases in circulating ANF were measured and compared to increases in sodium excretion in each group. Right atrial appendectomy resulted in an attenuated increase in ANF in response to volume expansion with subsequent blunted increase in sodium excretion. These studies strongly support a physiologic role for ANF as a hormonal link between atrial endocrine and renal excretory function. Hirth and colleagues reported that the renal natriuretic response was abolished in the presence of infusion of monoclonal antibodies to exogenous ANF.[36] Such studies, taken together, support the interpretation that ANF is a physiologic hormone. Its physiologic role is to modulate intravascular volume, specifically central cardiopulmonary volume, by an increase in sodium excretion and a decrease in venous return in association with inhibition of the renin-angiotensin-aldosterone system.

III. PLASMA AND CARDIAC ANF IN CONGESTIVE HEART FAILURE

Congestive heart failure is a syndrome characterized by elevated atrial pressures with avid sodium retention in association with activation of the renin-angiotensin-aldosterone system. Chimoskey and co-workers speculated that failure to produce sufficient ANF by degenerating hearts in heart failure may contribute to salt and water retention.[37] These

TABLE 1B
Effects of ANF Infusion on Renal Function

ANF dose (μg/kg/min)	V (ml/min)	GFR (ml/min)	$U_{Na}V$ (μeq/min)	FE_{Na} (%)	U_KV (μeq/min)	FE_K (%)	RBF (ml/min)	RVR (mmHg/ml·min^{-1})	FE_{Li} (%)	UOsm (mosmol/kg H_2O)
Control	0.16 ± 02	37.6 ± 1.4	22 ± 6	0.41 ± 0.11	29 ± 3	20 ± 2	147 ± 12	0.90 ± .08	0.21 ± .02	1292 ± 136
.0025	0.38 ± .08[a]	34.5 ± 2.5	66 ± 15[a]	1.30 ± 0.33[a]	32 ± 3	27 ± 4	144 ± 9	0.90 ± .05	0.32 ± .03[a]	994 ± 137[a]
.005	0.72 ± .15[a]	36.3 ± 2.9	131 ± 26[a]	2.61 ± 0.55[a]	39 ± 4[a]	30 ± 2[a]	148 ± 7	0.88 ± .05	0.43 ± .06[a]	741 ± 86[a]
.01	0.94 ± .14[a]	31.7 ± 1.5	171 ± 26[a]	3.76 ± 0.54[a]	37 ± 2[a]	34 ± 2[a]	143 ± 9	0.91 ± .07	0.50 ± .09[a]	608 ± 52[a]
.3	2.66 ± .46[a]	38.2 ± 3.9	397 ± 151[a]	6.81 ± 0.60[a]	56 ± 6[a]	42 ± 4[a]	166 ± 11	0.70 ± .06	0.67 ± 18[a]	431 ± 30[a]
Recovery	0.40 ± .06[a]	38.2 ± 4.0	70 ± 9[a]	1.31 ± 0.41[a]	29 ± 3	22 ± 3	136 ± 14	1.01 ± .11	0.32 ± .08	743 ± 50[a]

Note: ANF, atrial natriuretic factor; V, urine flow; GFR, glomerular filtration rate; $U_{Na}V$, absolute sodium excretion; U_KV, absolute potassium excretion; FE_K, fractional excretion of potassium; RBF, renal blood flow; RVR, renal vascular resistance; FE_{Li}, fractional excretion of lithium; UOsm, urine osmolality.

[a] $p < 0.05$, compared to control.

TABLE 1C
Hormonal Effects of ANF Infusion

ANF dose (μg/kg/min)	ANF (pg/ml)	Aldo (ng/dl)	PRA (ng/ml/h)
Control	68 ± 8	5.7 ± 0.9	3.6 ± 1.3
.0025	100 ± 8[a]	5.5 ± 0.7	2.9 ± 1.0
.005	164 ± 18[a]	5.1 ± 0.6	2.2 ± 0.8[a]
.01	282 ± 22[a]	5.0 ± 0.7	1.5 ± 0.5[a]
.3	519 ± 34[a]	5.3 ± 0.9	1.4 ± 0.5[a]
Recovery	70 ± 10	6.0 ± 0.7	2.7 ± 0.7

Note: ANF, atrial natriuretic factor; Aldo, aldosterone; PRA, plasma renin activity.

[a] $p < 0.05$, compared to control.

investigators based this conclusion upon the observation that atrial content of ANF was decreased in hamsters with familial cardiomyopathy and congestive heart failure. Rector and colleagues determined the ANF content in the atria of rats with chronic congestive heart failure which had been produced by experimental myocardial infarction.[38] These experimental rats had reduced ANF activity within the atria, as compared with sham-operated rats. Although these investigators suggested that an ANF deficiency may account for the sodium retention observed in conjunction with congestive heart failure, they cautioned that the atrial content may not reflect the circulating levels of ANF and that the importance of their findings must await concomitant assessment of both atrial content and circulating ANF.

In studies by Edwards et al., the relationship between immunoreactive ANF granularity within the atria and circulating ANF was examined in normal hamsters and in hamsters with familial cardiomyopathy and congestive heart failure.[39] Consistent with previous studies, a decreased atrial ANF was observed in congestive heart failure. However, coincident with the reduced atrial granularity, an increase in circulating immunoreactive ANF was reported. These two observations provide insight into the dynamics of the storage and release of ANF. The best explanation for the reduction in atrial granularity and the elevated circulating ANF is a stimulated system in which the atrial peptide is synthesized and released into circulation and the storage of ANF is minimal.

Studies in humans with congestive heart failure have provided further support for congestive heart failure as a state characterized by increased circulating ANF.[5,10,11] Burnett and co-workers determined circulating concentrations of ANF in normal human volunteers with no history of cardiovascular disease, patients with cardiovascular disease but normal cardiac filling pressures, patients with cardiovascular disease and markedly elevated cardiac filling pressures but without congestive heart failure, and patients with cardiovascular disease, markedly elevated cardiac filling pressures, and congestive heart failure (Table 2).[10] These investigations and those of other laboratories demonstrate that marked elevation of cardiac filling pressure associated with congestive heart failure is associated with increased circulating ANF. Thus, the sodium retention and edema formation characteristic of congestive heart failure occurs despite increased circulating ANF levels. Indeed, in these later studies, the patients with the highest concentrations of circulating ANF had symptoms of biventricular failure, which is consistent with recent animal studies that have reported an attenuated natriuretic response to exogenously administered ANF in experimental heart failure. Thus, these studies from various laboratories establish that in human subjects, congestive heart failure reflects not an ANF deficiency state, but rather a compensatory increase in peptide release.

While these previous investigators have demonstrated elevation of plasma alpha-human

TABLE 2
Individual Patient Profile, Hemodynamic and Atrial Natriuretic Peptide Data

Patient	Age (years)	Sex	MAP (mmHg)	HR (bpm)	CFP (mmHg)	ANP (pg/ml)	Clinical diagnosis

Group 2: Normal Cardiac Filling Pressure without Congestive Heart Failure (n = 11)

Patient	Age (years)	Sex	MAP (mmHg)	HR (bpm)	CFP (mmHg)	ANP (pg/ml)	Clinical diagnosis
1	69	M	98	62	8	104	CAD
2	64	F	58	46	10	54	CAD
3	33	M	76	70	7	33	CAD
4	48	M	93	55	10	73	CAD
5	31	M	113	98	6	47	ACP,NCA
6	47	M	107	65	10	57	EH,CAD
7	60	M	89	70	8	63	CAD
8	41	M	105	76	9	37	CAD
9	43	M	94	65	7	22	CAD
10	65	M	65	90	5	33	CAD
11	49	F	79	63	7	47	CAD
Mean	—	—	89 ± 5	69 ± 4	7.9 ± 0.5	51.8 ± 6.9	—

Group 3: Elevated Cardiac Filling Pressure without Congestive Heart Failure (n = 6)

Patient	Age (years)	Sex	MAP (mmHg)	HR (bpm)	CFP (mmHg)	ANP (pg/ml)	Clinical diagnosis
12	74	M	107	57	25	316	CAD
13	54	M	83	46	31	126	EH,CAD
14	68	M	108	73	30	314	EH,CAD
15	73	M	92	63	28	323	CAD
16	75	M	97	90	29	140	CAD
17	82	M	109	73	22	173	CAD
Mean	—	—	99 ± 4	67 ± 6	27.5 ± 1.4[a]	232.0 ± 38.8[a]	—

Group 4: Elevated Cardiac Filling Pressure with Congestive Heart Failure (n = 6)

Patient	Age (years)	Sex	MAP (mmHg)	HR (bpm)	CFP (mmHg)	ANP (pg/ml)	Clinical diagnosis
18	76	M	105	.44	34	700	RC,CAD,EH
19	55	M	83	62	21	215	AS
20	68	F	68	68	23	746	IC
21	74	M	88	66	29	164	IC
22	66	F	94	67	33	162	IC
23	29	M	84	72	32	685	IDC
Mean	—	—	87 ± 5	63 ± 4	28.6 ± 2.2[a]	445.3 ± 119.0[a]	—

Note: MAP, mean arterial pressure; HR, heart rate; CFP, cardiac filling pressure; ANP, atrial natriuretic peptide; CAD, coronary artery disease; ACP, atypical chest pain; NCA, normal coronary arteries; EH, essential hypertension; RC, restrictive cardiomyopathy; AS, aortic stenosis; IC, ischemic cardiomyopathy, IDC, idiopathic dilated cardiomyopathy. All data were averaged and expressed as means ± SE.

[a]   indicates p <.005 and is calculated from comparisons for the value in Group 3 or Group 4 against Group 2, employing the Behrens-Fisher test.

ANF representing the biologically active C-terminal form (99 — 126) of the ANF molecule released from ANF granules, Itoh et al. have reported probable cosecretion of the N-terminal form of the ANF molecule (23 — 56) in humans with and without congestive heart failure.[40] Specifically, N-terminal concentrations were significantly increased in both normals and heart failure subjects, compared to the C-terminal form. The functional significance of N-terminal fragments of ANF must await further investigation. The striking sequence conservation of the N-terminal region among species raises the possibility of unknown biological action of N-terminal form. The simultaneous measurement of plasma N-terminal and C-terminal may also provide insight into the evaluation of the secretory function of the heart during the therapeutic administration of alpha-hANF or of possible pathophysiologic conditions producing the release of structurally abnormal ANF.

Studies have demonstrated the occurrence of ventricular deposits of ANF in primitive organisms and in neonatal mammalian ventricular cardiocytes.[41] The induction of ANF and increased quantities of ANF mRNA has been observed in ventricular tissue of rats subjected to chronic aortic constriction or dexamethasone.[42] Lattion and associates have reported an increase in ANF mRNA in the ventricle of rat hearts subjected to chronic volume overload.[43]

Recent studies by Edwards et al. have reported the existence of immunoreactive ANF within the ventricular myocardium of animals with familial cardiomyopathy and congestive heart failure[44] These studies also importantly extend this observation to demonstrate the occurrence of ventricular ANF in the human with congestive heart failure. The absence of ANF within the normal ventricle and the presence of ANF within the ventricle of the heart with congestive heart failure of various etiologies support the concept that heart failure is a stimulus for the production of ANF by the ventricle.

It is notable in heart failure that ANF granules are found within both right and left ventricles, predominantly in a subendocardial location. It has been demonstrated, using finite element analysis of myocardial stress/strain relationships, that intramural tension is greatest within the subendocardial region of the ventricle.[45] Increased intramural tension may represent the stimulating factor necessary for the ventricular synthesis of ANF. In addition, the subendocardial location makes it feasible that ventricular ANF may be identified in tissue obtained by endomyocardial biopsy.

Homogenates of cardiac and noncardiac tissue clearly demonstrate a significant quantity of ANF within ventricular tissue in animals with CHF. This ANF does not appear to be secondary to contamination from elevated circulating ANF since the heart failure group tissue from the diaphragm also subjected to increased circulating ANF does not contain an increased quantity of ANF. Further, atrial tissue in the heart failure group contains significantly less ANF than that observed in control animals. This observation is in agreement with prior studies in which atrial ANF was assessed semiquantitatively by means of immunohistochemical techniques.[39] While nonspecific immunoperoxidase activity may occur at the periphery of treated tissue, the quality of staining is markedly different from the definite granules observed within myocytes. Judging by the lack of immunoreactive ANF detected within the pericardial tissue, edge artifact did not appear to significantly alter the interpretation of the tissue. The immunoperoxidase reaction is specific for the cardiac myocyte as there as no evidence of immunoreactivity in noncardiac vascular smooth muscle or connective tissue.

The significance of ventricular ANF occurring in animals and humans with CHF is unclear at this time. However, this observation does provide support to the interpretation that in pathophysiologic states characterized by cardiac volume overload, the ventricle, as well as the atria, sense and participate in volume regulation. The findings of ANF within the ventricle of the failing mammalian heart, as well as its occurrence in more primitive ventricles, suggests that ANF may represent a fundamental regulatory peptide important to both ontogeny and phylogeny. According to de Bold "the finding of secretory-like morphological characteristics in heart muscle cells in all species studied, together with the highly conserved nature of the known sequence of ANF peptides, hints of a fundamental evolutionary strategy to maintain water and electrolyte balance".[46] The observations that the ventricle appears to be capable of producing ANF in response to the stress of chronic volume overload suggests that this peptide may play a very fundamental role in the maintenance and regulation of intravascular volume.

In summary, the present studies demonstrate that ANF is present in mammalian ventricular myocardium. Further, these studies establish that the presence of ventricular ANF is associated not with normal cardiac function, but with chronic volume overload and a failing myocardium.

IV. FUNCTIONAL SIGNIFICANCE OF ELEVATED ANF IN CONGESTIVE HEART FAILURE

The functional significance of elevated plasma concentrations of ANF in congestive heart failure is unclear. Inasmuch as heart failure may be associated with sodium retention and activation of the renin-angiotensin-aldosterone system, investigators speculated that ANF did not contribute to renal and endocrine regulation in heart failure. Such a conclusion may, however, be premature as studies readdress the question of the physiologic significance of elevated plasma ANF in acute and chronic heart failure.

Michel and colleagues examined the hormonal effects of congestive heart failure induced by myocardial infarction in the rat.[47] Plasma ANF and ANF mRNA were assessed and compared to other volume regulating hormones at 2 months. Surprisingly, plasma aldosterone was not elevated in infarcted rats. The investigators suggested that the lack of increase in the heart failure group may be related to ANF. Both plasma and cardiac mRNA ANF were increased. As ANF acts directly to inhibit aldosterone secretion, the enhanced synthesis and release of ANF could explain the suppression of aldosterone. In contrast to aldosterone, ANF seems to have been unable to totally suppress increases in renin, although renin release could have been limited.

In addition to possibly modulating renin and aldosterone in these correlative studies, rats with myocardial infarction were characterized by significant ventricular hypertrophy. In addition to enhanced ANF mRNA in atria in this group, ANF mRNA was increased in the hypertrophied ventricular myocardium as well. Michel et al. suggested that biosynthesis of ANF within the ventricular myocardium could be used as a qualitative marker for cardiac hypertrophy. Indeed, in all studies to date from various laboratories, the presence of ventricular ANF appears to be clearly associated and/or stimulated by the biochemical events of cardiac hypertrophy.

The studies of Michel et al. support a possible functional role for endogenous ANF as a modulator of renal, endocrine, and cardiovascular function in congestive heart failure. To date, three preliminary studies extend these previous investigations and further suggest an important compensatory role for ANF in both acute and chronic congestive heart failure.

Lee and colleagues investigated the role of endogenous ANF in acute congestive heart failure produced by rapid right ventricular pacing.[48] This model produces a decrease in cardiac output and arterial pressure with an increase in atrial pressures and circulating ANF. Despite the stimulus of arterial hypotension, sodium excretion was maintained and plasma renin and aldosterone did not increase. In marked contrast, reductions in arterial pressure to the same level in a low cardiac output model of heart failure produced by thoracic inferior vena cava constriction were unassociated with increases in atrial pressure or ANF. In association with arterial hypotension and no increase in ANF, plasma renin and aldosterone were markedly increased. When exogenous ANF was infused in dogs with acute caval constriction to mimic concentrations achieved in high ANF heart failure, renin and aldosterone were normalized and no sodium retention was observed. Thus, these studies support the interpretation for a role for increased endogenous ANF in acute congestive heart failure to limit activation of renin and aldosterone, as well as to maintain sodium excretion despite the stimulus of arterial hypotension.

To assess the functional role of ANF in chronic heart failure, Awazu et al. studied rats with heart failure produced by myocardial infarction of 4 weeks' duration in the presence and absence of infusion of anti-ANF antibody.[49] In response to anti-ANF antibodies, urine volume and sodium excretion markedly decreased in the absence of changes in glomerular filtration rate. Thus, these studies also support a functional role for elevated endogenous ANF in chronic heart failure in maintaining sodium and water excretion.

In a similar study, Drexler and colleagues employed monoclonal ANF antibodies in rats with chronic heart failure also produced by myocardial infarction and examined cardiovascular hemodynamic responses.[50] In response to ANF antibodies, rats with heart failure were characterized by an increase in systemic vascular resistance, decrease in cardiac output, and increase in cardiac filling pressures. These preliminary studies support a vasodilatory role of endogenous ANF in chronic heart failure. Thus, these studies, taken together, support the conclusion that elevated endogenous ANF in acute and chronic heart failure serve to maintain sodium excretion and limit activation of the renin-angiotensin-aldosterone system, as well as to oppose the vasoconstrictor stimuli also increased in the syndrome of congestive heart failure.

Despite this beneficial compensatory action of the atrial peptide system in acute and chronic heart failure, the renal natriuretic response to exogenously administered ANF is blunted, compared to control animals. Scriven and Burnett reported that intrarenal infusion of ANF in control dogs and those with low-output heart failure resulted in a significant increase in glomerular filtration rate and a decrease in proximal tubule reabsorption, as estimated by changes in lithium excretion.[51] ANF significantly decreased arterial pressure, as well as renin secretory rate, in both groups. Despite similar alterations in glomerular filtration rate, proximal tubular reabsorption, and renin release in the two groups, the natriuretic and diuretic response to ANF was markedly attenuated in animals with acute low-output heart failure, as compared with that in control dogs (Table 3). Such a response is similar to the excretory response to acute volume expansion previously observed in animals with experimental heart failure. These latter studies in dogs with heart failure demonstrated that acute saline volume expansion, a physiologic maneuver recently reported to be associated with increased levels of immunoreactive atrial natriuretic factor, is characterized by an increase in glomerular filtration rate and a decrease in proximal tubule reabsorption with a blunted natriuresis. The blunted natriuresis was attributed to enhanced solute reabsorption beyond the proximal tubule, perhaps in part mediated by enhanced circulating levels of aldosterone, which are known to be elevated in models of low-output heart failure, and/or alterations in physical factors, which occur during perturbations in renal perfusion and venous pressures. The present studies further support the hypothesis that the defect in the renal handling of sodium in heart failure may be mediated by factors that act beyond the proximal tubule and are therefore independent of the action of atrial natriuretic peptide on glomerular filtration rate and proximal tubular reabsorption. Thus, the present studies provide further insight into the understanding of heart failure by focusing on the importance of nephron segments beyond the proximal tubule in the pathophysiology of congestive heart failure.

The mechanism of the attenuated natriuretic response to ANF in heart failure may be multifactorial. Shriffin et al. have reported down-regulation of ANF receptors in platelets of humans with chronic congestive heart failure.[52] In elegant studies by Tsunada et al., the relationships between ANF binding sites in the renal medulla, plasma ANF concentrations, and ventricular dysfunction were examined in rats with myocardial infarction-induced congestive heart failure of 4 weeks' duration.[53] Extensive myocardial infarction was associated with elevated concentrations of plasma ANF and decreased ANF receptor numbers in the inner medulla. These investigators suggested that this decrease in medullary ANF receptors may contribute to the blunted renal response to ANF.

Studies by Showalter and colleagues offer an additional physiologic mechanism.[54] While in heart failure exogenous ANF may decrease plasma renin activity, this decrease may not be normalized, which is compatible with a lack of normalization of intrarenal angiotensin II (AII). In these studies by Showalter et al., intrarenally infused and confined AII infusion in normal dogs resulted in a significant attenuation of the renal natriuretic response to ANF.

TABLE 3
Renal Hemodynamic and Excretory Response to Intrarenal Infusion of Synthetic Atrial Natriuretic Peptide in Control and Acute Low Output Failure Dogs

	MAP (mmHg)	IVCP (mmHg)	RBF (ml/min)	GFR (ml/min)	RVR (mmHg·ml·min^{-1})	V (ml/min)	$U_{Na}V$ (μeq/min)	FE_{Na} (%)	FE_{Li} (%)	RSR (ng/ml)
Control Group (n = 6)										
Baseline	120 ± 4	1.9 ± 0.4	157 ± 24	34.0 ± 3.9	0.88 ± 0.19	0.47 ± 0.15	29.9 ± 7.8	0.57 ± 0.13	29.8 ± 4.1	308.5 ± 84.5
ANF	114 ± 4[a]	1.8 ± 0.4	146 ± 21	45.3 ± 3.6[a]	0.84 ± 0.13	2.49 ± 0.44[c]	231.0 ± 42.5	3.42 ± 0.54[c]	44.1 ± 4.6	44.5 ± 27.5[a]
Acute Low Output Failure Group (n = 6)										
Baseline	113 ± 5	10.8 ± 1.2[d]	143 ± 21	23.3 ± 4.4	0.89 ± 0.16	0.11 ± 0.03	10.8 ± 2.3	0.42 ± 0.16	17.7 ± 3.1	852.8 ± 183.0[d]
ANF	107 ± 4 -	10.8 ± 1.3[d]	137 ± 23	33.9 ± 5.6[a]	0.91 ± 0.17	0.41 ± 0.10[b,d]	46.2 ± 12.3[b,d]	0.90 ± 0.13[b,d]	30.2 ± 4.3[a]	149.5 ± 73.7

Note: ANP, atrial natriuretic peptide; MAP, mean arterial pressure; IVCP, inferior vena cava pressure; RBF, renal blood flow; GFR, glomerular filtration rate; RVR, renal vascular resistance; V, urine flow; $U_{Na}V$, urinary sodium excretion; FE_{Na}, fractional excretion of sodium; FE_{Li}, fractional excretion of lithium; RSR, renin secretory rate.

[a] $p < 0.05$, paired *t*-test.
[b] $p < 0.02$, paired *t*-test.
[c] $p < 0.005$, paired *t*-test.
[d] $p < 0.05$, unpaired *t*-test.

Data from Scriven, T. A. and Burnett, J. C., Jr., *Circulation*, 72, 892, 1984. With permission.

These investigators advanced the additional speculation that in the pathophysiologic state of congestive heart failure, the renin-angiotensin and atrial peptide systems oppose one another. Central volume is markedly expanded with enhanced release of ANF. The kidney, however, perceives underfilling due to decreases in cardiac output and arterial pressure. Activation of the adrenergic nervous system and increased renal sympathetic nerve activity in association with decreases in renal baroreceptor activity within the kidney all serve to enhance intrarenal AII. Therefore, in this pathophysiologic state, the blunted renal response to exogenous ANF may be mediated in part by the opposing action of the intrarenal AII system.

While ANF is increased by chronic heart failure and may have a functional role, it remains unclear whether ANF secretion is appropriate for the magnitude of increase in atrial and ventricular filling pressures. Studies by Raine et al. suggest that the release of ANF in heart failure may be relatively attenuated.[55] These investigators examined the increase in ANF in response to exercise-induced increases in atrial pressure in subjects with and without CHF. Exercise in the subjects with normal atrial pressures produced a marked and rapid increase in the concentrations of ANF which was consistent with the increase in right atrial pressure. The converse was observed in heart failure in which exercise resulted in appropriately small increases in ANF in relation to a marked increase in atrial pressure. This and more recent preliminary studies suggest an attenuated capacity to increase ANF secretion in response to increments in atrial and/or ventricular pressure in heart failure.[56] Work by Ding et al. also supports the conclusion that chronic congestive heart failure may evolve to a deficiency state, based upon the observations of decreasing plasma levels of ANF in the terminal phases of heart failure in cardiomyopathic hamsters.[57]

V. THERAPEUTIC TRIALS IN HUMANS WITH CONGESTIVE HEART FAILURE

The integrated cardiovascular, endocrine, and renal actions of ANF support a therapeutic role for this peptide in sodium retaining states such as congestive heart failure. This is underscored by the additional activation of the renin-angiotensin-aldosterone system in heart failure and the preliminary studies supporting a relative deficiency of maximal plasma ANF achieved in response to chronically elevated cardiac filling pressures. To date, studies have conflicted in regard to the functional response of cardiovascular, endocrine, and renal systems to exogenous infusion of ANF.

Elegant human studies by Cody et al. reported the response to intravenous ANF infusion in normal subjects and in subjects with chronic heart failure.[5] In normals, ANF induced increases in absolute and fractional sodium excretion, urine flow rate osmolar and free-water clearances, and filtration fraction. Plasma renin and aldosterone decreased, respectively. Systolic blood pressure decreased in the seated position, but only left atrial pressure decreased in the supine position. In subjects with congestive heart failure, ANF increased the cardiac index and decreased systemic vascular resistance, left atrial pressure, and plasma aldosterone. Plasma renin did not significantly decrease nor was a significant natriuresis or diuresis observed.

Crozier et al. performed similar studies, but continued intravenous infusion of ANF in heart failure patients for 4 h, compared to 1 h in the Cody studies.[58] Both investigations utilized comparable doses of atrial peptide. In this second study, ANF increased cardiac output, but this returned to control by 4 h, although with persistent reduction in arterial pressure and cardiac filling pressures. Plasma aldosterone, but not plasma renin, was decreased. No increase in urine volume or sodium excretion was observed. Thus, similar observations were reported which demonstrated that intravenous infusions of ANF in heart failure at the dose concentrations employed resulted in a vasodilating action that at least transiently increased cardiac output by reducing the total calculated peripheral resistance, in association with an inhibition of renin release. No renal action to enhance glomerular filtration rate or sodium excretion was observed.

In a third investigation by Saito et al., similar observations were reported.[59] Intravenous infusion decreased arterial pressure in association with a decrease in systemic vascular resistance and an increase in cardiac output. Plasma aldosterone was decreased, but no increase in sodium excretion was noted. Thus, a consistent observation in human studies is the ability of exogenously administered ANF to decrease arterial pressure, which appears to be mediated by a reduction in systemic vascular resistance with an increase in cardiac output. Thus, a favorable vasodilating action is observed. While plasma renin is not inhibited in these acute studies, plasma aldosterone is suppressed, which must be secondary to a direct action on aldosterone secretion. Nevertheless, as other vasodilators commonly employed in heart failure increase plasma renin activity in response to peripheral vasodilation, the lack of increase in plasma renin activity during ANF infusion in heart failure in human studies may represent a relative inhibition of renin release.

In contrast to the reports during infusion of ANF in heart failure, Riegger et al. have reported that bolus injection of ANF is associated with a significant natriuresis and diuresis.[60] Like the continuous infusion studies, cardiac output was increased, in association with a reduction in systemic vascular resistance. Aldosterone, but not renin, was suppressed.

Recent preliminary studies from two laboratories may provide insight into the differential renal responses in the previously reported human studies, Firth et al. reported that bolus injection of ANF in heart failure was associated with a definite natriuresis.[61] In this investigation, the hemodynamic action of ANF on arterial pressure was short lived. Recent preliminary studies from our laboratory employing low-dose, continuous infusion of ANF in heart failure also demonstrated no reduction in arterial pressure, cardiac filling pressures, or systemic vascular resistance.[62] In these studies, low-dose ANF selectively vasodilated the kidney with an increase in both renal blood flow and glomerular filtration rate. This marked increase was associated with a decrease in aldosterone as well as renin. The mechanism of the renin inhibition may be explained by enhanced delivery of sodium to the macula densa, in association with the increased glomerular filtration rate. Although ANF served as a selective renal vasodilator and an inhibitor of renin and aldosterone, the renal natriuretic response was attenuated, manifesting enhanced reabsorption of sodium in the more distal nephron segments, consistent with animal studies.

A unifying understanding of these human studies may be explained by an antagonistic role of ANF-mediated reduction in arterial pressure upon renal function in congestive heart failure. In animal studies of rats with experimental cirrhosis and ascites with active sodium retention, exogenously administered ANF, which decreased arterial pressure markedly, augmented sympathetic nerve activity to the kidney, which was actually inhibited with normal rats without sodium retention. This increase in renal sympathetic nerve activity mediated by arterial hypotension could offset any favorable renal action of ANF.

Two therapeutic scenarios with exogenous ANF may exist in congestive heart failure. One scenario is high-dose ANF, which acts as a systemic vasodilator to increase cardiac output and inhibit aldosterone with no renal action. The second scenario is low-dose ANF, with selective renal vasodilation and inhibition of both renin and aldosterone. Further, studies comparing low- and high-dose ANF, as well as bolus versus continuous infusion, are required. Moreover, since studies by Scoggins et al. have reported a changing renal and cardiovascular action of ANF during long-term infusion of ANF in sheep, the long-term administration of ANF may result in actions significantly different from observations reported from acute study designs.[63]

VI. SUMMARY

In summary, the atrial peptide system is a physiologic hormonal system which serves

TABLE 4
Atrial Natriuretic Factor in Congestive Heart Failure

I.   Circulating concentrations are increased in CHF in response to cardiac volume overload.

II. Circulating concentrations are increased in early asymptomatic left ventricular dysfunction, thus serving as a marker for early CHF.

III. ANF is present in the ventricle of the failing heart and has biological activity.

IV. ANF is a selective renal vasodilator and renin inhibitor at low doses in CHF.

V.   An attenuated stimulus-release relationship for ANF may exist in chronic congestive heart failure, thus contributing to a relative deficiency state.

VI. The natriuretic response to ANF is attenuated in CHF; this attenuation is mediated by the offsetting action of antinatriuretic systems and receptor-down regulation.

VII. ANF in congestive heart failure may serve to offset the actions of the RAAS and thus protect the organism from progressive cardiopulmonary volume-pressure overload.

to defend the central circulation from acute volume and pressure overload by increasing sodium excretion, inhibiting the renin-angiotensin-aldosterone system (RAAS), and decreasing venous return. In congestive heart failure (Table 4), ANF is acutely and chronically increased secondary to increases in atrial pressure and stretch. ANF is present in the chronically failing heart and this ventricular ANF has physiologic activity. In acute heart failure, endogenous ANF serves to maintain sodium excretion and inhibit activation of the RAAS. In chronic CHF, these actions in part are attenuated by a blunted release of atrial peptide. In both acute and chronic CHF, the renal natriuretic response to ANF is attenuated in part due to receptor down-regulation, as well as to the offsetting action of the intrarenal renin-angiotensin system. From a therapeutic perspective, high-dose ANF administration results in systemic vasodilation, while low-dose ANF results in selective renal vasodilatation. Both concentrations result in aldosterone inhibition. Further, studies of both the physiology and therapeutics of ANF are required to fully elucidate the role of ANF in congestive heart failure.

REFERENCES

1. **Gauer, O. H. and Henry, J. P.**, Circulatory basis of fluid volume control, *Phys. Rev.*, 43, 423, 1963.
2. **de Bold, A. J., Borenstein, H. B., Veress, A. T. and Sonnenberg, H.**, A rapid and potent natriuretic response to intravenous injection of atrial myocardial extract in rats, *Life Sci.*, 28, 89, 1981.
3. **Burnett, J. C., Jr., Granger, J. P., Opgenorth, T. J.**, Effects of synthetic atrial natriuretic factor on renal function and renin release, *Am. J. Physiol.*, 247, F863, 1984.
4. **Maack, T., Marion, D. M., Camargo, M. J., Kleinert, H. D., Laragh, J. H., Vaughn, E. D., Jr., and Atlas, S. A.**, Effect of auriculin (atrial natriuretic factor) on blood pressure, renal function, and the renin-aldosterone system in dogs, *Am. J. Med.*, 77, 1069, 1984.
5. **Cody, R. J., Atlas, S. A., Laragh, J. H., Kubo, S. H., Covit, A. B., Ryman, K. S., Shaknovich, A., Pondolfino, K., Clark, M., Camargo, M. J. F., Scarborough, R. M., and Lewicki, J. A.**, Atrial natriuretic factor in normal subjects and heart failure patients. Plasma levels and renal, hormonal, and hemodynamic responses to peptide infusion, *J. Clin. Invest.*, 78, 1362, 1986.
6. **Goetz, K., Wang, D., Geer, P. G., Leadley, R. J., and Reinhardt, H. W.**, Atrial stretch increases sodium excretion independently of release of atrial peptides, *Am. J. Physiol.*, 250, R946, 1986.
7. **Zimmerman, R. S., Schirger, J., Edwards, B. S., Schwab, T. R., Heublein, D. M., and Burnett, J. C., Jr.**, Cardiorenal endocrine dynamics during step-wise infusion of physiologic and pharmacologic concentrations of atrial natriuretic factor in the dog, *Circ. Res.*, 61, 63, 1987.

8. **Burnett, J. C., Jr., Rubanyi, G. M., Edwards, B. S., Schwab, T. R., Zimmerman, R. S., and Vanhoutte, P. M.,** Atrial natriuretic peptide decreases arterial pressure in the absence of coronary vaso-constriction, *Proc. Soc. Exp. Med. Biol.,* 186, 313, 1987.

9. **Salazar, F. G., Romero, J. C., Burnett, J. C., Jr., Schryver, S., and Granger, J. P.,** Atrial natriuretic peptide levels during acute and chronic saline loading in the conscious dog, *Am. J. Physiol.,* 251, R499, 1986.

10. **Burnett, J. C., Jr., Kao, P. C., Hu, D. C., Heser, D. W., Heublein, D., Granger, J. P., Opgenorth, T. J., and Reeder, G. S.,** Atrial natriuretic peptide elevation in congestive heart failure in the human, *Science,* 231, 1145, 1986.

11. **Shenker, Y., Sider, R. S., Ostafin, E. A., and Grekin, R. J.,** Plasma levels of immunoreactive atrial natriuretic factor in healthy subjects and in patients with edema, *J. Clin. Invest.,* 76, 1684, 1985.

12. **Fried, T. J., and Stein, J.,** Effect of atrial natriuretic factor on glomerular function, *Am. J. Physiol.,* 250, F119, 1986.

13. **Ichikawa, S., Dunn, B. R., Troy, G. L., Maack, T., and Brenner, B. M.,** Influence of atrial natriuretic peptide on glomerular microcirculation in vivo, *Clin. Res.,* 33, 487A, 1985.

14. **Burnett, J. C., Jr., Opgenorth, T. J., and Granger, J. P.,** The renal action of atrial natriuretic peptide during control of glomerular filtration, *Kidney Int.,* 30, 16, 1986.

15. **Hammond, T. Yusufi, A., Knox, F., and Dousa, T.,** Administration of atrial natriuretic factor inhibits sodium transport in proximal tubules, *J. Clin. Invest.,* 75, 1983, 1985.

16. **Schwab, T. R., Edwards, B. S., Zimmerman, R. S., Heublein, D. M., and Burnett, J. C., Jr.,** Renal interstitial pressure increases during atrial natriuretic peptide-induced natriuresis, *Biologically Active Atrial Peptides,* Vol. 1, Brenner, B. M., and Laragh, J. H., Eds., 1987, 413.

17. **Ichikawa, S., Saito, t., Okada, K., Kuzuya, T., Kangawa, K., and Matsuo, H.,** Atrial natriuretic factor increases cyclic GMP and inhibits cyclic AMP in rat renal papillary collecting tubule cells in culture, *Biochem. Biophys. Res. Commun.,* 130, 1147, 1985.

18. **Ziedel, M. L., Seifter, J. L., Lear, S., Brenner, B. M., and Silva, P.,** Atrial peptides inhibit oxygen consumption in kidney medullary collecting duct cells, *Am. J. Physiol.,* 251, F379, 1986.

19. **Bornstein, H. B., Cupples, W., Sonnenberg, H., and Veress, A. J.,** The effect of a natriuretic atrial extract on renal hemodynamics and urinary excretion in anesthetized rats, *J. Physiol. (London),* 334, 133, 1983.

20. **Burnett, J. C., Jr., Haas, J. A., and Larson, M. S.,** Renal interstitial pressure in mineralocorticoid escape, *Am. J. Physiol.,* 249, F396, 1985.

21. **Zimmerman, R. S., Edwards, B. S., Schwab, T. R., Heublein, D. M., and Burnett, J. C., Jr.,** Atrial natriuretic peptide (ANP) during mineralocorticoid escape in the human, *J. Clin. Endocrinol. Metab.,* 63, 624, 1987.

22. **Schwab, T. R., Edwards, B. S., Zimmerman, R. S., Heublein, D. M., and Burnett, J. C., Jr.,** Role of renal interstitial hydrostatic pressure in atrial natriuretic factor-induced natriuresis, *Proc. BAAP,* 197A (Abstr), 1987.

23. **Opgenorth, T. J., Burnett, J. C., Jr., Granger, J. P., and Scriven, T. A.,** Effects of atrial natriuretic peptide on renin secretion in nonfiltering kidney, *Am. J. Physiol.,* 250, F798, 1986.

24. **Obana, K., Naruse, M., Naruse, K., Sakurai, H., Demura, H., Inagami, T., and Shizume, K.,** Synethetic rat atrial natriuretic factor inhibits *in vitro* and *in vivo* renin secretion in rats, *Endocrinology,* 117, 1282, 1985.

25. **Garcia, R., Thibault, G., Cantin, M., and Genest, J.,** Effect of a purified atrial natriuretic factor on rat and rabbit vascular strips and vascular beds, *Am. J. Physiol.,* 247, R34, 1984.

26. **Cody, R. J., Kubo, S. J., Atlas, S. A., Ryman, K. S., Shaknovich, A., and Laragh, J. H.,** Circulating atrial natriuretic factor and the response to synthetic atrial natriuretic factor in patients with chronic congestive heart failure, in *Biologically Active Atrial Peptides,* Vol. 1, Brenner, B. M. and Laragh, J. H., Eds., 1987, 97.

27. **Edwards, B. S., Schwab, T. R., Zimmerman, R. S., Heublein, D. M., Jiang, N. S., and Burnett, J. C., Jr.,** Cardiovascular, renal, and endocrine response to atrial natriuretic peptide in angiotensin II mediated hypertension, *Circ. Res.,* 59, 663, 1986.

28. **Trippodo, N., Cole, F., Frohlich, E., and MacPhee, A.,** Atrial natriuretic peptide decreases circulatory capacitance in areflexic rats, *Circ. Res.,* 49, 291, 1986.

29. **Chen, Y., Frohlich, E., and Trippodo, N.,** Atrial natriuretic peptide increases resistance to venous return, *Am. J. Physiol.,* 252, H894, 1987.

30. **Gardner, D. G., Deschepper, C. F. and Baxter, J. D.,** The gene for atrial natriuretic factor is expressed in the aortic arch, *Hypertension,* 9, 103, 1987.

31. **Thoren, P., Mark, A., Morgan, D., O'Neill, P., Needleman, P., and Brody, M.,** Activation of vagal depressor reflexes by atriopeptins inhibits renal sympathetic nerve activity, *Am. J. Physiol.,* 251, H1252, 1986.

32. **Wangler, R. D., Breuhaus, B. A., Otero, H. O., Hastings, D. A., Holzman, M. D., Saneii, H. H., Sparks, H. V., Jr., and Chimoskey, J. E.,** Coronary vasoconstrictor effects of atriopeptin II, *Science,* 230, 598, 1985.

33. **Bache, R., Dai, X., Schwartz, J., and Chen, D.,** Effects of atrial natriuretic peptide in the canine coronary circulation, *Circ. Res.,* 62, 178, 1988.

34. **Zimmerman, R. S., Edwards, B. S., Schwab, T. R., Heublein, D. M., Burnett, J. C., Jr.,** Cardiorenal-endocrine dynamics during and following volume expansion, *Am. J. Physiol.,* 252, R336, 1987.

35. **Schwab, T. R., Edwards, B. S., Heublein, D. M., and Burnett, J. C., Jr.,** The role of atrial natriuretic peptide in volume expansion natriuresis, *Am. J. Physiol.,* 251, R310, 1986.

36. **Hirth, C., Stasch, J., John, A., Kazda, S., Morich, F., Neuser, D., and Wohlfeil, S.,** The renal response to acute hypervolemia is caused by atrial natriuretic peptides, *J. Cardiovasc. Pharmacol.,* 8, 268, 1986.

37. **Chimoskey, J. E., Spielman, W. S., Brandt, M. A., and Heideman, S. R.,** Cardiac atria of bio 14.6 hamsters are deficient in natriuretic factor, *Science,* 223, 820, 1984.

38. **Rector, T. S., Carlyle, P., and Cohn, J.,** Reduced atrial natriuretic factor after coronary ligation of the left coronary artery in rats, *Am. Heart J.,* 110, 1197, 1985.

39. **Edwards, B. S., Ackermann, D. M., Schwab, T. R., Edwards, W. D., Wold, L. E., and Burnett, J. C., Jr.,** The relationship between atrial granularity and circulating atrial natriuretic peptide in hamsters with congestive heart failure, *Mayo Clin. Proc.,* 61, 517, 1986.

40. **Itoh, H., Nakao, K., Mukoyama, M., Sugawara, A., Saito, Y., Morii, N., Yamada, T., Shiono, S., Arai, H., and Imura, H.,** Secretion of N-terminal fragment of gamma-human atrial natriuretic polypeptide, *Hypertension,* 11, 152, 1988.

41. **Bloch, K., Seidman, J., Naftilan, J., Fallon, J., and Seidman, C.,** Neonatal atria and ventricles secrete atrial natriuretic factor via tissue-specific secretory pathways, *Cell,* 47, 695, 1986.

42. **Day, M. L., Schwartz, D., Wiegand, R., Standaert, D., and Needleman, P.,** Ventricular atriopeptin: unmasking of messenger RNA and peptide synthesis by hypertrophy or dexamethasone, *Hypertension,* 9, 485, 1987.

43. **Lattion, A. L., Michel, E., Arnauld, E., Corvol, P., and Soubrier, F.,** Myocardial recruitment during ANF mRNA increase with volume overload in the rat, *Am. J. Physiol.,* 25, H890, 1986.

44. **Edwards, B. S., Ackermann, D. M., Lee, M. E., Reeder, G. S., Wold, L. E., and Burnett, J. C., Jr.,** Identification of atrial natriuretic factor within ventricular tissue in hamsters and humans with congestive heart failure, *J. Clin. Invest.,* 81, 82, 1988.

45. **Ritman, E. L. and Pao, Y. C.,** Finite element analysis of myocardial diastolic stress and strain relationship in the intact heart, *Eur. J. Cardiol.,* 7, S105, 1978.

46. **de Bold, A. J.,** Atrial natriuretic factor: a hormone produced by the heart, *Science,* 230, 767, 1985.

47. **Michel, J., Lattion, A., Salzman, J., Cerol, M., Philippe, M., Camilleri, J., and Corvol, P.,** Hormonal and cardiac effects of converting inhibition in rat myocardial infarction, *Circ. Res.,* 62, 641, 1988.

48. **Lee, M. E., Edwards, B. S., Miller, W., and Burnett, J. C., Jr.,** Endogenous atrial natriuretic factor prevents sodium retention in acute congestive heart failure, *Kidney Int.,* 30, 272, 1988.

49. **Awazu, M., Imada, H., Kon, V., Inagami, T., and Ichikawa, I.,** Assessment of the functional role of endogenous atrial natriuretic peptide by purified anti-ANP antibody: study in rat model of congestive heart failure, *Kidney, Inc.,* 33, 253, 1988.

50. **Drexler, H., Hirth, C., Morich, F., Traub, C., and Maio, G.,** Vasodilatory action of endogenous ANP in chronic congestive heart failure as determined by monoclonal ANP-antibodies, *Circulation,* 76 (Suppl. 2), 532A, 1987.

51. **Scriven, T. A. and Burnett, J. C., Jr.,** Effects of synthetic atrial natriuretic peptide on renal function and renin release on acute experimental heart failure, *Circulation,* 72, 892, 1985.

52. **Shriffin, E., Deslongchamps, M., and Thibault, G.,** Platelet binding sites for atrial natriuretic factor in humans, *Hypertension,* 8 (Suppl. 2), 6, 1986.

53. **Tsunoda, K., Mendelsohn, F., Sexton, P., Chai, S., Hodsman, G., and Johnston, C.,** Decreased atrial natriuretic peptide binding in renal medulla in rats with chronic heart failure, *Circ. Res.,* 62, 155, 1988.

54. **Showalter, C. J., Zimmerman, R. S., Schwab, T. R., Edwards, B. S., Opgenorth, T. J., and Burnett, J. C., Jr.,** Renal response to atrial natriuretic factor is modulated by intrarenal angiotensin II, *Am. J. Physiol.,* 254, R453, 1988.

55. **Raine, A., Burgisser, E., Muller, F., Bolli, P., Burkart, F., and Buhler, F.,** Atrial natriuretic peptide and atrial pressure in patients with congestive heart failure, *N. Engl. J. Med.,* 315, 533, 1986.

56. **Edwards, B. S., Miller, W. L., Zimmerman, R. S., McGoon, M. D., and Burnett, J. C., Jr.,** Atrial natriuretic factor in acute and chronic congestive heart failure: variation in stimulus/release relationship and target organ effects, *Kidney Int.,* 33, 262, 1988.

57. **Ding, J., Thibault, G., Gutkowska, J., Garcia, R., Karabatsos, T., Jasmin, G., Genest, J., and Cantin, M.,** Cardiac and plasma atrial natriuretic factor in experimental congestive heart failure, *Endocrinology,* 121, 248, 1987.

58. **Crozier, I. G., Ikram, H., Gomez, H., Nicholls, M., Espiner, E., and Warner, N.,** Hemodynamic effects of atrial natriuretic peptide in heart failure, *Lancet,* 224, 1242, 1986.
59. **Saito, Y., Nakao, K., Nishimura, K., Sugawara, A., Okumura, K., Obata, K., Sonoda, R., Ban, T., Yasue, H., and Imura, H.,** Clinical application of atrial natriuretic polypeptide in patients with congestive heart failure: beneficial effects on left ventricular function, *Circulation,* 76, 115, 1987.
60. **Riegger, G., Elsner, D., Kromer, E., Daffner, C., Forssmann, W., Muders, F., Pascher, E., and Kochsiek, K.,** Atrial natriuretic peptide in congestive heart failure in the dog: plasma levels, cyclic guanosine monophosphate, ultrastructure of atrial myoendocrine cells, and hemodynamic, hormonal and renal effects, *Circulation,* 77, 398, 1988.
61. **Firth, B. G., Perna, R., Bellomo, J., and Toto, R.,** Renal and hemodynamic effects of low and high dose ANF bolus doses in congestive heart failure, *JACC,* 11, 118, 1988.
62. **Burnett, J. C., Jr., Edwards, B. S., Schwab, T. R., Zimmerman, R. S., Smith, R. D., Gersh, B. J., Heublein, D. M., and Puetz, P.,** Low dose atrial natriuretic factor is a selective renal vasodilator in humans with congestive heart failure, *JACC,* 11, 239, 1988.
63. **Parkes, D., Coughlan, J., McDougall, J. G., and Scoggins, B.,** Long-term hemodynamic actions of atrial natriuretic factor (99-126) in conscious sheep, *Am. J.Physiol.,* 253, H811, 1988.

INDEX

A

AI, see Angiotensin I
AII, see Angiotensin II
A23187, 55—56, 73
Acetylcholine, 67
ACTH, see Adrenocorticotropin
Adenosine, 135, 275
Adenylate cyclase, 29, 96, 99—101
ADH, 100
Adrenal
  actions, 251—253, 257
  cells, 88
  hormones, 52—54
  medulla, 192, 210, 257
Adrenalin, 192
Adrenocorticotropin (ACTH), 162
  ANP and, 185, 191—192, 225, 227, 236, 238,
    252—253, 257
  secretion, 236, 238
Age
  ANF and, 61, 266—269, 280
  ANP and, 114
AGPR-MCA, see Boc-Ala-Gly-Pro-Arg-MCA
  (AGPR-MCA) substrate
Aldosterone
  ANF and, 262—264, 274, 276, 279, 282—283,
    285—287
  ANP and, 78, 89, 98, 100, 184, 190, 210, 225, 227,
    248—249, 251—253, 257
  secretion of, 130, 139
  synthesis of, 86, 88
Alpha-ANP, 163
Alpha-hANF, 281, see also α-Human atrial natriuretic
  factor
Alpha-human ANP, 162; see also α-Human atrial
  natriuretic peptide
Alpha-methyl-para-tyrosine (ampt), 236—237
Alpha-rat ANP, 162; see also α-Rat atrial natriuretic
  peptide
Amiloride, 86
Amino acid sequence, 42, 44, 82
Aminomethylcoumarine (MCA), 44
ampt, see Alpha-methyl-para-tyrosine
Analogs of ANP, 80, 83, 88, 99
Androgen release, 184
ANF, see Atrial natriuretic factor
ANG II, see Angiotensin II
Angiotensin, 52, 68
Angiotensin I (AI), 162
Angiotensin II (AII), 98
  ANF and, 52, 55, 276, 283, 285
  ANP and, 113, 115—118, 120, 130, 136—139, 162,
    185, 190—191, 202—203, 210, 216, 223—
    228, 232, 235, 239, 248, 250, 252
Angiotensinogen, 52
ANP, see Atrial natriuretic peptide
ANP-LI, see ANP-like immunoreactivity

ANP-like immunoreactivity (ANP-LI), 222—223,
  225—226, 228, 232
Antinatriuresis, 150—151, 255, 287
Antiserum, 146—147
Aortic pressure (AP), 119, 152
AP, see Aortic pressure
Aprotinin, 46
Arginine residue, 3, 185, 222
Arginine vasopression, 115—116, 162, 257
Arterial pressure
  ANF and, 268, 274—277, 282—283, 285—286
  ANP and, 121—122, 225, 245, 247—250, 255
  atriopeptin and, 151—152
Asialoglycoprotein receptor, 11—12
Astroglial cells, 200—201, 203
Atenolol, 268
Atrial appendages, 147, 157
Atrial cardiocytes, 4—5, 34, 37, 66—68
  ANF and, 20, 22—24, 26—28
  ANP and, 244
  IR-ANF and, 20
Atrial distension, 146, 149, 151
Atrial myocardium, 184
Atrial myocytes, 42, 58—61, 244
Atrial natriuretic factor (ANF), 130, 233—234, 236—
  237
  AII and, 52, 55, 276, 283, 285
  A23187 and, 55—56
  adenosine and, 275
  adenylate cyclase and, 29
  adrenal effects of, 264
  age and, 61, 266—269, 280
  aldosterone and, 262—264, 274, 276, 279, 282—
    283, 285—287
  amino acid sequence of, 44
  analysis of, 36
  angiotensinogen and, 52
  arterial pressure and, 268, 274—277, 282—283,
    285—286
  atenolol and, 268
  atrial cardiocytes and, 66—68
  atrial myocytes and, 42, 58—61
  atrial peptides and, 146
  atrial pressure and, 276—277, 282, 285, 287
  atrial stretch and, 66, 274, 287
  in the atrio-ventricular node, 22—23, 25, 28
  baroreceptors and, 263, 268, 274, 285
  BAY K8644 and, 55
  beta blockers and, 268
  binding sites, 190—191
  biochemistry of, 25
  biosynthesis of, 52—54, 57—61, 282
  blood flow and, 264, 275, 278, 284, 286
  blood pressure and, 52, 262—269, 285
  blood volume and, 264, 268
  body fluid and, 274
  bradycardia and, 262—264
  in Brattleboro rats, 20